Lower Extremity Amputation

Wesley S. Moore, M.D.

Professor of Surgery
Chief, Vascular Surgery
UCLA School of Medicine
The Center for the Health Sciences
Los Angeles, California

James M. Malone, M.D.

Chairman, Department of Surgery
Maricopa Medical Center
Phoenix, Arizona

1989
W.B. SAUNDERS COMPANY
Harcourt Brace Jovanovich, Inc.

Philadelphia   London   Toronto   Montreal   Sydney   Tokyo

W. B. SAUNDERS COMPANY
Harcourt Brace Jovanovich, Inc.

The Curtis Center
Independence Square West
Philadelphia, PA 19106

Library of Congress Cataloging-in-Publication Data

Lower extremity amputation.

1. Amputations of leg.   2. Artifical legs.   I. Moore,
Wesley S.   II. Malone, James M. (James Michael),
1946–   . [DNLM: 1. Amputation. 2. Leg—surgery.
WE 850 L9168]

RD560.L68   1989   617'.58059   88–6671

ISBN 0–7216–6485–7

Editor: Edward Wickland
Developmental Editor: David Kilmer
Designer: Dorothy Chattin
Production Manager: Bob Butler
Manuscript Editor: David Indest
Illustration Coordinator: Brett MacNaughton
Indexer: Sally Burke

Lower Extremity Amputation   ISBN 0–7216–6485–7

Last digit is the print number: 9   8   7   6   5   4   3   2   1

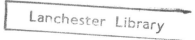

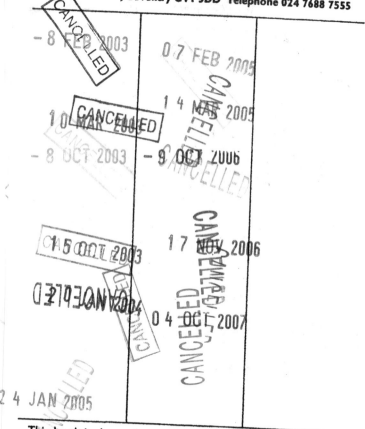

Contributors

SAMUEL S. AHN, M.D.
Assistant Professor of Surgery, UCLA School of Medicine, Los Angeles, California; Attending Surgeon, UCLA Center for the Health Sciences, Los Angeles, California; Consulting Surgeon and Chief of Vascular Surgery Section, Olive View Medical Center, Sylmar, California

JEFFREY BALLARD, M.D.
Resident in General Surgery, Maricopa Medical Center, Phoenix, Arizona

J.H. BOWKER, M.D.
Professor, Department of Orthopaedics and Rehabilitation, University of Miami School of Medicine, Miami, Florida; Medical Director, Rehabilitation Center, University of Miami/Jackson Memorial Medical Center, Miami, Florida

BURNELL R. BROWN, Jr., M.D., Ph.D.
Professor and Head of Anesthesiology, Professor of Pharmacology, University of Arizona Health Sciences Center, Tucson, Arizona; Chief of Clinical Anesthesiology, Medical Director of Operating Room, University Medical Center, Tucson, Arizona

ERNEST M. BURGESS, M.D.
Clinical Professor of Orthopedic Surgery, University of Washington School of Medicine, Seattle, Washington; Director and Principal Investigator of Prosthetics Research Study, Seattle, Washington; Distinguished American Physician, United States Veterans Administration; Surgeon, University of Washington School of Medicine–Affiliated Hospitals, Seattle, Washington

RICHARD CHAMBERS, M.D.
Clinical Assistant Professor of Orthopaedics, University of Southern California, Los Angeles, California; Chief of Amputee Service, Rancho Los Amigos Medical Center, Downey, California

JOSEPH A. GALLO, Jr., M.D.
Clinical Assistant Professor, University of Arizona Medical School, Tucson, Arizona; Director of Cardiac Anesthesia and Associate Head of Anesthesiology, University Medical Center, Tucson, Arizona

FRANK L. GOLBRANSON, M.D.
Clinical Professor of Surgery, UCSD, San Diego, California; Attending Surgeon, UCSD Hospital, San Diego California; Consulting Surgeon, Naval Medical Center, San Diego, California; Consulting Surgeon, Veterans Administration Medical Center, La Jolla, California.

ZANE GRIMM, M.S., C.C.T.
Retired, Private Practice, San Francisco, California

G. ALLEN HOLLOWAY, Jr., M.D.
Associate Professor of Bioengineering, University of Washington, Seattle, Washington; Staff, Orthopaedics, Veterans Administration Medical Center, Seattle, Washington; Director of Vascular Laboratory, Maricopa Medical Center, Phoenix, Arizona

ROBERT P. IACONO, M.D.
Assistant Professor of Surgery and Director of Pain Clinic, University of Arizona, Tucson, Arizona; Head of Neurosurgery, Veterans Administration Medical Center, Tucson, Arizona

M. KAZIM, M.B., B.S., F.R.C.S.(C)
Attending Orthopaedic Surgeon, Howard University Hospital, Washington, D.C.

RICHARD F. KEMPCZINSKI, M.D.
Professor of Surgery, University of Cincinnati, Cincinnati, Ohio; Chief of Vascular Surgery, University of Cincinnati Hospital, Cincinnati, Ohio

STANLEY R. KLEIN, M.D.
Assistant Professor of Surgery, UCLA School of Medicine, Los Angeles, California; Chief of Trauma Surgery, Harbor-UCLA Medical Center, Torrance, California

STEPHEN G. LALKA, M.D.
Assistant Professor of Surgery, Indiana University School of Medicine, Indianapolis, Indiana; Attending Vascular Surgeon, Indiana University Medical Center, Wishard Memorial Hospital, and Richard L. Roudebush Veterans Administration Medical Center, Indianapolis, Indiana

JENNIFER LINFORD, Pharm.D.
Assistant Professor, College of Pharmacy, University of Arizona, Tucson, Arizona; Medical Student, University of Arizona, Tucson, Arizona

JAMES M. MALONE, M.D.
Clinical Professor of Surgery, University of Arizona, Tucson, Arizona; Chairman, Department of Surgery, Maricopa Medical Center, Phoenix, Arizona

KENNETH E. McINTYRE, Jr., M.D.
Assistant Professor of Surgery, Section of Vascular Surgery, University of Arizona, Tucson, Arizona; Director of Traumatic Service, University of Arizona Health Sciences Center, Tucson, Arizona

WESLEY S. MOORE, M.D.
Professor of Surgery, UCLA School of Medicine, Los Angeles, California; Chief of Vascular Surgery, UCLA Center for the Health Sciences, Los Angeles, California

JACQUELIN PERRY, M.D.
Professor of Orthopaedics, University of Southern California, Los Angeles, California; Chief of Pathokinesiology Laboratory, Rancho Los Amigos Medical Center, Downey, California

JOHN C. RACY, M.D.
Professor of Psychiatry, College of Medicine, University of Arizona, Tucson, Arizona; Attending Psychiatrist, University Medical Center, Veterans Administration Medical Center, and Palo Verde Hospital, Tucson, Arizona

JEFFREY R. RUBIN, M.D.
Assistant Professor of Surgery, Case Western Reserve University, Cleveland, Ohio; Chief of Vascular Surgery, Veterans Administration Medical Center, Cleveland, Ohio

DAVID G. SILVERMAN, M.D.
Associate Professor and Director of Clinical Research, Department of Anesthesiology, Yale University School of Medicine, New Haven, Connecticut; Attending Anesthesiologist, Yale–New Haven Hospital, New Haven, Connecticut

TIMOTHY B. STAATS, M.A., C.P.
Director of UCLA Prosthetics Education Program and Adjunct Assistant Professor of Orthopedic Surgery, UCLA School of Medicine, Los Angeles, California

JAN J. STOKOSA, C.P.
Director of Institute for the Advancement of Prosthetics, Lansing, Michigan

PAUL H. SUGARBAKER, M.D.
Director of Surgical Oncology, Emory University School of Medicine, Atlanta, Georgia

JOSÉ J. TERZ, M.D.
Chairman, Division of Surgery, City of Hope National Medical Center, Duarte, California

LAWRENCE D. WAGMAN, M.D.
Senior Surgeon, Department of General Oncologic Surgery, City of Hope National Medical Center, Duarte, California

F. WILLIAM WAGNER, Jr., M.D.
Clinical Professor of Orthopaedic Surgery, School of Medicine, University of Southern California, Los Angeles, California; Chief of Foot and Ankle Service, University of Southern California Medical Center, Los Angeles, California; Chief Consultant of Ortho-Diabetes Service, Rancho Los Amigos Medical Center, Downey, California

ROBERT L. WATERS, M.D.
Clinical Professor of Orthopaedics, University of Southern California, Los Angeles, California; Chairman, Department of Surgery, Rancho Los Amigos Medical Center, Downey, California

RODNEY A. WHITE, M.D.
Associate Professor of Surgery, UCLA School of Medicine, Los Angeles, California; Chief of Vascular Surgery, Harbor-UCLA Medical Center, Torrance, California

JOSEPH H. ZETTL, C.P.
Clinical Assistant Professor, University of Washington, Orthotic-Prosthetic Education, Department of Physical Medicine and Rehabilitation, Seattle, Washington; Staff Privileges, Providence Hospital and Virginia Mason Hospital, Seattle, Washington

Preface

With advances in the medical and surgical management of the various diseases that lead to amputation, progress is being made toward improving limb salvage. However, for those patients in whom aggressive efforts at saving an extremity are unsuccessful, amputation will be required. The ultimate fate of the patient, including survival, freedom from pain, emotional stability, ambulation, and successful rehabilitation, is entirely dependent on the skill, judgment, and dedication of the team effort directed toward bringing the patient through this period of crisis.

Amputation involves several surgical specialties, including orthopedics, general surgery, vascular surgery, and surgical oncology. This book is organized to encompass all aspects of amputation management, irrespective of the specialty of the reader.

Introductory chapters survey the various disease processes and the aspects of patient preparation required before amputation can proceed. For those patients who require amputation for ischemia, several approaches to level selection are described by advocates in individual chapters.

The physiological impact of amputation and prosthetic rehabilitation at each amputation level is outlined to provide a basis for understanding the problems associated with higher amputation levels and to orient the surgeon toward realistic expectations of ambulation on the basis of the patient's age, general physical condition, and factors of comorbidity.

The technical aspects of amputation are discussed in individual chapters dedicated to specific levels; these provide both narrative discussion as well as detailed illustration in order to achieve the qualities of a surgical atlas with respect to the technical aspects of amputation.

Since the ultimate objective of amputation is to return the patient to the highest level of ambulation possible, there is an extensive discussion of prosthetics fitting and fabrication—past, present, and future. In addition, the important aspects of physical therapy and rehabilitation are discussed.

It is the hope of the editors that the presentation of this information in a sequential and comprehensive manner will meet the needs of the surgeon caring for patients who require amputation and will ensure the health and optimal ambulatory rehabilitation of patients who will possess the maximal length of residual extremity.

WESLEY S. MOORE
JAMES M. MALONE

Acknowledgment

The editors would like to acknowledge the valuable role of the Veterans Administration (Division of Rehabilitation Engineering Research and Development) in advancing the fields of prosthetics and amputation surgery. The Veterans Administration and its various clinical and research divisions have played an important part in funding past research for both the editors. In large part, this book would not have been possible without that support. In addition, the Veterans Administration has played a major role in advancing the art and science of prosthetics and surgery for amputations, and this book reflects a multitude of ideas and thoughts that have arisen from that support, from ourselves and other contributing authors.

WESLEY S. MOORE
JAMES M. MALONE

Contents

1

Management of Acute and Chronic Ischemia

Richard F. Kempczinski, M.D.

Lower extremity arterial occlusion is one of the most common clinical manifestations of atherosclerosis. A review of the Vascular Registry of the author's institution showed that more than one half of all arterial reconstructions performed over the past 6 years were for the treatment of lower extremity ischemia and its complications.

In the early 1950s, vascular surgery began to emerge as a distinct surgical subspecialty. Over the ensuing 35 years, there have been numerous technological developments that have equipped today's vascular surgeons with a bewildering array of diagnostic and therapeutic options in the management of lower extremity ischemia.

The evolution of noninvasive diagnostic techniques in the late 1960s permitted the physiological assessment of extremity arterial hemodynamics heretofore lacking. These techniques facilitated the classification of patients into categories based on objective measurements rather than clinical symptoms and made possible the documentation of the results of medical or surgical therapy. During the postoperative period, they could be used not only to monitor graft function but also to provide valuable information on the nat-

ural history of atherosclerotic disease progression.

Parallel advances in the field of diagnostic radiology permitted visualization of the most distal arborizations of the arterial tree with striking clarity, and computer-enhanced technology promised comparable resolution without the risk and discomfort of intra-arterial injection of contrast materal.[1] After the introduction of percutaneous transluminal angioplasty more than 20 years ago, vascular radiologists, emboldened by their successes in catheterizing diseased distal vessels, assumed a more aggressive therapeutic role in the management of patients with extremity ischemia. Although the original technique was not generally accepted because of the high complication rate with the prototype coaxial catheters, results improved significantly after the development of special double-lumen balloon catheters, which are now widely used.[2]

Since thrombosis is one of the most common complications of arterial occlusive disease, vascular surgeons, of necessity, have become experienced in manipulation of the patient's coagulation system. The introduction of heparin by Howell in 1918 represented the first in a series of steps taken to alter intravascular coagulation.[3] Recognition of the central role of platelets in arterial thrombosis naturally led to the discovery of numerous drugs, such as aspirin, sulfinpyrazone, and dipyridamole, that have potent antiplatelet properties. More recently, thrombolytic agents, such as streptokinase, urokinase, and tissue plasminogen activator, have permitted the lysis of intra-arterial thrombi and restoration of circulation without operative intervention. Organizing this complex array of diagnostic and therapeutic options into a cohesive treatment plan is both the challenge and the reward of modern vascular surgery.

Depending on the clinical stage at which patients present with arterial occlusive disease, the goals of therapy may vary. However, foremost among these are relief of patients' symptoms and preservation of limb function, i.e., maintenance of painless bipedal gait. Clearly, salvage of the affected extremity is high on this list of priorities. However, when limb salvage conflicts with the primary goal of therapy, preservation of function, primary amputation may be the most appropriate treatment. This chapter will review the clinical features of acute and chronic lower extremity ischemia, discuss the diagnostic modalities currently used to define the underlying pathophysiological condition, and present the various medical and surgical options available to deal with them. Since arterial occlusive disease is a progressive, often unrelenting, process and limb loss may occur despite the most aggressive efforts by vascular surgeons to prevent limb-threatening ischemia, a discussion of these subjects is most apropos in a monograph on lower extremity amputations.

CLINICAL FEATURES

Since lower extremity arterial occlusive disease is merely a local manifestation of a generalized arterial degenerative disease, the history and physical examination of affected patients must be comprehensive. Although patients frequently present with complaints limited to their lower extremities, more serious, potentially life-threatening, manifestations of atherosclerosis, such as abdominal aortic aneurysm or coronary artery disease,

may deserve priority in treatment. Appropriate evaluation of such patients frequently involves a coordinated effort between vascular surgeon, cardiologist, and pulmonary specialist. Such a thorough and thoughtful evaluation is essential if perioperative morbidity and mortality are to be minimized.

History

The most common manifestation of extremity arterial occlusive disease is pain. The severity of this complaint and the urgency of the efforts to relieve it depend greatly on the rapidity with which the arterial occlusion developed. Patients with acute arterial insufficiency, without previous chronic ischemia, typically present with the sudden onset of severe pain and coldness of the extremity. If the ischemia is not relieved promptly, they may develop anesthesia, paralysis, and ultimately gangrene in the affected limb. Characteristically, the symptomatic manifestations are most severe in the distal extremity owing to the cumulative impact of multiple, serial arterial occlusions and the inadequate early development of collateral circulation. In less severe cases, in which limb viability is not jeopardized and extension of the original thrombosis can be prevented, the patients' acute complaints may improve over the course of days to weeks, leaving them with symptoms of chronic arterial insufficiency.

The manifestations of chronic limb ischemia can run the gamut from exercise-related muscle pain to frank tissue necrosis. However, its most common manifestation is a pain syndrome called *intermittent claudication*. The term derives from the Latin word meaning "to limp" and aptly describes the appearance of these patients' gait. Intermittent claudication is one of the most distinctive symptom complexes in clinical medicine. Characteristically, the pain is confined to a definable muscle group, most commonly the calf muscles, and is precipitated by a reproducible amount of exercise. By clinical convention, the maximum walking distance on level ground is used to define and follow the severity of each patient's disease. The one remaining essential element in the diagnosis is the consistent and prompt relief of pain after cessation of exercise. Typically, patients obtain complete relief of the pain within minutes of stopping exercise and are then able to walk again for a comparable distance. The presence of this triumvirate of complaints, i.e., extremity pain in a definable muscle group, precipitated by exercise and promptly relieved by rest, is diagnostic of intermittent claudication.

As arterial insufficiency becomes more severe, the patient may begin to experience early manifestations of *rest pain*. Typically, these first occur when the patient goes to bed at night and assumes a supine position. Within 20 to 30 minutes, such patients often awaken with numbness and dysesthesias in their feet and toes. Unlike the situation with intermittent claudication, such complaints are localized to the metatarsal heads or proximal forefoot and do not involve muscles. The patients frequently seek relief by massaging their feet or, more characteristically, by placing them in a dependent position over the side of the bed. With more advanced rest pain, the patients may find it impossible to sleep supine and may be forced to spend the night in a sitting position.

As rest pain becomes more severe, it may begin to occur even when the feet are in a dependent position and increasing amounts of analgesics may be required for relief. This represents a severe pregangrenous manifestation of arterial occlusive disease and deserves prompt and aggressive treatment. Finally, in its most advanced stage, arterial occlusive disease can cause frank *tissue necrosis* or *gangrene*. This may vary from a focal area of necrosis on the tip of a single digit, the "blue toe" syndrome,[4] to complete necrosis of an entire limb. Such severe manifestations of arterial occlusion are unusual in the chronic form of this disease and are more often seen in patients with major arterial emboli.

Although there are a number of nonarterial causes of extremity pain (Table 1–1), these can usually be easily distinguished on the basis of a careful clinical history and physical examination. Foremost among these

Table 1–1. DIFFERENTIAL DIAGNOSIS OF INTERMITTENT CLAUDICATION

Neurospinal compression
Musculoskeletal disorders
Venous "claudication"
Popliteal artery entrapment
Muscle cramps
Chronic anterior tibial compartment syndrome
McArdle's syndrome

is *neurospinal compression*, whose presentation may closely mimic vascular claudication. Although burning, tingling, and numbness are frequent complaints in such patients, similar symptoms may occur in patients, especially diabetics, with arterial occlusive disease. However, there are several distinguishing features that should arouse clinical suspicion. Characteristically, patients with neurospinal compression become symptomatic merely upon standing, and exercise may not be necessary to provoke their complaints. Furthermore, the pain often follows a dermatomal pattern on the anterolateral aspect of the thigh and is not confined to a definable muscle group. Frequently, these patients find it necessary to sit or lie down for extended periods in order to obtain relief. Vascular noninvasive testing, as explained later in this chapter, is particularly important in confirming this diagnosis.[5]

Patients with iliofemoral venous thrombosis may present many years later with *venous claudication*, which might initially be confused with intermittent claudication; however, the extremities in such patients are usually edematous and warm. The pain is characteristically described as being of a "bursting" quality and involves the entire leg rather than a definable muscle group. Symptoms may appear after prolonged standing as well as after exercise, and affected patients typically have to lie down and elevate their extremities to obtain relief. Although peripheral pulses may be difficult to palpate because of extremity edema, the Doppler velocity meter can be used to confirm the presence of normal arterial blood flow.

One of the most frequent and puzzling causes of extremity pain in patients seen by vascular specialists is *diabetic neuropathy*. This condition may be especially confusing when arterial occlusion is also present in the affected extremity. Typical neuropathic pain is often a severe burning dysesthesia or paresthesia that follows a dermatomal distribution rather than being confined to a specific muscle group. The pain is usually constant and unrelated to exercise and may be associated with alterations in vibratory sensation and loss of proprioception. Although it is generally not difficult to recognize the presence of neuropathy, a greater challenge for the vascular surgeon is determining to what extent coexisting arterial disease threatens limb viability and is responsible for the patient's resting symptoms. Once again, physiological testing by the vascular diagnostic laboratory is useful in making this distinction.

Rarely, young athletes, especially men, may present with complaints of calf muscle pain after vigorous exercise; this sounds typical of intermittent claudication, yet, on routine physical examination, peripheral pulses may be normal, even immediately after exercise. In this setting, the possibility of *popliteal artery entrapment* must be considered. Affected individuals will usually have an anomalous origin of the medial head of their gastrocnemius muscle, which compresses the popliteal artery during exercise. Diagnosis can be confirmed by palpation of distal pulses or measurement of pulse volume waveforms[6] while forcefully dorsiflexing the foot. Other interesting, but unusual, causes of limb pain include nocturnal muscle cramps, chronic anterior tibial compartment syndrome, and McArdle's syndrome, an inherited disorder of muscle phosphorylation.

Physical Examination

The physical findings in the extremities of individuals with arterial occlusive disease can be grouped into three broad categories: those due to acute arterial occlusion, those consistent with chronic arterial disease, and those caused by coexisting nonarterial conditions.

The acutely ischemic lower extremity may, on initial inspection, be either pale, violaceous, or cyanotic, depending on the degree of arterial spasm. Rubor or cyanosis is especially pronounced when the extremity is in the dependent position, whereas pallor is more characteristic on elevation. The extremity is cool, and peripheral pulses are absent or severely diminished. With more advanced limb-threatening ischemia, cutaneous anesthesia may be present. Paresis or frank paralysis may herald impending gangrene. An important finding of advanced, and probably irreversible, extremity ischemia is marked rigidity and tenderness of the muscles. If gangrene is present when the patient is first seen, its extent may, to a large degree, determine the subsequent course of therapy. For example, if the entire foot is nonviable but the more proximal skin and muscles are adequately perfused, a primary amputation may be the preferred mode of treatment, without the need for angiography and futile attempts at arterial reconstruction.

Patients with chronic lower extremity ischemia may have limbs that, at first glance, appear normal; however, when the extremity is placed in a dependent position, rubor may develop (Fig. 1–1). This change reverses with elevation, during which the ischemic extremity may become paler than its normal counterpart. Similarly, peripheral pulses are absent or diminished, and there may be cutaneous changes consistent with chronic ischemia, such as dry, scaling skin, thickening of the nail beds, absence of hair on the more distal portions of the extremity, and subcutaneous atrophy (Fig. 1–2). In the absence of rest pain, the color changes may be negligible, and motion and sensation are intact.

Manifestations of associated conditions, such as peripheral neuropathy or hypercholesterolemia, should be sought. Fine two-point discrimination, vibratory sensation, and proprioception may be absent in the feet of patients with diabetic neuropathy. This is a particularly important observation in a patient with absent peripheral pulses who is complaining of extremity pain at rest, which might otherwise be misinterpreted as advanced arterial insufficiency. The presence of cutaneous xanthomas suggests unrecognized hyperlipidemia. The feet should be carefully inspected for evidence of infection or focal areas of cyanosis that might be found in patients with atheromatous emboli.

In addition to the routine laboratory tests, such as chest X-ray films, electrocardiogram,

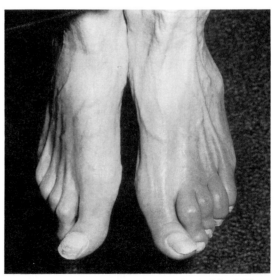

FIGURE 1–1. Patient with rest pain in the left foot. When such an extremity is placed in the dependent position, it becomes red or bluish-red in color.

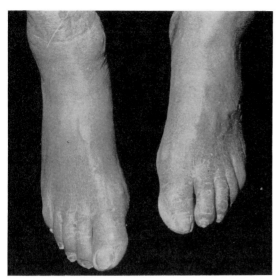

FIGURE 1–2. This patient had severe, bilateral lower extremity ischemia. Note the dry, scaling skin, the subcutaneous atrophy, the thickening of the nails, and the absence of hair.

complete blood count, and renal profile, patients with lower extremity arterial occlusive disease should also undergo a coagulation screening panel, which includes prothrombin time, activated partial thromboplastin time, and a platelet count. A lipid profile and 24-hour creatinine clearance test can detect hyperlipidemia and renovascular insufficiency. Perhaps the most important aspect of the assessment of patients with lower extremity arterial occlusive disease is the cardiovascular evaluation. Since the clinical history and physical examination are poor screening tools for significant coronary artery disease, an exercise multigated angiogram (MUGA) or a thallium scan after the intravenous injection of dipyridamole provides a more accurate assessment of cardiovascular reserve and determines the extent of any previous myocardial damage before major arterial reconstructive surgery is undertaken.[7]

DIAGNOSIS

Noninvasive Testing

The need for noninvasive hemodynamic tests to evaluate patients with extremity arterial occlusive disease remains controversial. In most patients, the absence of pulses, a classic history of intermittent claudication, and the physical appearance of the extremity are frequently all the experienced clinician needs to establish the diagnosis and predict the approximate level of arterial occlusion. However, simple clinical examination may be misleading, for example, when there is concomitant arterial occlusion and neuropathy. Furthermore, since many patients with extremity pain are initially seen by clinicians who are inexperienced in the management of these problems, the noninvasive laboratory tests can provide objective diagnostic confirmation and ensure prompt and appropriate triage of such patients.

Apart from the mere confirmation of arterial insufficiency, noninvasive testing is also useful in correlating an anatomical lesion with its resulting functional derangement. This is especially important in patients with diabetes mellitus; in such cases, hemodynamic data may be critical in categorizing the severity of resting extremity complaints.[8] It may also be useful in directing subsequent angiography by identifying probable areas of arterial occlusion. Finally, it is important in establishing a hemodynamic baseline with which the postoperative results can be compared.

Segmental limb pressures can be easily obtained using standard pneumatic cuffs and a simple Doppler velocity meter (Fig. 1–3). This is probably the most widely used technique for evaluation of extremity arterial disease. It is quite accurate in categorizing the extent of overall hemodynamic impairment. On the basis of this simple test alone, patients with exercise-related complaints can be reliably separated from those with more severe degrees of ischemia (Table 1–2). However, in order to more accurately localize the level of occlusion and to better evaluate the presence or absence of aortoiliac or "inflow" arterial occlusive disease, some additional testing, such as Doppler velocity or pulse volume waveforms, is necessary. Using a combination of segmental limb pressure and pulse volume recordings, aortoiliac disease can be identified with acceptable reliability and distinguished from coexisting femoropopliteal occlusive disease.[9] Duplex scanning, which has been widely used for cerebrovascular evaluation, is now being applied to the study of extremity arterial disease and may further refine the ability to identify or exclude the presence of aortoiliac lesions.[10]

In those patients who present with exercise-related complaints, a period of standard-

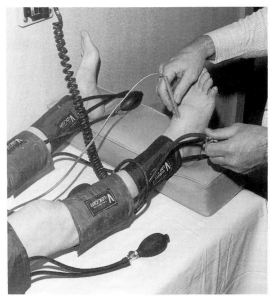

FIGURE 1–3. Technique for measurement of segmental limb blood pressures: Three standard pneumatic cuffs are placed on each extremity, and a Doppler velocity meter is used to insonate one of the pedal arteries. As the cuffs are, in turn, inflated above systolic pressure and then gradually deflated, the Doppler signal initially disappears and then returns as the cuff pressure falls below that in the underlying arteries. This pressure is noted on the sphygmomanometer and recorded as the systolic pressure for that limb segment.

ized treadmill exercise after completion of the baseline segmental limb pressure and pulse volume recordings is useful in objectively documenting the extent of their disability and reproducing their symptoms under physiological conditions. The author has found this particularly important in identifying those patients who may be more limited by coexistent cardiovascular or pulmonary disease and for whom arterial reconstruction might not result in any functional improvement. Once the patient completes the standardized period of treadmill exercise or is forced to stop because of the onset of symptoms, repeat ankle pressure determinations

Table 1–2. RELATIONSHIP BETWEEN ANKLE SYSTOLIC PRESSURE AND CLINICAL SEVERITY OF DISEASE

Disease	Ankle Systolic Pressure (mm Hg)
Claudication	70–100
Rest pain	< 50
Gangrene	0–30

will confirm the presence of additional hemodynamic impairment and relate the patient's symptoms to the appropriate physiological alterations.

Radiological Evaluation

Once the need for either reconstructive or ablative surgery is established by the clinical history and physical examination, all patients with arterial extremity disease should undergo a comprehensive radiological assessment. A biplanar aortogram is essential to evaluate the aortoiliac segment, since the traditional uniplanar view frequently underestimates the presence of iliac artery disease.[11] In addition, multilevel femoral shift study is necessary to evaluate the infrainguinal segment. Since patients with multisegmental arterial occlusions may have very poor perfusion of the distal extremity, adequate visualization of patent infrapopliteal vessels may be extremely difficult. In such patients, the use of computer-enhanced digital subtraction angiography has greatly facilitated the demonstration of suitable outflow vessels before distal bypass.[12] Even in situations in which such an examination has failed to demonstrate a patent distal vessel, a prereconstructive, "on-the-table" arteriogram of the patient's extremity should be considered before concluding that it is nonreconstructible and requires amputation. In one study, Ricco and colleagues[13] reported nonvisualization or inadequate visualization in 42% of conventional preoperative arteriograms. Without prebypass arteriography, the majority of such patients might have had an unnecessary amputation.

The use of computed axial tomography of the abdomen has added yet another dimension to the evaluation of the abdominal aorta and iliac arteries. It is useful in identifying unsuspected aneurysmal changes within the vessel wall as well as in more accurately diagnosing the presence of extraluminal blood in cases of unsuspected rupture or the presence of periaortic inflammation in patients with inflammatory aneurysms.[14] The use of computed tomographic scanning or B-mode ultrasound in patients with absent popliteal pulses and distal ischemia may be the only satisfactory means of documenting the presence of a thrombosed popliteal aneurysm as the cause of the patient's symptoms.

INDICATIONS
Arterial Revascularization

Patients with disabling claudication have only a relative indication for arterial revascularization. Since intermittent claudication rarely jeopardizes the future viability of the symptomatic extremity, revascularization is not required as prophylaxis against gangrene. In one study by Imparato and associates, 80% of patients with intermittent claudication treated medically remained stable or actually improved over a 2- to 5-year period without the need for revascularization.[15] In order to accurately assess the degree of disability, one may have to consider the patient's occupational status, age, and potential for rehabilitation; the presence or absence of coexisting cardiopulmonary diseases; and the economic and recreational impact of the patient's disability. In addition, since proximal reconstructions, such as aortofemoral grafts, are generally more durable than infrainguinal reconstructions, patients with claudication secondary to inflow lesions may be considered for revascularization more readily than those who would require a distal bypass.

Patients with severe, progressive claudication, especially those limited to less than 50 feet of walking, have a more urgent indication for revascularization. Characteristically, such patients, if untreated, will progress to limb-threatening ischemia. In a similar sense, patients with severe, dependent rubor or rest pain already have advanced ischemia and require more urgent angiography and, if appropriate, revascularization. If evidence of atheromatous embolization is seen on physical examination, such patients are generally considered at risk for limb loss and should undergo appropriate angiography before removal of the embolic source, since this condition characteristically recurs, with increasing jeopardy for extremity survival.[16] Focal digital or forefoot gangrene represents the most pressing indication for revascularization, since amputation in such patients with proximal, uncorrected arterial occlusion rarely heals and may require even more proximal major amputations.

Primary Amputation

In patients with limb-threatening arterial insufficiency or established gangrene who have severe coexisting medical problems that either make arterial reconstruction inappropriately hazardous or severely limit the patient's life expectancy, primary amputation, without prior angiography and attempts at revascularization, may be the most appropriate therapeutic alternative.

Certainly, patients who present with established gangrene that is so extensive as to preclude salvage of a useful extremity require a major amputation regardless of any attempts at arterial reconstruction. Not infrequently, the surgeon must decide whether the proposed amputation will heal at the below-knee level without a proximal revascularization. In such cases, the vascular diagnostic laboratory may document the adequacy of proximal perfusion and avoid unnecessary arteriography, which can define only the anatomical, not physiological, status of the patient's extremity circulation.[17] In more difficult cases in which the vascular laboratory findings may be equivocal, measurement of the disappearance of intradermal radioactive xenon (see Chapter 5) or the noninvasive, transcutaneous measurement of oxygen (see Chapter 6) has been useful in predicting the healing potential of proximal amputations. If either or both of these techniques document that a below-knee amputation is likely to heal in a patient with foot gangrene so extensive that it precludes limb salvage, there appears to be little rationale for arteriography or attempts at revascularization.

Certainly, an unsuccessful attempt at arterial reconstruction may further compromise the collateral circulation and raise the subsequent amputation level. Although several authors have presented data supporting this contention,[18-20] the question remains unsettled. If bypass surgery is attempted, careful planning and execution of the operation greatly reduce the risk of more proximal amputation. The incisions for harvesting the saphenous vein and exposing the arteries should be located with the subsequent amputation in mind. Care should be taken to preserve collateral blood flow and avoid wound infection and skin necrosis.

THERAPEUTIC ALTERNATIVES
Acute Extremity Ischemia

The distinction between acute arterial thrombosis and embolization is an important one, since the subsequent management of affected patients will vary depending on the pathophysiology. Characteristically, patients without an antecedent history of intermittent claudication who present with the sudden onset of extremity ischemia and have an appropriate embolic source, such as a cardiac arrhythmia, a recent myocardial infarction, rheumatic valvular disease, or an abdominal aortic aneurysm, are likely to have an arterial embolus. On the other hand, patients with a history of intermittent claudication who manifest extremity changes consistent with chronic arterial insufficiency and who may have absent pulses in the contralateral extremity are more likely to have acute arterial thrombosis. The urgency of initiating appropriate therapy depends on the severity of the patient's ischemia. Those patients who present with sensory loss or muscle weakness have an advanced stage of arterial insufficiency that must be reversed within 4 to 6 hours if a functional extremity is to be preserved. By contrast, in patients with ischemic but viable extremities, the responsible physician has more time to make a precise diagnosis and plan appropriate treatment. Regardless of the cause of acute arterial insufficiency, most patients should be started on full-dose, intravenous heparin as soon as the diagnosis is confirmed. This not only prevents extension of thrombosis in the stagnant distal vessels but may also reverse the vasospasm induced by the intra-arterial thrombus.[21] Frequently, within hours of initiating appropriate anticoagulation, extremity pain may decrease, and the appearance of the limb may improve.

Depending on the urgency of the clinical situation, appropriate arteriograms are usually necessary to help plan the operative approach. In patients with obvious distal arterial emboli and palpable proximal pulses, an appropriate intraoperative arteriogram is often more expeditious. When patients present with acute limb-threatening ischemia secondary to arterial emboli, prompt removal of the emboli with a balloon catheter rapidly restores normal circulation and reverses the ischemia.[22] In patients who seek medical help 12 to 24 hours after the onset of severe ischemia, restoration of circulation may result in the release of metabolic and toxic by-products from the ischemic extremity, which can have severe systemic side effects.[23] In such situations, the operating surgeon may

wish to anticipate this complication by suitably increasing urine output with osmotic agents, such as mannitol; by systemic alkalinization of the blood to reverse the effects of the anticipated lactic acidosis; or, perhaps, by discarding the initial 200 to 300 ml bolus of venous effluent after restoration of arterial flow to prevent a shower of microthrombi and toxic by-products from reaching the systemic circulation.

The introduction of thrombolytic agents, such as streptokinase and urokinase, raised expectations that acute arterial thrombi and, in some cases, emboli could be satisfactorily lysed without the need for arterial surgery. Unfortunately, thrombolytic agents currently in use usually require 12 to 36 hours to lyse extensive thrombi. This delay precludes their use in individuals with severe limb-threatening ischemia who require immediate revascularization. Since patients with arterial emboli can generally be treated most expeditiously with a simple balloon catheter embolectomy, thrombolytic therapy seems ill-advised in such cases. Furthermore, despite the acute onset of the patient's symptoms, the embolic material is old and may be less amenable to lysis by thrombolytic drugs. In some high-risk patients with acute arterial thrombosis in whom the degree of extremity ischemia allows sufficient time for such agents to act, thrombolytic therapy might be considered appropriate. In one series, complete or partial thrombolysis was achieved in 81% of arterial occlusions and was accompanied by significant clinical benefit in roughly 70% of patients in the entire series.[24] Ultimate clinical benefit was greatest in patients with arterial thrombosis in whom 90% of thrombi were successfully removed with lytic therapy. If thrombolysis is continued beyond 36 to 48 hours, systemic bleeding complications become more frequent and may outweigh the advantages of this approach. The development of more specific thrombolytic agents, such as tissue plasminogen activator, which works directly on the plasminogen already bound within the thrombus, may eventually reduce hemorrhagic complications and ensure a more important role for lytic therapy in the treatment of thromboembolic occlusive disease.

An alternative, albeit controversial, approach to the treatment of patients with lower extremity arterial thromboembolism and viable limbs is the use of high-dose heparin therapy. This approach has been championed by Blaisdell and colleagues, who note that the use of balloon catheter thromboembolectomy has failed to reduce the mortality or morbidity of patients with arterial embolism.[25] They recommend that such patients be started on high doses of intravenous heparin, which should be rapidly increased until the patient's symptoms are relieved. After an appropriate in-hospital period of treatment, patients can be considered for long-term oral anticoagulation or possibly delayed, elective surgical revascularization, if chronic disabling symptoms persist.[21]

Chronic Arterial Insufficiency

Patients who present with appropriate indications for arterial reconstruction to relieve the symptoms of chronic arterial insufficiency need a comprehensive diagnostic evaluation, as described earlier, before revascularization. Often, those who are most symptomatic have multiple, serial occlusions causing severe distal extremity ischemia, thus forcing the operating surgeon to decide which lesions to correct to relieve the patient's symptoms. In general, a choice has to be made between performing an "inflow" precedure, such as aortoiliac endarterectomy or aortofemoral grafting, as opposed to an "outflow" procedure, such as infrainguinal bypass.

Inflow Operations

Two broad types of surgical technique are available for most vascular reconstructions: thromboendarterectomy and bypass grafting. Although *aortoiliac thromboendarterectomy* was among the first procedures described for restoration of arterial circulation in ischemic extremities, it has been largely replaced by bypass operations, such as aortoiliac or aortofemoral grafting, because of their greater simplicity, broader applicability, and reduced operating time.[26] A small subset of patients, who are generally younger than typical patients with atherosclerosis and whose disease is localized to the distal aorta and common iliac arteries, may be considered candidates for thromboendarterectomy.

However, in most situations, the disease is more extensive, and the patient requires a prosthetic bypass graft to restore circulation. Patients with arterial occlusive disease are less

often candidates for aortoiliac grafting, since subclinical disease of the external iliac arteries is often present and may limit the postoperative hemodynamic improvement or subsequently be the site of disease progression. Consequently, most patients who require aortoiliac arterial reconstruction for occlusive disease should be considered for *aortofemoral bypass grafts.* These are generally performed with knitted Dacron prostheses inserted between the juxtarenal abdominal aorta and both common femoral arteries. Although the debate between proponents of proximal end-to-end anastomoses and end-to-side anastomoses continues, there appears to be little evidence that the function and potential complications of either technique significantly differ.[27] Distal anastomosis must be performed to a suitable infrainguinal vessel to ensure adequate perfusion of the deep femoral artery. When orificial stenosis is present in this vessel, the tip of the distal anastomosis should be carried sufficiently far down the deep femoral artery to ensure adequate unobstructed outflow.[28]

Younger patients with unequivocally unilateral symptoms in whom the contralateral iliac artery is free of hemodynamically significant occlusion may be considered for either a unilateral iliofemoral reconstruction through an extraperitoneal approach or a "crossover" graft from the contralateral iliac or femoral artery. Although such a reconstruction is generally referred to as an "*extra-anatomical bypass,*" this term is a misnomer, but one that is widely accepted. The inflow vessel may be either the contralateral common femoral artery or the common or external iliac artery, depending on the surgeon's preference. Such grafts can be tunneled in either a subcutaneous or a retrorectus plane and have proved to be both durable and hemodynamically satisfactory.[29] In a small subset of patients who require lower extremity revascularization for limb-threatening arterial insufficiency in whom intra-abdominal conditions preclude either aortoiliac thromboendarterectomy or aortofemoral bypass grafting, an additional extra-anatomical reconstruction is available. With a suitable axillary artery, a long prosthesis can be tunneled in a subcutaneous plane to the appropriate femoral artery. When contralateral disease is present and both legs require revascularization, a femorofemoral graft, originating from the axillofemoral graft, may be added. Although this reconstruction provides satisfactory early inflow and can result in extremity salvage, the hemodynamic benefits of axillofemoral grafts are less satisfactory than direct, in-situ aortic reconstruction and expose the patient to a significantly higher risk of graft thrombosis, requiring late thrombectomy and reoperation.[30]

Percutaneous transluminal angioplasty is yet another means of improving inflow in the ischemic leg. It is most effective when used to dilate short stenoses in an otherwise undiseased common iliac artery. When there are multiple stenoses in a diffusely diseased vessel or when external iliac lesions are dilated, the result is less satisfactory (Table 1–3).

Infrainguinal Reconstruction

The same two alternatives, thromboendarterectomy and bypass grafting, must be considered for infrainguinal arterial reconstruction. Thromboendarterectomy is less widely applied and less suitable in most patients, except those who require revascularization of the deep femoral artery. Those most likely to benefit from such a *profundaplasty* typically have a superficial femoral artery occlusion and associated infrapopliteal lesions. Inflow into the common femoral artery must be satisfactory, and a high-grade proximal stenosis or occlusion of the deep femoral artery must be present. If the distal deep femoral artery is open, especially if the popliteal artery is patent, a good result can be anticipated.[31]

Inahara and Scott have documented that femoral and popliteal thromboendarterectomies provide suitable long-term alternatives to bypass grafting in carefully selected patients. Those most likely to benefit from thromboendarterectomy have short segmental occlusions or stenoses with relatively undiseased vessels on either side of the lesion. Appropriate endarterectomy and vein patch angioplasty in such patients result in restoration of arterial flow, with long-term patency comparable with that of bypass grafts.[32]

Perhaps the most widely applied procedures for infrainguinal arterial reconstruction are *femoropopliteal* and *femorotibial bypass grafts*. A number of factors influence the long-term patency of such reconstructions. Among the most important are the choice of conduit, indications for operation, site of

Table 1–3. RESULTS OF INFLOW LOWER EXTREMITY ARTERIAL RECONSTRUCTIONS

Procedure*	Operative Mortality (%)	5-Yr Patency (%)
AI-TEA[52]	1	95
AIFG[26]	1–2	90
AxFG[53]	8	33
FFG[29, 54]	2–6	73
Iliac PTA[47]	0	61†

*See numbered references for details.
†3-yr results.
AI-TEA = aortoiliac thromboendarterectomy, AIFG = aortoiliofemoral grafting, AxFG = axillofemoral grafting, FFG = femorofemoral grafting, Iliac PTA = iliac percutaneous transluminal angioplasty.

distal anastomosis, quality of runoff, and continued use of tobacco products postoperatively.[33, 34] Also important, but of lesser influence, are the age of the patient and the use of antiplatelet drugs postoperatively.[35, 36]

The most important factor determining long-term patency of infrainguinal reconstructions is the choice of conduit. Although some authors[37] have suggested that prosthetic grafts composed of polytetrafluoroethylene (PTFE) are comparable to the autogenous saphenous vein, a prospective, multicenter trial has failed to support this opinion.[38] Certainly, in most studies, the autogenous saphenous vein remains the most durable conduit for lower extremity revascularization. Traditionally, this vein has been surgically removed and reversed before its use as a bypass graft. However, interest has revived in the in-situ use of this vein for extremity revascularization.[39] With the development of suitable miniaturized valvulotomes to render the vein valves incompetent and permit retrograde flow, the saphenous vein can be left in its subcutaneous bed with preservation of the vasa vasorum, helping to maintain an intact endothelial lining. In addition, it offers the potential hemodynamic advantages of a suitably tapered conduit (Fig. 1–4). Furthermore, vein utilization appears to be significantly increased by the use of the in-situ technique, making more patients candidates for autogenous reconstruction.[40] When prosthetic grafts must be used for infrainguinal bypass, significantly decreased patency can be anticipated if the site of distal anastomosis is below the knee. However, the patency of prosthetic grafts above the knee appears comparable with that of autogenous recon-

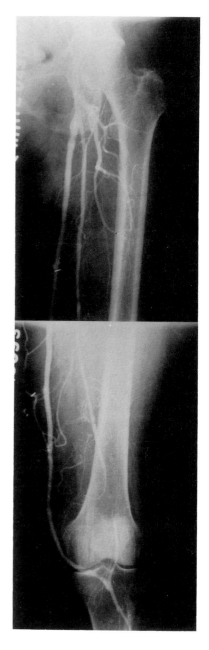

FIGURE 1–4. Postoperative angiogram of a left femoropopliteal graft using the in situ saphenous vein. Note the gradual taper in graft diameter.

structions.[41] Consequently, in such situations, the saphenous vein should be preserved for either subsequent downstream reconstruction or coronary artery bypass grafting.[42]

Prosthetic grafts to the tibial arteries currently carry unacceptable occlusion rates and should be used only when no suitable autogenous tissue is available and the alternative would be a major amputation. If the ipsilateral or contralateral greater and lesser saphenous veins have either been harvested for previous lower extremity revascularization or

damaged by disease, the arm vein provides an alternative autogenous conduit that has recently been shown to provide excellent long-term patency.[43] Certainly, if reconstruction is to be carried below the knee, this conduit is preferable to the nonbiologic prostheses currently in use. Other factors that affect the long-term patency of prosthetic bypass grafts, such as the quality of the distal runoff and the indication for operation, may further influence the choice of conduit (Fig. 1–5). Patients with rest pain

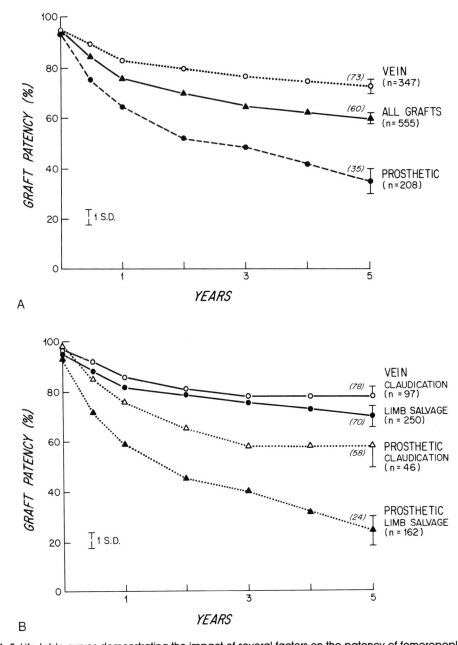

FIGURE 1–5. Life table curves demonstrating the impact of several factors on the patency of femoropopliteal grafts: *A,* Autogenous vein grafts vs prosthetic grafts, *B,* indication for operation, *C,* location of distal anastomosis, *D,* the combined impact of the site of distal anastomosis and the quality of runoff for prosthetic grafts. (*From* Brewster DC, LaSalle A J, Robison JG, et al: Factors affecting patency of femoropopliteal bypass grafts. Surg Gynecol Obstet 157:437, 1983. *By permission of* Surgery, Gynecology & Obstetrics.)

who require revascularization, especially if the subsequent angiogram demonstrates poor runoff, should generally undergo infrainguinal reconstruction with one of the available autogenous conduits, since long-term durability of prosthetic reconstruction in such patients is poor. If prosthetic conduits must be used below the knee, some means of augmenting the velocity of graft flow, such as the creation of a distal arterial venous fistula[44] or sequential distal anastomosis,[45] should be considered to try to reduce the risk of graft thrombosis.

The realization that most graft failures are

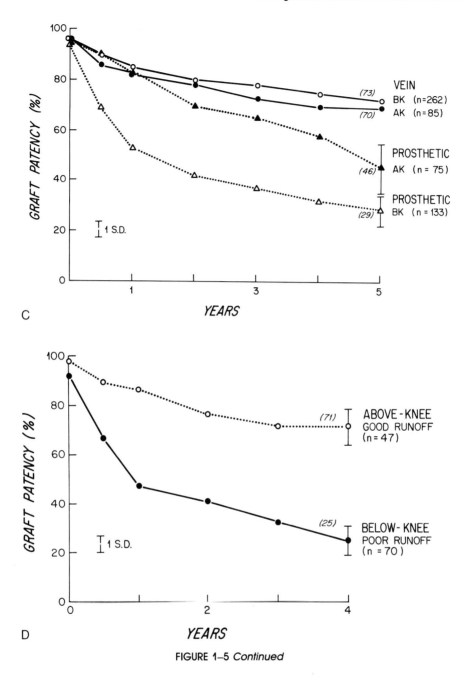

C

D

FIGURE 1–5 *Continued*

due to progression of the patient's atherosclerosis rather than to any defect in the prosthesis is less well recognized but no less important. Accordingly, every effort should be made to prevent the postoperative use of tobacco and control those medical conditions, such as hypertension, hyperlipidemia, and obesity, that are known to accelerate disease progression.

Another therapeutic alternative that may permit extremity revascularization without direct arterial surgery is *percutaneous transluminal angioplasty*. This technique was originally introduced by Dotter[46] but did not initially enjoy widespread popularity. After the development of suitable balloon catheters by Gruntzig,[2] there was a resurgence of interest in the technique. Short stenoses or occlusions of the superficial femoral artery are the lesions most likely to respond to this technique.[47] Transluminal angioplasty of the popliteal or tibial arteries has not been widely successful in most institutions. In patients with multiple, serial lesions, correction of one or more of these lesions may increase circulation sufficiently to relieve rest pain although patients may continue to experience disabling claudication. This technique should generally be reserved for either patients with short, localized lesions or those whose medical condition precludes more durable forms of arterial reconstruction.

RESULTS
General Considerations

Numerous factors must be considered in determining the "success" of various types of arterial reconstruction. Since the goals of lower extremity arterial surgery are limb salvage and preservation of normal function, long-term patency should not be the only parameter by which they are judged. For example, general applicability of a particular technique and ease of performance are both factors that are rarely mentioned in most reports and yet significantly influence the number of patients who are likely to benefit from a given procedure. Furthermore, some patients in whom an arterial reconstruction has thrombosed do not revert to their preoperative condition but, instead, maintain a viable, pain-free, functional extremity. Thus, limb salvage usually exceeds graft patency for each procedure by 10 to 15%.[48] Should the vascular reconstruction in such patients be considered a "failure"?

Cumulative life-table patency is the most recognized and widely used parameter by which the results of arterial reconstructions are judged. However, many factors extrinsic to the procedure itself affect patency and may explain the wide variations in results reported in the surgical literature. Since life-table analysis includes only those patients in whom the particular procedure was actually performed, results can vary significantly, depending on the stringency of the selection criteria used by the individual surgeons reporting their results. If patency is the criterion by which reconstructions are to be judged, the indications for operation, duration of follow-up, demographic characteristics of the patient population, presence of

associated risk factors, site of distal anastomosis, postoperative management, and quality of angiographic runoff must all be standardized before a valid comparison can be made. Since this is rarely possible, attempts at comparing various reconstructions, solely on the basis of cumulative life-table patency, are fraught with potential for misinterpretation.

The problem is further compounded by the manner in which some centers have reported "patency." Reconstructions that thrombosed but were successfully salvaged by thrombectomy have occasionally been reported as continuously patent.[49] This so-called "functional patency" can result in an apparent 10 to 15% improvement in patency at each interval.

Finally, postoperative management appears to influence patency significantly. The use of agents to inhibit platelet aggregation has been shown experimentally to reduce the incidence of neointimal fibroplasia significantly and may theoretically increase long-term patency.[50] However, a prospective study failed to show any improvement in graft patency when aspirin and dipyridamole were compared with a placebo.[51] Certainly, the success of individual surgeons in getting their patients to stop smoking can have a significant impact on the success of arterial reconstructive procedures.[34]

Inflow Arterial Reconstructions

The results of inflow, i.e., suprainguinal, arterial reconstructions are summarized in Table 1–3. Although very different results could have been presented merely by choosing other reports from the surgical literature, the series cited were selected because they represented the experience of recognized experts with each of these procedures and were performed for generally accepted indications. Thus, they represent the "gold standard" against which all surgeons should measure their own results. Clearly, direct aortic reconstructions, such as thromboendarterectomy or aortoiliofemoral grafting, are superior to extra-anatomical reconstructions, such as axillofemoral or femorofemoral grafting. The increased mortality rate cited for the latter procedures is a reflection of patient selection, since these procedures are typically reserved for individuals who are too ill to undergo standard, direct reconstructions. The inferior patency quoted for axillofemoral grafting indicates the *primary* patency of this procedure in patients requiring limb salvage surgery.

Outflow Arterial Reconstructions

The results of outflow, i.e., infrainguinal, arterial reconstructions are summarized in Table 1–4. Since there are so many variables that influence patency of these procedures, there are wide variations in the results reported in the surgical literature, depending on patient selection, variations in operative technique, and type of bypass graft chosen. Operative mortality for patients undergoing infrainguinal reconstruction generally averages 1 to 3% regardless of the type of procedure used. Accordingly, only 5-year cumulative life-table patency rates are given. The figures presented in Table 1–4 are reasonable averages for these procedures.

The results given for profundaplasty are achievable when the procedure is performed for claudication. If limb salvage is the indication for operation, a 5-year patency of 30

to 40% is more typical.[55] Clearly, the choice of prosthesis has the most significant impact on infrainguinal bypass grafting. The autogenous saphenous vein remains the preferred conduit for such distal bypasses. This is true for both femoropopliteal and femorotibial bypasses. Depending on whether the saphenous vein is used in a reversed or in-situ fashion, the reported patency for grafts with an infrapopliteal distal anastomosis varies between 40 and 60% at 5 years. Although prosthetic grafts function satisfactorily in the femoropopliteal position as long as the distal anastomosis is placed above the knee joint, they are clearly less satisfactory than the autogenous saphenous vein when used below the knee. In infrapopliteal bypasses, the results with both PTFE and human umbilical vein (HUV) are significantly disappointing. Percutaneous transluminal angioplasty of the superficial femoral artery has a 3-year patency, which is inferior even to that of prosthetic grafting and, accordingly, is not widely used in most vascular centers.

SUMMARY

Physicians treating patients with lower extremity arterial occlusive disease have a wide variety of diagnostic and therapeutic alternatives at their disposal. Since atherosclerosis, which is the underlying disease process in the majority of such patients, is a diffuse, systemic condition, the diagnostic evaluation of these patients must be appropriately comprehensive. Because the prognosis for limb survival is excellent in patients with intermittent claudication, indications for therapeutic intervention are relative, and surgical intervention should be reserved for patients with significant disability who are good operative risks and have favorable anatomical lesions. With more advanced degrees of arterial insufficiency, indications can be appropriately liberalized in an effort to salvage extremities and preserve bipedal gait. On the basis of appropriate physiological data obtained through noninvasive vascular testing and the anatomical correlation provided by high-quality angiograms, satisfactory arterial reconstruction can be performed in most patients requiring revascularization. Proper utilization of the alternative procedures requires a broad familiarity with the principles of

Table 1–4. RESULTS OF OUTFLOW LOWER EXTREMITY ARTERIAL RECONSTRUCTIONS

Procedure*	5-Yr Patency (%)
Infrainguinal TEA	
Profundaplasty alone[55]	77
SFA-TEA[56]	57
Popliteal TEA[57]	59
Bypass Grafting	
FPG	
ASV[38, 58, 59]	67–77
PTFE[36, 38, 60–62]	30–70
HUV[60, 63]	50–70
FTG	
ASV[38, 59, 64]	40–62
Prosthetic[36, 38, 60, 65]	12–40
Femoral PTA[47]	45†

*See numbered references for details.
†3-yr results.
TEA = thromboendarterectomy, SFA = superficial femoral artery, FPG = femoropopliteal grafting, ASV = autogenous saphenous vein, PTFE = polytetrafluoroethylene, HUV = human umbilical vein, FTG = femorotibial grafting, PTA = percutaneous transluminal angioplasty.

vascular reconstruction and the requisite technical skills to apply them correctly.

REFERENCES

1. Crummy AB, Strother CM, Lieberman RP: Digital subtraction angiography for evaluation of peripheral vascular disease. Radiology 141:22, 1981.
2. Gruntzig A, Kumpe DA: Technique of percutaneous transluminal angioplasty with the Gruntzig balloon catheter. AJR 132:547, 1979.
3. Howell WH: Two new factors in blood coagulation. Heparin and proantithrombin. Am J Physiol 47:328, 1918.
4. Karmody AM, Powers SR, Monaco VJ, et al: "Blue toe" syndrome: An indication for limb salvage surgery. Arch Surg 111:1263, 1976.
5. Goodreau JJ, Creasy JK, Flanigan DP, et al: Rational approach to the differentiation of vascular and neurogenic claudication. Surgery 84:749, 1978.
6. Darling RC, Buckley CJ, Abbot WM, et al: Intermittent claudication in young athletes: Popliteal artery entrapment syndrome. J Trauma 14:543, 1974.
7. Brewster DC, Okada RD, Strauss HW, et al: Selection of patients for preoperative coronary angiography: Use of dipyridamole-stress–thallium myocardial imaging. J Vasc Surg 2:504, 1985.
8. Marinelli MR, Beach KW, Glass MJ, et al: Noninvasive testing vs clinical evaluation of arterial disease. A prospective study. JAMA 241:2031, 1979.
9. Kempczinski RF: Segmental volume plethysmography in the diagnosis of lower extremity arterial occlusive disease. J Cardiovasc Surg 23:125, 1982.
10. Kohler TR, Martin RL, Strandness, DE Jr: Duplex scanning for extremity arterial occlusive disease. In Kempczinski RF, Yao JST (eds): Practical Noninvasive Vascular Diagnosis, 2nd Ed. Chicago, Year Book Medical Publishers, 1987, pp 178–209.
11. Moore WS, Hall AD: Unrecognized aortoiliac stenosis: A physiologic approach to the diagnosis. Arch Surg 103:633, 1971.
12. Dardik H, Miller N, Adler J, et al: Primary and adjunctive intra-arterial digital subtraction arteriography of the lower extremities. J Vasc Surg 3:599, 1986.
13. Ricco JB, Pearce WH, Yao JST, et al: The use of pre-bypass arteriography and Doppler ultrasound recordings to select patients for extended femorodistal bypass. Ann Surg 198:646, 1983.
14. Larsson EM, Albrechtsson U, Christenson JT: Computed tomography versus aortography for preoperative evaluation of abdominal aortic aneurysm. Acta Radiol 25:95, 1984.
15. Imparato AM, Kim GE, Davidson T, et al: Intermittent claudication: Its natural course. Surgery 78:795, 1975.
16. Kempczinski RF: Lower-extremity arterial emboli from ulcerating atherosclerotic plaques. JAMA 241:807, 1979.
17. Nicholas GG, Myers JL, DeMuth WE: The role of vascular laboratory criteria in the selection of patients for lower extremity amputation. Ann Surg 195:469, 1982.
18. Kazmers M, Satiani B, Evans WE: Amputation level following unsuccessful distal limb salvage operations. Surgery 87:683, 1980.
19. Szilagyi DE, Hageman JH, Smith RF, et al: Autogenous vein grafting in femoropopliteal atherosclerosis: The limits of its effectiveness. Surgery 86:836, 1979.
20. Dardik H, Kahn M, Dardik II, et al: Influence of failed vascular bypass procedures on conversion of below-knee to above-knee amputation levels. Surgery 91:64, 1982.
21. Blaisdell FW: Use of anticoagulants in the ischemic lower extremity: An alternate perspective. In Kempczinski RF (ed): The Ischemic Leg. Chicago, Year Book Medical Publishers, 1985, p 247.
22. Kendrick J, Thompson BW, Read RC, et al: Arterial embolectomy in the leg: Results in a referral hospital. Am J Surg 142:739, 1981.
23. Haimovici H: Muscular, renal and metabolic complications of acute arterial occlusions: Myonephropathic-metabolic syndrome. Surgery 85:461, 1979.
24. Berkowitz HD, Hargrove WC, Roberts B: Thrombolytic therapy for arterial occlusion. In Kempczinski RF (ed): The Ischemic Leg. Chicago, Year Book Medical Publishers, 1985, p 255.
25. Blaisdell FW, Steele M, Allen RE: Management of acute lower extremity arterial ischemia due to embolism and thrombosis. Surgery 84:822, 1978.
26. Brewster DC, Darling RC: Optimal methods of aortoiliac reconstruction. Surgery 84:739, 1978.
27. Rutherford RB, Jones DN, Martin MS, et al: Serial hemodynamic assessment of aortobifemoral bypass. J Vasc Surg 4:428, 1986.
28. Welch P, Repetto R: Revascularization of the profunda femoris artery in aortoiliac occlusive disease. Surgery 78:389, 1975.
29. Dick LS, Brief DK, Alpert J, et al: A 12-year experience with femorofemoral crossover grafts. Arch Surg 115:1359, 1980.
30. Donaldson MC, Louras JC, Bucknam CA: Axillofemoral bypass: A tool with a limited role. J Vasc Surg 3:757, 1986.
31. Mitchell RA, Bone GE, Bridges R, et al: Patient selection for isolated profundaplasty. Am J Surg 138:912, 1979.
32. Inahara T, Scott CM: Endarterectomy for segmental occlusive disease of the superficial femoral artery. Arch Surg 116:1547, 1981.
33. Brewster DC, LaSalle AJ, Robison JG, et al: Factors affecting results of femoropopliteal bypass grafts. Surg Gynecol Obstet 157:437, 1983.
34. Couch NP: On the arterial consequences of smoking. J Vasc Surg 3:807, 1986.
35. Martin P: Relationship between age and success of arterial operations. J Cardiovasc Surg 16:155, 1975.
36. Veith FJ, Gupta SK, Samsom RH, et al: Progress in limb salvage by reconstructive arterial surgery combined with new or improved adjunctive procedures. Ann Surg 194:386, 1981.
37. Quinones-Baldrich WJ, Martin-Paradero V, Baker JD, et al: PTFE grafts as the arterial substitute of first choice in femoral-popliteal revascularization. Arch Surg 119:1238, 1984.
38. Veith FJ, Gupta SK, Ascer E, et al: Six-year prospective multicenter randomized comparison of autologous saphenous vein and expanded polytetrafluoroethylene grafts in infrainguinal arterial reconstructions. J Vasc Surg 3:104, 1986.
39. Leather RP, Powers SR, Karmody AM: A reappraisal of the in-situ saphenous vein arterial bypass. Surgery 86:453, 1979.
40. Leather RP, Shah DM, Buchbinder D, et al: Further

experience with the saphenous vein used in situ for arterial bypass. Am J Surg 142:506, 1981.

41. Kempczinski RF: Infrainguinal arterial bypass using prosthetic grafts. *In* Kempczinski RF (ed): The Ischemic Leg. Chicago, Year Book Medical Publishers, 1985, p 255.

42. Sterpetti AV, Schultz RD, Feldhaus RJ, Peetz DW: Seven-year experience with polytetrafluoroethylene as above-knee femoropopliteal graft. Is it worthwhile to preserve the autologous saphenous vein? J Vasc Surg 2:907, 1985.

43. Harris RW, Andros G, Dulawa LB, et al: Successful long term limb salvage using cephalic vein bypass grafts. Ann Surg 200:785, 1984.

44. Dardik H, Sussman B, Ibrahim IM, et al: Distal arteriovenous fistula as an adjunct to maintaining arterial and graft patency for limb salvage. Surgery 94:478, 1983.

45. Hadcock MM, Ubatuba J, Littooy F, et al: Hemodynamics of sequential grafts. Am J Surg 146:170, 1983.

46. Dotter CT, Judkins MP: Transluminal treatment of arteriosclerotic obstruction: Description of a preliminary report of its application. Circulation 30:654, 1964.

47. Johnson KW, Colapinto RF, Baird RJ: Transluminal dilation: An alternative? Arch Surg 117:1604, 1982.

48. Hobson RW, Lynch TG, Jamil Z, et al: Results of revascularization and amputation in severe lower extremity ischemia: A five-year clinical experience. J Vasc Surg 2:174, 1985.

49. Sladen JG, Maxwell TM: Experience with 130 polytetrafluoroethylene grafts. Am J Surg 141:546, 1981.

50. Gloviczki P, Hollier LH, Dewanjee MK, et al: Quantitative evaluation of ibuprofen treatment on thrombogenicity of expanded polytetrafluoroethylene vascular grafts. Surgery 95:160, 1984.

51. Kohler TR, Kaufman JL, Kacoyanis G, et al: Effect of aspirin and dipyridamole on the patency of lower extremity bypass grafts. Surgery 96:462, 1984.

52. Quarfordt PG, Stoney RJ: Aortoiliac thromboendarterectomy. *In* Kempczinski RF (ed): The Ischemic Leg. Chicago, Year Book Medical Publishers, 1985, p 291.

53. Eugene J, Goldstone J, Moore WS: Fifteen-year experience with subcutaneous bypass grafts for lower-extremity ischemia. Ann Surg 186:177, 1976.

54. Plecha FR, Plecha FM: Femorofemoral bypass grafts: Ten-year experience. J Vasc Surg 1:555, 1984.

55. Towne JB, Bernhard VM, Rollins DL, Baum PL: Profundaplasty in perspective: Limitations in the long-term management of limb ischemia. Surgery 90:1037, 1981.

56. Ouriel K, Smith CR, DeWeese JA: Endarterectomy for localized lesions of the superficial femoral artery at the adductor canal. J Vasc Surg 3:531, 1986.

57. Inahara T, Toledo AC: Endarterectomy of the popliteal artery for segmental occlusive disease. Ann Surg 188:43, 1978.

58. Ricotta JJ, DeWeese JA: Femoropopliteal/tibial bypass grafting using the reversed autogenous saphenous vein. *In* Kempczinski RF (ed): The Ischemic Leg. Chicago, Year Book Medical Publishers, 1985, p 386.

59. Leather RP, Shad DM, Corson JD, Karmody AM: Instrumental evolution of the valve incision method of in situ saphenous vein bypass. J Vasc Surg 1:113, 1984.

60. Cranley JJ, Hafner CD: Revascularization of the femoropopliteal arteries using saphenous vein, polytetrafluoroethylene, and umbilical vein grafts. Arch Surg 117:1543, 1982.

61. Julian TB, Loubeau JM, Stremple JF: Polytetrafluoroethylene or saphenous vein as a femoropopliteal bypass graft? J Surg Res 32:1, 1982.

62. LaSalle AJ, Brewster DC, Corson JD, Darling RC: Femoropopliteal composite bypass grafts: Current status. Surgery 92:36, 1982.

63. Dardik H, Baier RE, Meenaghan M, et al: Morphologic and biophysical assessment of long term human umbilical cord vein implants used as vascular conduits. Surg Gynecol Obstet 154:17, 1982.

64. Kacoyanis GP, Whittemore AD, Couch NP, Mannick JA: Femorotibial and femoroperoneal bypass vein grafts. A 15-year experience. Arch Surg 116:1529, 1981.

65. Ricco JB, Flinn WR, McDaniel MD: Objective analysis of factors contributing to failure of tibial bypass grafts. World J Surg 7:347, 1983.

2

The Diabetic Foot and Management of Infectious Gangrene

Kenneth E. McIntyre, Jr., M.D.

Each year, thousands of diabetic patients are hospitalized with foot infections. The infections may stem from trauma, ischemia, neuropathy, poor control of diabetes, or a combination of these elements. Regardless of the inciting factor, the diabetic foot does not tolerate infections well. Many infections become relentlessly progressive, and this leads to a high rate of limb amputation. In contrast to nondiabetics, diabetic patients are 17 times more likely to develop gangrene.[22] In addition, five of six major limb amputations occur in diabetic patients.[22] This chapter will attempt to identify those factors that predispose the diabetic patient to serious limb-threatening foot infections. On the basis of an understanding of the factors involved in diabetic foot infections that are addressed in this chapter, a rational algorithm is presented for the care of these difficult patients.

SCOPE OF THE PROBLEM

Diabetes affects approximately 5% of the United States' population (10 to 12 million people).[17, 22] Advances in treatment have contributed to increased survival among diabetic patients. Unfortunately, as these patients live longer, the complications of long-standing illness become more apparent. There is an increased incidence of all complications of diabetes mellitus, especially cardiovascular, eye, renal, cerebrovascular, and peripheral vascular problems. These problems, as well as lower extremity infections, lead to many hospitalizations during the diabetic patient's life. Ischemic foot lesions are generally seen in elderly patients with adult-onset diabetes, whereas patients with neuropathic lesions usually have juvenile or early-onset insulin-dependent diabetes. Although careful personal hygiene and attention to diabetic management (diet, insulin, and exercise) may postpone foot problems, such care probably will not prevent them.[22]

In 1980, direct hospital costs alone for diabetic care in the US exceeded 200 million dollars.[22] This figure does not include lost productivity, disability pay, unemployment, or other indirect medical costs.

During a 12-month period at New England Deaconess Hospital, 22% of diabetic patients were admitted because of gangrene and lower extremity infections.[36] Whitehouse and colleagues reported that of 640 diabetic patients hospitalized during a 6-month period from 1966 to 1967, 10.5% were admitted because of an infection.[51] Of those patients, 75% had infections involving the lower extremity, lower respiratory tract, or upper urinary tract. Thirty-eight percent of the patients with lower extremity infections underwent amputations.[51] In a similar time period from 1969 to 1970, Whitehouse and colleagues noted that 22% of diabetic patients admitted to the hospital had a serious infection, and one half of these infections involved the foot. Of the patients with a foot infection, 56% required an amputation before leaving the hospital.[51]

Many large clinics have reported amputation rates of greater than 50% in diabetic patients with foot infections.[38, 41, 51, 52] Schalt reported a 5-year follow-up study of 25 diabetic patients with major arterial occlusions who developed gangrene. Thirteen (52%) of those patients required leg amputations.[41] The estimated incidence of major lower limb amputation in a high-risk diabetic patient ranges from 6 to 12% per year.[25]

The mortality rate among diabetic patients with lower extremity infection is also impressive. Review of the literature reveals mortality rates of 2.7 to 25% for infection and gangrene of the lower extremity in surgically treated diabetic patients.[5, 10, 18, 28, 30, 45, 52] In addition, the diabetic has a limited life expectancy after amputation.[5, 45] Joslin and associates reported that "among 206 gangrene cases, 48 died in the first year after operation, but the average length of life was 2.9 years after operation."[17] Whitehouse observed 67 diabetic patients who had lost one leg to gangrene. By 3 years, only 50% of the amputees survived, and by 5 years, only 36% were alive.[50] Similar data were reported by Roon and coworkers, who noted that the age-adjusted 5-year survival in nondiabetic patients after major lower limb amputation was almost normal (75 versus 85%), whereas it was only 39% in diabetic patients.[37]

Other authors have examined the fate of the remaining leg in the diabetic amputee. Silbert and Haimovici observed that 40% of diabetic patients who survived for 3 years after the loss of one leg would require amputation of the second leg within that period.[43, 44] These findings were also supported by Goldner, who noted that 50% of diabetic patients who had undergone amputation for gangrene developed lesions of the remaining leg within 2 years after involvement of the first leg.[14] In Mazet and associates'[29] study of geriatric patients from Veterans Administration and county hospitals, 18 to 28% of the patients had lost their opposite limb within 2 years, with little difference between diabetic and nondiabetic patients. However, by 5 years after amputation, significantly more diabetics than nondiabetics had lost their opposite limb in both the VA series (66 versus 28%) and the county series (46 versus 28%). Whitehouse, however, felt that the diabetic amputee would likely die from complications of atheroclerosis before losing the remaining leg.[50]

HISTORICAL PERSPECTIVE

Bell's study of atherosclerotic gangrene in 1957 reviewed the autopsy records of 2130 diabetics and 59,733 nondiabetics.[2] He found that the incidence of gangrene increased with age and that gangrene of the lower extremities was 156 times more common in diabetics than in nondiabetics in the fifth decade, and 85 and 53 times more common in the sixth and seventh decades, respectively.

Considering the high morbidity and mortality in diabetic patients undergoing amputation for infectious gangrene, it is no surprise that this problem is of utmost concern to surgeons. A brief look at the history of management of diabetic gangrene will give better insight into the limited progress made over the past 50 years.

As early as 1935, Levin and Dealy recognized that surgical procedures in diabetic patients were associated with a high incidence of complications.[23] Even with the advent of insulin in the 1930s, the mortality rate of diabetics undergoing amputation was reported to be 50%.[23] Before that time, it was assumed that diabetics who did not receive insulin treatment usually died before surgical intervention could proceed. Antibiotics ushered in a new era in the 1940s; however, the mortality rate for amputation in diabetics remained at 32%.[28] With improved antibiotics and better surgical and anesthetic techniques, the mortality rate continued to fall in the 2 decades between 1940 and 1960 but remained above 20%.[5, 10, 16, 17, 35] Since then, the mortality rate has continued to decline but has remained about 5 to 10% for below- and 13 to 35% for above-knee amputations.[8, 18, 21, 30, 31, 34]

Even though many advances in the diagnosis and management of diabetic vascular disease have been made over the past 50 years, limb loss in the diabetic patient is still, unfortunately, a common problem.

ETIOLOGY OF FOOT LESIONS

Ischemia

Of the recognized factors contributing to the development of foot lesions in diabetics, vascular impairment may be the only one that is treatable. In a survey by Delbridge and associates, large vessel vascular disease was found in all patients with diabetic foot lesions and was not present in a control group of diabetics without foot lesions.[9] Atherosclerosis tends to occur with greater frequency and severity and appears earlier in diabetics than in age-matched controls.[12] Strandness and colleagues[48] reported that 81% of diabetics have stenosis or occlusion of the tibial trifurcation vessels, whereas only 57% of nondiabetics have similar disease. The severity of large vessel lesions, however, seems unrelated to the duration or management of diabetes.[13]

Diabetics characteristically have two different types of arterial changes: large vessel (macroangiopathy) and small vessel (microangiopathy). There are no distinctive histopathological lesions of diabetic macroangiopathy; however, there are qualitative differences in mucopolysaccharides, calcium, cholesterol, and ash compared with nondiabetics.[13] Regardless of these qualitative changes, it must be emphasized that the macrovascular lesion is, for practical purposes, "garden variety" atherosclerosis. Importantly, however, the disease is much more extensive and more commonly associated with medial calcific sclerosis in diabetics than in nondiabetics.[20] Diabetic microangiopathy involves arteries smaller than 115 mμ in diameter. The severity and extent of the small vessel lesion distinguish diabetics from nondiabetics.[20] The arteriolar lesion consists of thickening of the vessel wall with material

that stains with periodic acid–Schiff (PAS) stain, proliferation of the intima and endothelium, pericyte proliferation, collagen deposition, and irregular basement membrane thickening. However, a given arteriole from a diabetic with hyaline sclerosis is morphologically indistinguishable from a given arteriole of a nondiabetic, in whom the disease may be due to age or hypertension.[20] The hallmark of diabetic microangiopathy is PAS-positive thickening of the capillary wall, the most advanced degree occurring in the most dependent areas of the body—the lower extremity vessels. Unfortunately, only the macroangiopathy, atherosclerosis, can be treated directly with surgery. Although meticulous management of diabetes may delay or postpone microangiopathy and its complications, such careful treatment will not prevent the complications, and the vessels involved are beyond surgical therapy owing to their exceedingly small size.[22]

There are a multiplicity of pathogenic factors that account for an increased frequency of atherosclerosis in diabetic patients; they include hyperlipidemia, hypertension, smoking, the secondary consequences of hyperglycemia, obesity, genetic factors, and hypercoagulability. One of the peculiar features of diabetic vascular disease is that this type of complication is not restricted to any one type of diabetes. Instead, the complications tend to be a function of both the duration and severity of hyperglycemia over years.[22] Therefore, vascular complications tend to be more common in patients with Type I diabetes. On the other hand, macrovascular complications are frequently unrelated to the severity or duration of diabetes. The lipid disturbances reported with diabetes mellitus include elevated levels of low-density lipoprotein (LDL) cholesterol, low concentrations of high-density lipoprotein (HDL) cholesterol, and elevated levels of very low-density lipoprotein (VLDL) triglyceride. The incidence of hyperlipidemia varies between 25 and 75% depending on the type and severity of diabetes, glycemic control, age, nutritional status, and other factors.[12, 13] Many hematological disturbances leading to hypercoagulability have been demonstrated in diabetic patients, including enhanced platelet aggregation and release; excess fibrinogen; decreased fibrolytic activity; elevated serum viscosity; elevated levels of clotting factors V, VII, VIII, and X; and hypertriglyceridemia.[13]

Diabetic patients who present with foot lesions need careful evaluation of their peripheral vasculature to ensure adequate healing of foot lesions or when debridements or amputations are necessary. In one study of gangrenous extremities in diabetic patients, Collens and associates found that 73% of patients had objective evidence of peripheral atherosclerosis obliterans.[7] In a study of transmetatarsal amputations in diabetic patients, Wheelock found that only 40% of patients with gangrene had a palpable popliteal pulse and less than one third were deemed fit for arterial reconstruction after arteriography.[49] Pearse and Ziegler also found that most (67%) of 277 diabetic patients admitted to the hospital with foot infections had some serious impairment in their peripheral circulation.[35]

A careful history and physical examination usually provide an accurate assessment of the status and location of occlusive lesions within the arterial tree of the lower extremity. Symptoms of intermittent claudication and rest pain are typical of moderate and severe ischemia, respectively. Findings of hair loss, hypertrophic nails, or decreased pulses are indicative of mild to moderate arterial insufficiency. The absence of pulses indicates more severe, but not necessarily limb-threatening, ischemia, whereas evidence of dependent rubor or elevation pallor clearly suggests limb-threatening ischemia. Finally, tissue gangrene clearly indicates areas that are not amenable to salvage and suggests that the entire limb may be in jeopardy. The noninvasive vascular laboratory may provide adjunctive data that are useful for evaluating and following up patients, especially after surgical reconstructions, but noninvasive data should not replace a careful history and physical examination.

It is generally accepted that in diabetic patients with normal distal circulation, foot wounds heal after local debridement and do not require higher amputation. In those patients with palpable pedal pulses, foot salvage with local debridement should always be attempted first. If healing occurs, the need for higher amputation is obviated. Occasionally, foot wounds do not heal and continue to suppurate in the presence of pedal pulses. It is unclear whether this is due to microcirculatory impairment, abnormal glucosylation of collagen, or inability of diabetic's phagocytes to function properly.[1, 4, 42] In that setting, an aggressive posture toward arteriography and

vascular reconstruction is appropriate. Many legs are lost because revascularization is not considered or undertaken soon enough.

A complete discussion of the indications, techniques, and results of lower extremity revascularization are beyond the scope of this chapter; however, several factors regarding vascular reconstruction in diabetic patients are important when considering surgical therapy. First, the long-term success rates for certain lower extremity vascular reconstructions are worse in diabetic than nondiabetic patients.[26, 27, 37] Second, vascular disease appears earlier in diabetics than does similar disease in nondiabetics, and it tends to be of greater severity. Third, the extent of the atherosclerotic lesions tends to be more diffuse and widespread and often involves blood vessels that are uncommonly involved in nondiabetics, such as the deep femoral artery. Fourth, the hallmark of diabetic peripheral vascular disease is extensive involvement of the tibial trifurcation vessels, precisely the vessels that are needed to allow satisfactory patency for lower extremity vascular reconstructive procedures. Finally, vascular disease affects young and old female diabetics with equal severity compared with nondiabetics, among whom premenopausal women are relatively free of atherosclerosis. The mechanism of diabetic women's increased propensity for vascular disease has not been defined at the present time.

In summary, the diabetic patient suffers from both large vessel atherosclerosis and microangiopathy. The severity and extent of these two pathological processes varies from patient to patient, and their onset may be quite insidious, the first manifestation being tissue loss or gangrene.

Neuropathy

Neuropathy is an important factor in the development of diabetic foot problems. Unlike ischemia, which may develop despite the duration or control of diabetes, peripheral neuropathy may well be related to the quality of glycemic control.[22]

The neuropathic foot has poor sensation and good circulation. All problems related to neuropathic feet are based on those two facts. Loss of sensation makes the feet vulnerable to trauma, yet good circulation makes them able to heal wounds or minor infections; however, even though pulses may be present, indicating acceptable large vessel circulation, there may be microvascular disease, leaving the skin and other tissues more vulnerable than usual to infection or injury. The diabetic patient with a neuropathic foot usually has an antecedent history of paresthesias and pains in the feet or legs. The usual clinical findings include calluses on pressure points; a tendency for hammer toes and high arches; diminished or absent sensation, vibratory sense, or Achilles' tendon reflex; good dorsalis pedis and posterior tibial pulses; well-nourished subcutaneous tissue; and, in more severe cases, Charcot's deformities, drop foot, and superimposed infections including ulcers and osteomyelitis.

In addition to sensation, the peripheral neuropathy also affects muscle receptors, causing atrophy of some muscle groups in the leg and foot. The muscle atrophy results in disproportionate muscle tone in the feet, causing cavus deformities as well as drop foot in advanced cases. Although the foot develops calluses on pressure points to protect itself, the trauma to the underlying tissues may cause deep ulcers or abscesses, the latter of which may extend into joints and bones, causing osteomyelitis. Neuro-osteoarthropathy is characterized by joint swelling and bone disruption and absorption with fractures. That process leaves disrupted joints, collapsed arches, and shortened toes, and the resultant wide deformed foot is subject to calluses and ulcers because of its irregular contour (Charcot's foot).

Hyaline arteriosclerosis has been found in intraneural arterioles in diabetics. That finding has prompted some investigators to suggest that angiopathy is the basic lesion of neuropathy.[22] However, current work tends to support the hypothesis that diabetic peripheral neuropathy is a primary metabolic problem.[6, 12, 13] There is degeneration of non-myelinated nerve fibers and foci of demyelination and degeneration of myelinated nerve fibers. Whether or not the demyelination represents a primary vascular problem due to ischemic damage or is unrelated and due to a primary metabolic problem will undoubtedly continue to be debated. Nevertheless, the primary concern is prevention of the problem. In reality, however, meticulous management of diabetes will not prevent neuropathy but will, in all likelihood, postpone or delay its appearance.[22]

The neuropathic diabetic foot is at great risk for several reasons. First, there is no protective sensation; therefore, minor trauma may go relatively unnoticed until there is significant ulceration, infection, or bone injury. This observation may explain why putrid, necrotic foot lesions go virtually undetected by patients until they smell them. Second, because of intrinsic foot muscle atrophy and secondary foot deformities, there is an alteration in the weight distribution and biomechanics of foot function that leads to pressure points, callus formation, and skin breakdown.[15, 46] The combination of bony foot deformity and the lack of protective sensation leads to abnormal skin problems due to friction, pressure, and shear forces.[46] The classic diabetic neuropathic foot has bounding pedal pulses and therefore a presumably "normal" arterial circulation. However, the presence of microangiopathy lessens the ability of skin to resist these abnormal biomechanical forces; therefore, microvascular disease or macrovascular disease, if it exists, forms the final part of the triad in the evolution of diabetic foot problems.

For those patients with diabetic sympathetic dystrophy, the lack of sympathetic tone causes lower extremity skin to become dried, thinned, and cracked. Small areas of skin breakdown then become an entry site for bacteria and subsequent infection. Sympathetic dystrophy, therefore, worsens or may lead directly to diabetic foot problems when it is added to the triad of neuropathy, ischemia, and biomechanical changes in the foot.

Neither neuropathy nor ischemia is totally responsible for gangrene of the foot in diabetics. Careful glycemic control may improve neuropathy, thereby making the foot less unstable. It is the neuropathic unstable diabetic foot, with or without macro- or microangiopathy, that is susceptible to gangrene, plantar infection, and limb loss.

Infection

Although it has been stated that diabetics are more prone to infection than nondiabetics, there is little clinical evidence to support this hypothesis. Perhaps such thinking evolved from the recognition of the hyperglycemia associated with necrotic diabetic foot infections. Infection affects glycemic control, and uncontrolled diabetes affects infection. Polymorphonuclear leukocytes obtained from both diabetic patients with ketoacidosis and diabetic patients under good glycemic control demonstrate a marked difference in their ability to phagocytize and destroy bacteria.[1, 4] With insulin therapy, the abnormality in phagocytosis is reversed, but the leukocytes of diabetics still have an abnormal capacity to kill bacteria.[1] Owing to the absence of protective sensations and symptoms, the lack of adequate blood supply to allow healing or fighting of infection, and the immunological impairment, minor foot infections can quickly progress to an unsalvageable state in diabetics with neuropathy and ischemia. Neuropathy, foot deformity, sympathetic dystrophy, and ischemia set the stage for a diabetic foot infection. Infection per se is merely the final insult to an already compromised unstable foot.

MICROBIOLOGY OF DIABETIC FOOT INFECTIONS

Historically, the most common organism cultured from diabetic foot infections was *Staphylococcus aureus*. It was apparent, however, that serious limb-threatening infections had many of the characteristics of anaerobic infections, such as putrid odor, gas in the tissues, necrosis of fascia, and virulent progression.[3] As better culture techniques were employed, it became clear that the predominant cause for gangrenous diabetic foot infections was a multiplicity of mixed aerobic and anaerobic organisms.[3, 11, 40, 47] Louie and colleagues[24] cultured 20 diabetic foot ulcers and noted anaerobic bacteria in 18 patients, with an average of 5.8 species isolated per foot infection. The common isolates, in order of decreasing frequency, were *Bacteroides, Peptococcus, Proteus,* enterocci, *S. aureus,* clostridia, and *Escherichia coli*.[24] In a similar study, Fierer and associates[11] reviewed 30 consecutive diabetics who required surgery for lower extremity infection and found that 17 of the infections were caused by a combination of obligate and facultative anaerobes, whereas only 20% were caused by *S. aureus* alone. The most common anaerobic organism isolated in that series was *Bacteroides fragilis*. In a similar study of 32 diabetic patients with infected feet, Sapico and coworkers[40] reported that the predominant culture was a mixture of aerobes and anaerobes. Importantly, in that

series, prior antibiotic therapy did not appear to influence the isolation of microorganisms.

There are certain clinical features that are commonly associated with mixed aerobic-anaerobic tissue infections. Characteristically, the infections are foul smelling. Soft tissue gas or liquifying fascial necrosis is often found. Stone and Martin have described that syndrome as synergistic necrotizing cellulitis.[47] In their patients with diabetes mellitus, the mortality rate was 85%, as compared with 44% for the nondiabetic patients. They described a symbiotic relationship between one or more species of gram-negative aerobic bacteria and an obligate or facultative anaerobe, such as streptococcus or bacteroides, in most of their diabetic patients.

In order to ensure the recovery of anaerobic organisms, adequate culture techniques must be employed. Ideally, these should include deep curettage of the ulcer/wound base. Surface swabs and Gram's stains of material taken from ulcers give unreliable data and have the least chance of recovering anaerobic organisms.[40]

The choice of initial antibiotic therapy for diabetic foot problems is influenced by many variables, including the likely pathogens, local bacterial resistance patterns, pre-existing renal or hepatic dysfunction, prior antibiotic therapy, and severity of the infection. In previously untreated patients with mild infections, a broad-spectrum third-generation cephalosporin may be adequate. It is important to note, however, that although third-generation cephalosporins do provide broader protection against gram-negative bacteria, they do so at the expense of a relative loss of potency against gram-positive organisms.[11] Since there are presently no data to support the superiority of third-generation cephalosporins over second-generation cephalosporins or combination therapy with less expensive drugs, the routine use of these more costly drugs cannot be recommended at the present time. In patients with severe or rapidly progressing infections and a recent history of antibiotic therapy or in those strongly suspected of having a major anaerobic infection, high-dose broad-spectrum intravenous antibiotic coverage is appropriate. One commonly used regimen is clindamycin with an aminoglycoside. Because of the evidence that tobramycin may be less nephrotoxic than gentamicin and because of the former's greater activity against *Pseudomonas aeruginosa*, tobramycin may be preferable to gentamicin. However, in diabetic patients, some of whom may already have renal impairment, aminoglycosides must be used with the utmost caution. Neither cephalosporins alone nor clindamycin plus an aminoglycoside provides adequate coverage for enterococci; therefore, an argument can be made for triple therapy using ampicillin or penicillin to cover enterococcus. At the author's institution, until culture-specific results are available, the broad-spectrum therapy of choice for life- and limb-threatening infections is a combination of intravenous penicillin and chloramphenicol.

MANAGEMENT OF DIABETIC GANGRENE

There are four principles of successful management of infectious gangrene in the diabetic foot: aggressive debridement, evaluation of perfusion, antibiotic therapy, and, most importantly, functional restoration of the limb. An algorithm of the author's management approach for diabetic foot problems is shown in Table 2–1.

First, aggressive surgical debridement of

necrotic, infected, and devitalized tissue is mandatory. The debridement should extend to clean tissue margins and may need to include musculoskeletal components in order to drain the wound adequately and prevent spread of the infection. Usually, inadequate debridement results in a further delay in healing and advancement of the infection. If the tissue margins do not bleed or if thrombosed veins are present within the proximal margin, one can assume that the debridement is not adequate. Surgical exploration should be performed in an operating room, with adequate anesthesia, in order to optimize assessment of the extent of the infection and involvement of vital structures. Once the infected tissue has been adequately debrided and drained, the next step is to establish the need for revascularization.

An adequate physical examination should include the status of all peripheral pulses, documentation of the presence or absence of femoral bruits, and notation of the palpable quality of the femoral and lower limb pulses. The lower limb and foot should be examined for hair distribution, temperature demarcation, sensory and motor function, elevation pallor, dependent rubor, cellulitis, edema, ulceration, deep infection, gangrene, emboli, and bone abnormalities. Dependent rubor,

Table 2–1. ALGORITHM FOR TREATMENT OF DIABETIC FOOT PROBLEMS*

Mild	Moderate	Severe
Superficial infection/ulcer	Deep ulcer	Deep ulcer or infection
No cellulitis	Cellulitis	± Bone involvement
No bone involvement	± Bone involvement	Pedal edema
No systemic signs	Pedal edema	Ascending cellulitis
	± Deep infection	Systemic toxicity
	± Systemic toxicity	Threatened limb loss
	± Threatened limb loss	
Trial of ambulatory care†	Hospital admission†	Same as Moderate Category, but:
Rest injured area	Control hyperglycemia	
Culture and sensitivity testing	Initial broad-spectrum	Initial drainage may
Broad-spectrum followed by	followed by culture-specific	require guillotine,
culture-specific oral	high-dose antibiotics	partial or complete
antibiotics	Surgical debridement and	foot amputation
Local wound care	drainage	Early and aggressive
Podiatric prosthetic shoe or	Aggressive wound care	consideration for
modification	Selective arteriography,	vascular
Careful follow-up	revascularization, and	reconstruction
Careful documentation of	conservation amputations	
vascular examination	Podiatric/prosthetic shoe/	
	appliance	
	Careful follow-up	

*All groups receive patient education on diabetic management and foot care.
†If the treatment fails, the patient is moved up one category in severity.

venous troughing, hair loss, and trophic skin changes are all indicators that the foot may be chronically ischemic. Neurological dysfunction may indicate diabetic neuropathy or acute ischemia. Peripheral emboli, dependent rubor, elevation pallor, tissue loss, and nonhealing lesions all indicate limb-threatening ischemia and mandate early and aggressive consideration for arterial reconstruction. Besides physical examination, the noninvasive vascular laboratory may provide useful information in quantitating the extent of arterial insufficiency. Doppler-derived ankle/arm indices may or may not be helpful in assessing the severity of ischemia, depending on whether or not calcified lower extremity vessels are present. In the presence of large vessel calcification, the pressure cuffs used for Doppler-derived blood pressure measurements cannot adequately compress the arteries. Therefore, the pressures that are recorded are artificially high, giving an artificially elevated ankle/arm index, which suggests that arterial perfusion is acceptable while in fact it may be abnormal. This phenomenon is readily apparent when suprasystolic pressures are recorded in lower extremities or when foot or lower limb X-ray films reveal calcified arterial walls in the distal lower limb and pedal arch. In the presence of calcified arterial walls, new techniques—such as Doppler-derived toe, transcutaneous oxygen, and transcutaneous carbon dioxide pressure determinations; intradermal xenon-133 clearance; and fiberoptic fluorometry—may be useful in more accurately assessing the exact degree of ischemia and the quality of local tissue perfusion.[25, 25a] Most of these tests do not appear to be affected by the presence of diabetes since their ability to predict successful healing of amputations is not significantly different between diabetic and nondiabetic populations.[25]

In any patient under consideration for arterial reconstruction, arteriography is mandatory. If there have been no antecedent symptoms of intermittent claudication and if the femoral pulses are normal, evaluation of the aortoiliac system may not be required. If, however, there is a decreased femoral pulse, the presence of femoral bruits, or a history of claudication, the arteriogram must include evaluation of the aortoiliac system. Visualization of the lower extremity requires complete views of the thigh, lower limb, and pedal arch. Unfortunately, diabetics with large vessel occlusive disease generally have a characteristic "tandem" occlusive pattern that makes lower extremity revascularization extremely difficult. This tandem lesion consists of deep femoral artery stenosis or diffuse occlusive disease (in the presence of prior superficial femoral artery occlusion) and severe infrapopliteal or tibial trifurcation occlusive disease. The other pattern typically seen in diabetics is that of relatively normal superficial femoral, deep femoral, and popliteal arteries with basically no major identifiable tibial or peroneal artery present in the lower limb or foot. In general, it is unusual to see tissue loss with only one level of occlusion; therefore, diabetics presenting with gangrene or nonhealing lesions most probably have two or three levels of occlusive disease. Careful evaluation of the arteriogram and the patient's clinical findings will be helpful in assessing the possibility of successful lower extremity arterial reconstruction.

Although profundaplasty has been advocated by some authors as a substitute for distal femoral bypasses, this author has been disappointed in his results with profundaplasty for limb salvage in patients presenting with tissue loss. Profundaplasty may be helpful in patients presenting with early rest pain or in patients with nonhealing lesions, but it probably is not a satisfactory procedure by itself for patients with established gangrene or severe limb-threatening ischemia. In these latter patients, the best long-term results for limb salvage are found with femoral distal bypasses. A complete discussion of lower limb revascularization is well beyond the scope of this chapter, and the interested reader is referred to the appropriate references.[19, 33, 39] In general, the best long-term results for limb salvage are seen when saphenous vein is used as a prosthetic conduit. Whether the saphenous vein should be reversed, translocated, or used in situ is still controversial. In the absence of usable saphenous vein, the present graft of choice is polytetrafluoroethylene. Saphenous vein is the best conduit for reconstruction in the face of distal ipsilateral soft tissue infection.

In addition to adequate surgical debridement and evaluation of the patient's vascular status with or without subsequent vascular reconstruction, high-dose intravenous antibiotic therapy is important. As discussed in a previous section, moderate or severe diabetic foot problems (see Table 2–1) should be viewed as limb threatening; therefore, initial broad-spectrum followed by culture-specific intravenous antibiotic coverage is appropriate. The rationales for specific antibiotic therapies have been previously discussed and will not be repeated in this section. However, regardless of the choice of antibiotics, antibiotic therapy must be deemed adjunctive to adequate surgical debridement and, if appropriate, vascular reconstruction. Antibiotic therapy merely helps to control sepsis and reduce localized cellulitis. Antibiotic therapy cannot take the place of adequate surgical debridement and drainage.

Finally, although the author has stated that aggressive debridement is important in the management of diabetic foot problems, that procedure must be carefully performed with the goal of treatment in mind: the primary healing of the most functional extremity possible. In that light, as much tissue and limb length as possible should be saved.

Conservative amputations and limited partial foot amputations should be considered first when trying to achieve adequate debridement or drainage of a deep forefoot infection in a diabetic patient. Such amputations usually heal if the infected tissue is appropriately debrided and drained and there is an adequate blood supply. Skin coverage can be obtained through the rotation of flaps or the application of skin grafts; however, skin grafts do not have the durability normally associated with plantar skin, and they may later break down as a result of prosthesis use. For patients with life- or limb-threatening situations, a guillotine amputation of the forefoot or foot may be required to achieve control of sepsis and adequately drain the foot infection. A guillotine amputation can be accomplished in a relatively short time, and that maneuver alone may be lifesaving. In a prior series of diabetic patients who presented with septic foot problems, McIntyre and associates found that ankle guillotine amputation followed by definitive below-knee amputation at a later date (a two-stage amputation) significantly reduced the chance of residual limb infection (3%) when compared with the one-stage below-knee amputation (22%).[30]

In the author's experience, toe, ray transmetatarsal, below-knee, and above-knee amputations have all been durable and reliable for subsequent prosthetic rehabilitation in diabetic patients. However, the author has been uniquely disappointed with Syme's amputations in diabetic patients; in a review of the author's series of diabetic patients, it is apparent that in many cases a Syme's amputation was performed in patients with present but *diminished* sensation. These patients later returned with an insensate distal limb and gradually had breakdown of the Syme's stump, ultimately requiring below-knee amputation. It is, therefore, the author's preference not to perform Syme's amputation in diabetic patients unless their foot sensation is *normal*. In this light, it is interesting that the author has seen few problems (2.3% late failure) with below-knee amputation residual limbs in diabetic patients who have neuropathy below the knee.

Amputation in a diabetic patient should be coupled with aggressive prosthetic rehabilitation. The techniques of prosthetic rehabilitation are addressed in Chapters 16, 19, and 23, to which the interested reader is referred.

SUMMARY

It is difficult to identify the one factor that is responsible for diabetic foot problems. Rather, such foot problems are the result of an interplay between diabetic neuropathy, macro- and microvascular disease, trauma, and infection. Unfortunately, excellent diabetic management and good patient hygiene will not prevent the occurrence of diabetic foot problems; however, such care may clearly postpone or minimize the problems. Owing to the inability of diabetic patients to handle infection well, aggressive management of seemingly innocuous infections is appropriate to prevent limb loss. An algorithm for the author's suggested management of diabetic foot problems is shown in Table 2–1.

REFERENCES

1. Bagdade J, Nielson K, Root R, et al: Host defense in diabetes mellitus: The feckless phagocyte during poor control and ketoacidosis. Diabetes 19:364, 1970.
2. Bell ET: Atherosclerotic gangrene of the lower extremities in diabetic and non-diabetic persons. Am J Clin Pathol 28:27, 1957.
3. Bessman AN, Wagner W: Nonclostridial gas gangrene. Report of 48 cases and review of the literature. JAMA 233:958, 1975.

4. Bybee JD, Rogers DE: The phagocytic activity of polymorphonuclear leukocytes obtained from patients with diabetes mellitus. J Lab Clin Med 64:1, 1964.
5. Cameron HD, Lennard-Jones JE, Robinson MP: Amputations in the diabetic (outcome and survival). Lancet 2:605, 1964.
6. Chopra JS, Hurwitz LJ, Montgomery DAD: The pathogenesis of sural nerve changes in diabetes mellitus. Brain 92:391, 1969.
7. Collens WS, Vlahos E, Dobbin GB, et al: Conservative management of gangrene in the diabetic patient. JAMA 181:692, 1962.
8. Colt JD, Lee PY: Mortality rate of above-the-knee amputation for arteriosclerotic gangrene: A critical evaluation. Angiology 23:205, 1972.
9. Delbridge L, Appleberg M, Reeve TS: Factors associated with development of foot lesions in the diabetic. Surgery 93:78, 1983.
10. Ecker ML, Jacobs BS: Lower extremity amputation in diabetic patients. Diabetes 19:189, 1970.
11. Fierer J, Daniel D, Davis C: The fetid foot: Lower-extremity infections in patients with diabetes mellitus. Rev Infect Dis 1:210, 1979.
12. Ganda OP: Pathogenesis of macrovascular disease in the human diabetic. Diabetes 29:931, 1980.
13. Ganda OMP: Pathogenesis of accelerated atherosclerosis in diabetes. In Kozak GP, Campbell D, Hoar CS Jr, et al (eds): Management of Diabetic Foot Problems. Philadelphia, WB Saunders Co, 1984.
14. Goldner MG: The fate of the second leg in the diabetic amputee. Diabetes 9:100, 1960.
15. Habershaw G, Donovan JC: Biomechanical considerations of the diabetic foot. In Kozak GP, Campbell D, Hoar CS Jr, et al (eds): Management of Diabetic Foot Problems. Philadelphia, WB Saunders Co, 1984.
16. Hoar CS, Torres J: Evaluation of below-the-knee amputation in the treatment of diabetic gangrene. N Engl J Med 266:440, 1962.
17. Joslin E, Root H, White P, et al: The Treatment of Diabetes Mellitus. Philadelphia, Lea & Febiger, 1946.
18. Kahn O, Wagner W, Bessman AN: Mortality of diabetic patients treated surgically for lower limb infection and/or gangrene. Diabetes 23:287, 1974.
19. Kempczinski R (ed): The Ischemic Limb. Chicago, Year Book Medical Publishers, 1985.
20. Khettry V: Pathology of the diabetic foot. In Kozak GP, Campbell D, Hoar CS Jr, et al (eds): Management of Diabetic Foot Problems. Philadelphia, WB Saunders Co, 1984.
21. Kihn RB, Warren R, Beebe GW: The "geriatric" amputee. Ann Surg 176:305, 1972.
22. Kozak GP, Rowbotham JL: Diabetic foot disease: A major problem. In Kozak GP, Campbell D, Hoar CS Jr, et al (eds): Management of Diabetic Foot Problems. Philadelphia, WB Saunders Co, 1984.
23. Levin CM, Dealy FN: The surgical diabetic, a five year survey. Ann Surg 102:1029, 1935.
24. Louie TJ, Bartlett JG, Tally FP, et al: Aerobic and anaerobic bacteria in diabetic foot ulcers. Ann Intern Med 85:461, 1976.
25. Malone JM, Goldstone J: Lower extremity amputation. In Moore WS (ed): Vascular Surgery: A Comprehensive Review. New York, Grune & Stratton, 1984.
25a. Lalka SG, Malone JM, Anderson GG, et al: Trans-

cutaneous oxygen and carbon dioxide pressure monitoring to determine severity of limb ischemia and to predict surgical outcome. J Vasc Surg 7:507, 1988.
26. Malone JM, Moore WS, Goldstone J: The natural history of bilateral aortofemoral bypass grafts for ischemia of the lower extremities. Arch Surg 110:1300, 1975.
27. Malone JM, Goldstone J, Moore WS: Autogenous profundaplasty: The key to long-term patency in secondary repair of aortofemoral graft occlusion. Ann Surg 188:817, 1978.
28. Mandelberg A, Sheinfeld W: Diabetic amputations; Amputation of lower extremity in diabetics—analysis of 128 cases. Am J Surg 71:70, 1946.
29. Mazet R Jr, Schiller FJ, Dunn OJ, et al: The influence of prosthesis wearing on the health of the geriatric patient. Project 431, Department of Health, Education, and Welfare, Office of Vocational Rehabilitation, Washington, DC, March 1963, unpublished.
30. McIntyre KE, Bailey SA, Malone JM, et al: Guillotine amputation in the treatment of nonsalvageable lower-extremity infections. Arch Surg 119:450, 1984.
31. Moore WS, Hall AD, Lim RC: Below the knee amputation for ischemic gangrene. Am J Surg 124:127, 1972.
32. Moore WS, Malone JM: Vascular reconstruction in the diabetic patient. Angiology 29:741, 1978.
33. Moore WS (ed): Vascular Surgery: A Comprehensive Review. New York, Grune & Stratton, 1984.
34. Otteman JG, Stahlgren LH: Evaluation of factors which influence mortality and morbidity following major lower extremity amputation for arteriosclerosis. Surg Gynecol Obstet 120:1217, 1965.
35. Pearse HE, Ziegler HR: Is the conservative treatment of infection or gangrene in diabetic patients worthwhile? Surgery 8:72, 1940.
36. Pratt TC: Gangrene and infection in the diabetic. Med Clin North Am 49:987, 1965.
37. Roon AJ, Moore WS, Goldstone J: Below knee amputation: A modern approach. Am J Surg 134:153, 1977.
38. Root HF: Collected study of 9 hospitals in Boston area. N Engl J Med 253:685, 1955.
39. Rutherford R (ed): Vascular Surgery. Philadelphia, WB Saunders Co, 1984.
40. Sapico FL, Witte JL, Canawati HN, et al: The infected foot of the diabetic patient: Quantitative microbiology and analysis of clinical features. Rev Infect Dis 6(Suppl 1):S171, 1984.
41. Schalt DC: Chronic atherosclerotic occlusion of femoral artery. JAMA 175:937, 1961.
42. Schnider SL, Kohn RR: Glucosylation of human collagen in aging and diabetes mellitus. J Clin Invest 66:1179, 1980.
43. Silbert S: Midleg amputation for gangrene in the diabetic. Ann Surg 27:503, 1948.
44. Silbert S, Haimovici H: Results of midleg amputations for gangrene in diabetics. JAMA 144:454, 1950.
45. Smith BC: A twenty-year follow-up in below-knee amputations for gangrene in diabetes. Surg Gynecol Obstet 103:625, 1956.
46. Stokes IAF, Faris IB, Hutton WC: The neuropathic ulcer and loads on the foot in diabetic patients. Acta Orthop Scand 46:839, 1975.

47. Stone HH, Martin JD: Synergistic necrotizing cellulitis. Ann Surg 175:702, 1972.
48. Strandness DE Jr, Priest RE, Gibbons GE: Combined clinical and pathologic study of diabetic and nondiabetic peripheral arterial disease. Diabetes 13:366, 1964.
49. Wheelock FC: Transmetatarsal amputations and arterial surgery in diabetic patients. N Engl J Med 264:316, 1961.
50. Whitehouse FW: Infections that hospitalize the diabetic. Geriatrics 28:97, 1973.
51. Whitehouse FW, Jurgensen C, Block MA: The later life of the diabetic amputee. Diabetes 17:520, 1968.
52. Williams HTG, Hutchinson KJ, Brown GD: Gangrene of the feet in diabetics. Arch Surg 108:609, 1974.

3

General Principles of Amputation Level Selection

Wesley S. Moore, M.D.

Amputation level selection depends, in large part, on the indication for amputation. For example, the lower extremity amputation level for a tumor depends on the location or extent of the neoplasm. In the case of ischemia, the amputation level is the most distal level that encompasses the ischemic process, but the primary determinant or limiting factor in ultimate level selection is the adequacy of skin blood flow at the level selected.

OBJECTIVES OF AMPUTATION LEVEL SELECTION

Ablation of Pathology

The primary objective of amputation is to remove the diseased tissue, whether tumor, ischemic gangrene, or devitalized tissue resulting from trauma.

Primary Healing

The next objective of amputation level selection is to pick the most distal level that will result in primary healing. This minimizes morbidity and hospitalization time and provides the most expeditious pathway to bipedal ambulation with a prosthesis.

The criteria for distal amputation level selection are most critical in cases of trauma, infection, and ischemia.

Best Level for Prosthetic Fitting and Function

Although it might be possible to achieve primary healing at certain unusual distal levels, these sites may not be the best locations for prosthetic fitting. For example, an amputation of the first metatarsal head leaves an unstable foot; in contrast, a well-performed transmetatarsal amputation of the entire foot can be fitted with a custom shoe and provides a good gait pattern. A below-knee amputation just above the malleoli may heal but presents a difficult fitting problem for the prosthetist in contrast to a below-knee amputation at a more acceptable level.

Best Level for Ambulation

In general, the more distal the lower extremity amputation, the better the prospects for ambulation, provided that proper prosthetic fitting can be achieved. Exceptions to this rule include a transmetatarsal or Syme's amputation in a patient with sensory neuropathy. Amputations under these conditions ultimately lead to skin breakdown. For patients with sensory neuropathy of the foot, a below-knee amputation is a better choice. Another exception to the previous rule occurs in patients with either severe knee flexion contracture or a stiff knee joint. A below-knee amputation may heal, but the patient will lack the knee joint mobility required to enjoy the benefits of a below-knee amputation. In this case, a knee disarticulation provides the best opportunity for ambulation.

OPTIONS FOR LEVEL SELECTION IN THE ISCHEMIC EXTREMITY

Clinical Criteria

The most common method of evaluating the level of a proposed amputation has been to rely on the experienced surgeon's judgment. This was true in the past and probably continues to be true. Unfortunately, this often leads to the decision to amputate at an unacceptably high level. In the past, a supracondylar above-knee amputation was erroneously recommended for all patients requiring amputation for ischemic gangrene. The basis for this recommendation was that this level could always be expected to heal and that prosthetic fitting and ambulation were not considered to be major objectives. Over the past 20 years, such thinking has proved fallacious, particularly with the recognition of the importance of knee joint preservation.

Currently, a surgeon is likely to assess the ischemic process so as to include the extent of the gangrene. If there is dependent rubor present in the extremity, a level above the point of rubor must be selected for amputation. Skin temperature of the extremity, determined subjectively, often entered into the decision-making process. Finally, the presence of lower extremity pulses and the quality of the pulse were also considered. It used to be stated that a palpable pulse had to be present at the level immediately above the proposed amputation level. This implies that a popliteal pulse must be present in order for a below-knee amputation to be performed. This, too, has been shown to be fallacious. There are many examples of successful below-knee amputations in the absence of a popliteal pulse and even in the absence of a femoral pulse. Therefore, the patterns of collateral blood flow are more important than the presence or absence of a palpable pulse.

Although the clinical determination of amputation level selection lacks quantitation and may underestimate or overestimate skin blood flow, it can be a reasonably reliable method in the hands of a highly experienced surgeon. The importance of the knee joint is well recognized, and surgeons will often be inclined to try amputation at the below-knee level and will accept an occasional failed amputation, requiring higher revision, as a price for not underestimating a patient's potential to heal at the below-knee level and enjoy the benefits of a knee joint.

Angiographic Patterns of Disease

It was hoped that arteriography might aid in the quantitation of amputation level selection. Unfortunately, this is not the case. Although the angiogram provides static information concerning the availability of blood vessels, it gives no dynamic information with respect to the physiology or pathology of blood flow.

Quantitation of Skin Blood Flow

Over the past few years, a number of methods have been applied in an attempt to more accurately quantify skin blood flow and predict success of amputation healing. These techniques will be covered in detail in subsequent chapters and include segmental blood pressure determination using the Doppler flowmeter; documentation of skin blood flow quality by transcutaneous oxygen tension; and determination of skin blood flow by quantitative skin fluorescence, isotope clearance, laser Doppler, and maintenance of normal skin temperature.

SUMMARY

Although many factors enter into amputation level selection, the objective of amputation level selection is to choose the most distal amputation that encompasses the pathological process, is consistent with primary healing, produces a residual limb that can be fitted with an appropriate prosthesis, and provides the patient with the maximum opportunity to return to bipedal ambulation.

4

Amputation Level Selection by Doppler Assessment

James M. Malone, M.D.
Stephen G. Lalka, M.D.

The objective of preoperative amputation level selection is to determine the most distal site that will heal. Selection of the proper level is important not only to preserve the maximal length of the viable extremity but also to minimize morbidity and mortality. The general requirements for amputation level selection are (1) the amputation must remove all necrotic, painful, or infected tissue; (2) the residual limb must be able to be fitted with a functional prosthesis; and (3) the blood supply at the level of the proposed amputation must be sufficient to allow primary skin healing. Appropriate amputation level selection is critical. If too proximal an amputation site is selected, the patient may be deprived of the opportunity for subsequent ambulation and rehabilitation, although the amputation might heal without difficulty. If too distal an amputation site is selected, the blood supply may be inadequate for amputation healing, and further surgery may be required to achieve healing of an amputation at a higher level. The latter approach may result in increased morbidity and mortality and may ultimately result in a rehabilitation failure.[17]

It is usually possible for the surgeon to decide on an amputation level that will remove necrotic, painful or infected tissue as well as create a residual limb that can be fitted with a prosthesis. However, the decision regarding the adequacy of blood supply at the proposed level of amputation is one of the most difficult problems facing the amputation surgeon.

The most important goal for the amputation surgeon is salvage of a below-knee rather than an above-knee amputation. The inherent advantage of a below-knee amputation should be obvious. It is easier to ambulate on a below-knee prosthesis, a fact that is extremely important in geriatric (over 60 years of age) patients. In general, a unilateral below-knee amputee requires a 10 to 40% increase in energy expenditure for ambulation, compared with the energy required for walking with an intact extremity. In contrast, a unilateral above-knee amputee requires approximately a 50 to 70% increase in energy expenditure. For comparison's sake, crutch walking without a lower extremity prosthesis uses approximately a 60% increase in energy expenditure, whereas wheelchair use necessitates only a 9% increase in energy expenditure. The difference between the energy expenditure for walking after an above-knee versus a below-knee amputation may be the single most important factor in trying to rehabilitate a geriatric amputee who has decreased physiological reserve owing to associated medical problems and cardiovascular diseases. Such patients may be physically unable to provide the additional energy expenditure required for ambulation on an above-knee compared with a below-knee prosthesis.

The need for more sensitive and objective methods for preoperative amputation level selection has led to the development of numerous noninvasive techniques for assessing the adequacy of limb blood flow. The purpose of this chapter is to review and discuss the use of Doppler systolic blood pressure measurements as they apply to amputation level selection.

DOPPLER SYSTOLIC BLOOD PRESSURE MEASUREMENT

Unlike noninvasive methods such as intradermal xenon-133 clearance or transcutaneous oxygen pressure recording, Doppler segmental pressure measurement is a simple technique. The methods for toe, ankle, calf, popliteal, and thigh Doppler systolic blood pressure determinations have been previously well described and will not be covered in this chapter.[2, 7, 17]

The advantages of Doppler-derived blood pressure measurements are that they are easy to obtain, noninvasive, inexpensive, and good predictors of amputation healing. However, a major problem with Doppler segmental pressure measurements for amputation level selection is their relative inability to predict which amputations will not heal (negative predictive value).

Below-Knee Amputation

The success rates for amputation level selection using Doppler-derived pressures have varied with both the amputation level and the absolute pressure chosen as a selection point. Several studies have reported that primary healing of below-knee amputations can be expected in 88 to 100% of cases if the calf systolic pressure is greater than 50 mmHg (Table 4–1).[2, 7, 19] However, Barnes and associates[2] also noted that primary healing occurred in 10% of patients with calf systolic blood pressures less than 50 mmHg. In a more recent study, Barnes and associates[3] concluded that there was no significant difference in the mean blood pressure between groups with healed and failed amputations, irrespective of absolute pressure measurement. In addition, they observed healing in 90% of below-knee amputations in extremities with unobtainable pressures at the below-knee or ankle level. Similarly, Dean and colleagues[7] found no correlation between Doppler ankle systolic pressure measurements and successful healing of below-knee amputations, and 10 of 22 (46%) below-knee amputations with ankle systolic pressures less than or equal to 20 mmHg healed. On the other hand, Lepantalo and coworkers[14] reported 100% healing in 31 below-knee amputations when the calf systolic pressures were greater than or equal to 68 mmHg and the distal thigh systolic pressures were greater than or equal to 100 mmHg. In that particular study, when calf blood pressures were less than 35 mmHg and distal thigh

Table 4–1. HEALING OF BELOW-KNEE AMPUTATION

Level Selection Criteria	Reference	Healing Extremities	(%)
Doppler *ankle* systolic pressure ≥ 30 mmHg	Boeckstyns & Jensen,[4] Holstein[10]	66/70	(94)
Doppler *calf* systolic pressure ≥ 50 mmHg	Barnes et al,[3] Yao & Bergan[24]	64/67	(95)
≥ 68 mmHg	Baker & Barnes,[1] Holstein,[10] Nicholas et al[18]	96/97	(99)
Doppler *thigh* systolic pressure > 70 mmHg	Holstein et al[12]	12/14	(86)
Empiric BKA	Lee et al,[13] Lim et al,[15] Robbs & Ray[20]	209/260	(80)
Totals (excludes empiric BKA)		238/248	(96)

BKA = below-knee amputation.

pressures were less than 60 mmHg, all amputations failed to heal. Although it is generally recognized that Doppler systolic pressures may be falsely elevated in diabetic patients,[8, 14] Lepantalo and coworkers[14] also noted that diabetes mellitus had no effect on the rate of amputation healing. Their data coincide nicely with the report by Nicholas and associates[18] wherein 33 of 34 (97%) below-knee amputations healed when the calf systolic blood pressure was greater than 70 mmHg. However, Nicholas and associates[18] also reported that the false-negative rates for calf and ankle systolic blood pressure measurements were 32 and 40%, respectively. They concluded that Doppler systolic blood pressure measurements can predict successful amputation healing but cannot reliably predict amputations that will fail to heal. In a series of 66 patients who had major amputations, Dean and associates[7] used Doppler ankle systolic pressure; lower thigh Doppler systolic pressure; and recorded waveforms from posterior tibial, anterior tibial, and dorsal pedal arteries to determine level of amputation. Their data suggested that when there was no detectable flow in the popliteal artery, an above-knee amputation was advisable. With detectable flow in the popliteal artery and a distal thigh pressure greater than 50 mmHg, the authors suggested that a below-knee amputation should be attempted because the chances for success were quite high.[7] This latter observation has been reported by others.[2, 6, 13, 18] However, it is important to realize that Doppler-derived pressure measurements alone have a poor negative predictive value, and other important factors for successful amputation healing, which are not addressed by the use of Doppler pressures, include operative technique and the presence of ipsilateral distal limb infection.

For purposes of a reference standard, it must be pointed out that empiric below-knee amputation level selection has a high rate of success. A composite of reports from several authors (see Table 4–1)[13, 15, 20] suggests that 80% (209/260) of all limbs can heal below-knee amputations, even when objective non-invasive techniques are not used to select the amputation level.

An overview of the published data for Doppler-derived systolic pressure measurements for prediction of satisfactory healing of below-knee amputations is shown in Table 4–1. The composite data suggest that the overall accuracy is 96% (238/248).

Amputation Below the Ankle

Although Doppler systolic pressures are reasonably accurate for below-knee amputation level selection, they are less precise in predicting the success of forefoot or toe amputation. The use of ankle pressure measurement alone for prediction of toe or forefoot healing should be avoided, since ankle pressure does not necessarily reflect adequate perfusion through the pedal arch and digital arteries. This problem is particularly true in diabetics, although there is some controversy in the literature regarding the validity of ankle systolic pressure measurements in diabetic patients.[4, 10–12, 17, 21] Since ankle pressure measurements alone fail to indicate the patency of the pedal arch and digital arteries, a combination of Doppler systolic pressure and pulse volume (PVRs) recordings might be expected to provide improved criteria for objective amputation level selection. Although Raines and colleagues,[19] using a combination of ankle and calf blood pressure measurements with PVR, reported 100% successful healing of 27 below-knee amputations, Gibbons and associates[8] were unable to duplicate those results and concluded, in fact, that "there are no consistent criteria which are more accurate and reliable than clinical judgment and no ankle pressure above which primary healing was guaranteed." They found that forefoot PVRs predicted failure in 50% of diabetic patients whose amputations eventually healed at that level. Gibbons and associates[8] felt strongly that noninvasive studies should be used to supplement clinical judgment in selecting amputation level, not supplant it.

Foot and Forefoot Amputation

Barnes and colleagues[3] reported a failure rate of 24% in patients with a Doppler ankle pressure greater than 60 mmHg undergoing foot amputations; however, they also found that 33% of foot amputations healed despite a Doppler ankle pressure less than 60 mmHg. Bone and Pomajzl[5] found that primary healing occurred in all forefoot amputations with toe pressures in excess of 55 mmHg and that failure of forefoot amputation occurred in all limbs with toe pressures less than 45 mmHg. More recently, Boeckstyns and Jensen[4] reported that only 17 of 63 foot and

Table 4–2. HEALING OF FOOT AND FOREFOOT AMPUTATIONS

Level Selection Criteria	Reference	Healing Extremities	(%)
Doppler *ankle* systolic pressure			
≥ 40 mmHg or ABI > 0.43	Boeckstyns & Jensen,[4] Verta et al[23]	28/69	(41)
≥ 50 mmHg	Holstein[11]	14/21	(67)
≥ 70 mmHg	Baker & Barnes,[1] Nicholas et al[18]	70/93	(75)
Doppler *toe* systolic pressure			
≥ 30 mmHg	Holstein[11]	4/5	(80)
< 45 mmHg*	Bone & Pomajzl[5]	0/8	(0)
> 45 mmHg	Bone & Pomajzl[5]	6/8	(75)
> 55 mmHg	Bone & Pomajzl[5]	10/14	(71)
Totals (*excluded)		132/210	(63)

ABI = ankle/brachial index.

forefoot amputations healed when the systolic ankle blood pressure was greater than 40 mmHg. They also noted that there was no apparent correlation between diabetes mellitus and amputation healing.

The problems with Doppler-derived pressures for amputations below the ankle were nicely summarized by Verta and associates,[23] who noted that "for forefoot amputation, a high Doppler ankle blood pressure did not guarantee successful healing and a low ankle pressure did not contraindicate primary healing."

An overview of published data on the success rates for Doppler ankle systolic pressures as a predictor for healing of foot and forefoot amputations is shown in Table 4–2. The overall accuracy was 63% (132/210).

Toe Amputation

Holstein[10] suggested that digital systolic, rather than ankle systolic, blood pressure measurements might be more useful for distal forefoot and toe amputations. He reported a 78% (51/65) success rate for toe and forefoot amputation healing when the digital systolic blood pressure was greater than 30 mmHg but only a 72% (47/65) success rate when the ankle systolic blood pressure was greater than 100 mmHg. Holstein also noted that diabetes did not seem to have an effect on the success rates of digit and transmetatarsal amputations.[10] Verta and coworkers[23] found that toe amputations healed in patients with ankle pressures greater than 40 mmHg if there was no invasive sepsis. However, Baker and Barnes[1] reported that even with ankle pressures in excess of 60 mmHg, only 83% of toe amputations healed and if amputation was attempted at pressures less than 60 mmHg, all failed.

An overview of the published data on the success rates for Doppler digit systolic pressure as a predictor for healing of toe amputations is shown in Table 4–3. The overall accuracy was 88% (111/126).

Overview

The authors' greatest experience with noninvasive tests for objective amputation level selection is with the use of xenon-133 skin clearance[17] and Doppler segmental systolic blood pressure measurements. With xenon-133, the authors have been consistently able to achieve an overall accuracy rate of 92 to 97%,[6] and the test is accurate at all levels of lower extremity amputation, although there are some problems at the transmetatarsal and toe levels. Although xenon-133 skin clearance has provided reliable data in a few other centers,[9, 22] its use has been limited owing to cost and test complexity. In order to evaluate other methods of objective amputation level selection, the authors completed a prospective study in 1987 at the Tucson Veterans Administration Medical Center, comparing transcutaneous oxygen pressure, transcutaneous carbon dioxide pressure, xenon-133 skin clearance, Doppler popliteal systolic pressure, and the ankle/brachial index for preoperative amputation level selection in patients undergoing major elective lower extremity amputations. Surgical decisions regarding amputation level were based on xenon-133 skin clearance. The study included 52 patients: 23 above-knee, 21 below-knee, and 8 transmetatarsal amputees. The overall data are shown in Table 4–4. These data demonstrate that xenon-133 skin clearance, the ankle/brachial index, and Doppler popliteal systolic pressures are not reliable for objective amputation level selection; how-

Table 4–3. HEALING OF TOE AMPUTATION

Level Selection Criteria	Reference	Healing Extremities	(%)
Doppler *toe* systolic pressure ≥ 30 mmHg	Schwartz et al[21]	47/60	(78)
Doppler *ankle* systolic pressure ≥ 35 mmHg	Malone & Goldstone[17]	44/46	(96)
Photoplethysmographic digit or TMA systolic pressure ≥ 20 mmHg	Verta et al[23]	20/20	(100)
Totals		111/126	(88)

TMA = transmetatarsal amputation.

Table 4–4. PROSPECTIVE COMPARISON OF NONINVASIVE TECHNIQUES FOR AMPUTATION LEVEL SELECTION

Test	Healed		Failed		p Value*
	Mean ± SD	n	Mean ± SD	n	
Overall					
$P_{TC_{O_2}}$ (torr)	32.5 ± 8.1	40	11.8 ± 5.6	11	0.001
$P_{TC_{CO_2}}$ (torr)	32.2 ± 4.9	40	37.8 ± 4	11	0.001
$P_{TC_{O_2}}$ to $P_{TC_{CO_2}}$	1.04 ± 0.36	40	0.32 ± 0.16	11	0.001
Foot to chest $P_{TC_{O_2}}$	0.80 ± 0.75	40	0.29 ± 0.14	11	0.001
Xenon-133 (ml/100 g tissue/min)	5.1 ± 2.9	35	7.5 ± 7.1	6	NS
ABI	0.74 ± 0.4	35	0.78 ± 0.4	11	NS
POP (mmHg)	134 ± 74	25	124 ± 42	9	NS
Above-Knee					
$P_{TC_{O_2}}$	34.7 ± 9.3	20	12.6 ± 0.9	2	0.005
$P_{TC_{CO_2}}$	32.2 ± 5.3	20	36.5 ± 0.7	2	NS
$P_{TC_{O_2}}$ to $P_{TC_{CO_2}}$	1.12 ± 0.4	20	0.34 ± 0.01	2	0.025
Foot to chest $P_{TC_{CO_2}}$	0.9 ± 0.3	19	0.34 ± 0.08	2	0.025
Xenon-133	—	13	—	0	—
ABI	0.65 ± 0.46	17	0.91 ± 0.80	2	NS
POP	94 ± 60	13	60	1	NS
Below-Knee					
$P_{TC_{O_2}}$	30.6 ± 6.7	16	12.4 ± 5	5	0.001
$P_{TC_{CO_2}}$	32.3 ± 4.5	16	40.2 ± 3.6	5	0.005
$P_{TC_{O_2}}$ to $P_{TC_{CO_2}}$	0.98 ± 0.32	16	0.31 ± 0.13	5	0.001
Foot to chest $P_{TC_{O_2}}$	0.72 ± 0.18	16	0.29 ± 0.13	5	0.001
Xenon-133	5.3 ± 2	16	3.7 ± 1.8	3	NS
ABI	0.76 ± 0.3	14	0.7 ± 0.28	5	NS
POP	179 ± 70	9	117 ± 35	4	NS
Transmetatarsal					
$P_{TC_{O_2}}$	28.8 ± 2.3	4	10.8 ± 8.2	4	0.010
$P_{TC_{CO_2}}$	32 ± 5.3	4	35.5 ± 4.2	4	NS
$P_{TC_{O_2}}$ to $P_{TC_{CO_2}}$	0.91 ± 0.15	4	0.32 ± 0.26	4	0.010
Foot to chest $P_{TC_{O_2}}$	0.675 ± 0.05	4	0.255 ± 0.19	4	0.010
Xenon-133	9.8 ± 4.9	4	11.2 ± 8.9	3	NS
ABI	1.05 ± 0.25	4	0.84 ± 0.26	4	NS
POP	170 ± 47	3	148 ± 37	4	NS

SD = standard deviation, $P_{TC_{O_2}}$ = transcutaneous oxygen pressure, $P_{TC_{CO_2}}$ = transcutaneous carbon dioxide pressure, NS = not significant, ABI = ankle-brachial index, POP = absolute popliteal artery Doppler systolic pressure.

*Student's t test and one-way analysis of variance.

From Malone JM, Anderson G, Lalka SG, et al: Prospective comparison of noninvasive techniques for amputation level selection. Am J Surg 154:179, 1987.

ever, both transcutaneous oxygen and transcutaneous carbon dioxide pressures are highly accurate overall ($p<0.001$), although transcutaneous carbon dioxide measurements alone are not accurate at the above-knee and transmetatarsal levels.[16]

SUMMARY

Doppler systolic blood pressures have been used for amputation level selection at the toe, forefoot, foot, below-knee, and above-knee levels with varying success rates, depending on the amputation level and the absolute pressure or calculated ratio. Amputation healing can be accurately predicted when the systolic pressure is above a predetermined number; however, Doppler systolic pressures do not appear to have accuracy in predicting those patients who will fail to heal their lower extremity amputation. On the basis of data reported in this chapter as well as further results from that ongoing study, the authors would suggest that transcutaneous oxygen pressure measurements appear to be better objective tests than Doppler systolic pressure measurements or calculated Doppler ratios for amputation level selection. Although the transcutaneous equipment is slightly more expensive and the test is more time consuming than Doppler testing, transcutaneous monitoring clearly provides a higher level of objective accuracy (see Table 4–4).

REFERENCES

1. Baker WH, Barnes RW: Minor forefoot amputation in patients with low ankle pressure. Am J Surg 133:331, 1977.
2. Barnes RW, Shanik GD, Slaymaker EE: An index of healing in below-knee amputation: Leg blood pressure by Doppler ultrasound. Surgery 79:13, 1976.
3. Barnes RW, Thornhill B, Nix L, et al: Prediction of amputation wound healing: Roles of Doppler ultrasound and digit photoplethysmography. Arch Surg 116:80, 1981.
4. Boeckstyns MEH, Jensen CM: Amputation of the forefoot: Predictive value of signs and clinical physiological tests. Acta Orthop Scand 55:224, 1984.
5. Bone GE, Pomajzl MJ: Toe blood pressure by photoplethysmography: An index of healing in forefoot amputation. Surgery 89:569, 1981.
6. Cederberg PA, Pritchard DJ, Joyce JW: Doppler-determined segmental pressures and wound-healing in amputations for vascular disease. J Bone Joint Surg 65:363, 1983.
7. Dean FH, Yao JST, Thompson RG, et al: Predictive value of ultrasonically derived arterial pressure in determination of amputation level. Am Surg 41:731, 1975.
8. Gibbons GW, Wheelock FC Jr, Siembieda C, et al: Noninvasive prediction of amputation level in diabetic patients. Arch Surg 114:1253, 1979.
9. Holloway GA Jr, Burgess EM: Cutaneous blood flow and its relation to healing of below-knee amputation. Surg Gynecol Obstet 146:750, 1978.
10. Holstein P: Distal blood pressure as guidance in choice of amputation level. Scand J Clin Lab Invest 31:Suppl 128:245, 1973.
11. Holstein P: The distal blood pressure predicts healing of amputations on the feet. Acta Orthop Scand 55:227, 1984.
12. Holstein P et al: Distal blood pressure in severe arterial insufficiency: Strain-gauge, radioisotopes, and other methods. In Bergan JJ, Yao JST (eds): Gangrene and Severe Ischemia of the Lower Extremities. New York, Grune & Stratton, 1978.
13. Lee BY, Trainer FS, Kavner D, et al: Noninvasive hemodynamic evaluation in selection of amputation level. Surg Gynecol Obstet 149:241, 1979.
14. Lepantalo MJA, Haajanen J, Linfors O, et al: Predictive value of preoperative segmental blood pressure measurements in below-knee amputations. Acta Chir Scand 148:581, 1982.
15. Lim RC Sr, Blaisdell FW, Hall AD, et al: Below-knee amputation for ischemic gangrene. Surg Gynecol Obstet 125:493, 1967.
16. Malone JM, Anderson G, Lalka SG, et al: Prospective comparison of noninvasive techniques for amputation level selection. Am J Surg 154:179, 1987.
17. Malone JM, Goldstone J: Lower extremity amputation. In Moore WS (ed): Vascular Surgery: A Comprehensive Review. New York, Grune & Stratton, 1983, pp 909–974.
18. Nicholas GG, Myers JL, Demuth WE: The role of vascular laboratory criteria in the selection of patients for lower extremity amputation. Am Surg 195:469, 1982.
19. Raines JK, Darling RC, Buth J, et al: Vascular laboratory criteria for the management of peripheral vascular disease of the lower extremities. Surgery 79:21, 1976.
20. Robbs JV, Ray R: Clinical predictors of below-knee stump healing following amputation for ischemia. S Afr J Surg 20:305, 1982.
21. Schwartz JA, Schuler JJ, O'Connor RJA, Flanigan DP: Predictive value of distal perfusion pressure in the healing of amputation of the digits and the forefoot. Surg Gynecol Obstet 154:865, 1982.
22. Silberstein EB, Thomas S, Cline J, et al: Predictive value of intracutaneous xenon clearance for healing of amputation and cutaneous ulcer sites. Radiology 147:227, 1983.
23. Verta MJ, Gross WS, van Bellen B, et al: Forefoot perfusion pressure and minor amputation for gangrene. Surgery 80:729, 1976.
24. Yao JST, Bergan JJ: Application of ultrasound to arterial and venous diagnosis. Surg Clin North Am 54:23, 1974.

5

Amputation Level Selection by Isotope Clearance Techniques

Samuel S. Ahn, M.D.
Wesley S. Moore, M.D.

The critical tissue for amputation healing is the skin.[1, 2] The condition of the deeper tissue has little influence on primary healing and ultimate residual limb function. Thus, the residual limb will heal satisfactorily for a prosthetic device if the skin is viable and its blood supply adequate at the proposed amputation level. This chapter will discuss the radioisotope clearance techniques that can be used to determine skin blood flow and thus predict the optimal level of amputation.

THE DEVELOPMENT OF XENON CLEARANCE TECHNIQUES

In 1949, Kety measured the disappearance of locally injected radioactive sodium as an indicator of blood flow in gastrocnemius muscle.[3] The local clearance of radioactive sodium followed a simple exponential curve that yielded a straight line when plotted semilogarithmically. The slope of this line, in turn, measured the ability of the local circulation to remove freely diffusible substances. However, this technique for quantitating tissue flow was not applicable to the skin, since the capillary permeability of radioactive sodium is limited and since this washout model depended on diffusion equilibrium between the tissues studied and the effluent venous blood.[4, 5] Lassen and associates overcame this problem by employing xenon-133, which diffuses freely across capillaries.[6] In 1973, Moore retrospectively applied Lassen's technique using xenon-133 to measure cutaneous skin blood flow in patients undergoing amputations and noted that amputation sites healed if skin blood flow at the level selected exceeded 2.4 ml/min/100 g tissue.[7] In 1981, Moore and colleagues studied 45 cases prospectively and confirmed that residual limb healing occurred only in patients with blood flow equal to or greater than 2.4 ml/min/100 g tissue.[8] Later in 1981, Malone and colleagues reported on 102 amputation patients and established xenon-133 clearance techniques as the "gold standard" for amputation level selection.[9]

T, the decay time of the radioactivity at the injection site.

BASIC PRINCIPLES

Xenon-133 is a lipophilic, metabolically inert gas that diffuses freely across the capillary cell membrane into the intravascular compartment; this passive diffusion is the only mechanism of removal from the injection site.[5, 6, 7] The rate of permeation therefore is directly proportional to the differential concentration of xenon on either side of the capillary wall (Fig. 5–1). Thus, the rate of removal, or clearance, is dependent on the flow rate within the capillary system.

If the partition coefficient for xenon between skin and blood is known, the clearance equation can be modified to express actual capillary blood flow as follows:

$$F = \log_e \times \lambda \times 100/\tfrac{1}{2}T = 48.51/\tfrac{1}{2}T$$

where

F = flow in ml/min/100 g tissue.
λ = blood/skin partition coefficient for xenon-133 = 0.7.
T = time for a complete decay of radioactivity at the injection site.[7]

Thus F, or flow, is directly dependent upon

TECHNIQUE

Each patient is examined carefully, and the most distal amputation level that encompasses the gangrenous or ischemic process is identified. Specifically, the midpoint on the anterior portion of the proposed skin incision is identified and marked for blood flow measurement using the xenon-133 technique (Fig. 5–2). Blood flow is generally determined at both the proposed site of amputation and one level lower.

The actual skin blood flow measurements are determined in the nuclear medicine department using a standardized gamma camera technique (Fig. 5–3). The patient is placed in a supine position and allowed to equilibrate with the room temperature for 15 minutes. The room temperature is generally regulated between 22 and 27°C, since temperature extremes in either direction alter xenon skin blood flow. Xenon-133 dissolved in saline (0.05 ml) is injected intradermally using a tuberculin syringe and a 26-gauge needle.[7] Two parallel injections 2 cm apart are made immediately at a point lateral to the one previously injected by the surgeon.

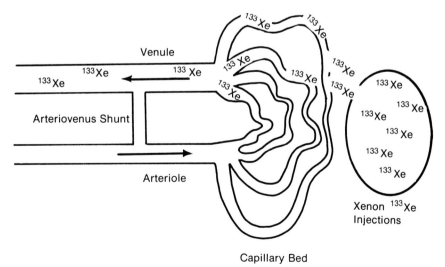

FIGURE 5–1. Artist's concept of a bolus of ^{133}Xe atoms in contact with the capillary bed. The rate of diffusion of ^{133}Xe atoms across the capillary cell membrane is a function of differential concentration, and therefore of blood flow rate through the capillary. Since ^{133}Xe is removed only by crossing the capillary cell membrane, flow that takes place through arteriovenous fistulas will not affect measurement of ^{133}Xe clearance. (*From* Moore WS: Arch Surg 107:798–802, 1973. *Copyright* 1973, American Medical Association.)

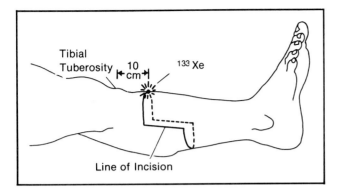

FIGURE 5–2. Outline of proposed incision used for below-knee amputation. An intradermal injection of ^{133}Xe is made in the midanterior portion of the proposed skin incision so nutritional blood flow can be measured in this critical location. (*From* Moore WS: Arch Surg 107:798–802, 1973. *Copyright* 1973, American Medical Association.)

After injection, the needle is kept in place for approximately 10 seconds, then slight pressure is applied over the injection point for 5 seconds in order to prevent leakage of radioactive material from the injection site. The patient's leg is covered with a sheet before and after injection to prevent convection heat loss. The gamma camera, with a low-energy parallel-hole collimator interfaced to a microcomputer, then monitors the xenon-133 activity for 10 minutes at four frames per minute. The injection sites are displayed on a computer cathode ray tube terminal, and the areas of interest limited to the injection sites are chosen to generate time activity curves (Fig. 5–4). Using a least square fit for monoexponential function, the slope constant for xenon washout is calculated for the first 6 minutes after injection (Fig. 5–5). This slope value provides the essential components for the Kety-Schmidt equation as follows:

$$F = 100 \times \lambda \times K/P$$

where

F = skin blood flow in ml/min/100 g tissue.
λ = blood/skin partition coefficient for xenon-133 = 0.7.

K = slope constant of xenon-133.
P = specific gravity of the skin = 1.05.

When a difference in flow rate between adjacent parallel injection sites occurs, the higher flow rate is accepted since injection error tends to result in an erroneously low flow rate.[14]

RESULTS

In 1973, Moore reported an excellent correlation of skin blood flow measured by xenon-133 clearance technique and the success rate of amputation healing in 31 patients undergoing 33 below-knee amputations.[7] The three amputations that failed to heal because of ischemic necrosis had the three lowest blood flows. In 1977, Roon and associates, in a prospective study using the same xenon-133 clearance technique, reported almost uniform healing at the below-knee level.[10] In 1981, Moore and colleagues demonstrated that the minimum criterion for adequate healing was skin blood flow of 2.4 ml/min/100 g tissue.[8] They further demonstrated that this same criterion was applicable

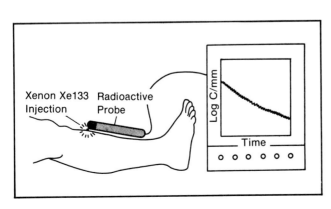

FIGURE 5–3. Diagrammatic representation of the method for measuring radioactive counts per minute and recording data on a strip chart recorder. (*From* Moore WS: Arch Surg 107:798–802, 1973. *Copyright* 1973, American Medical Association.)

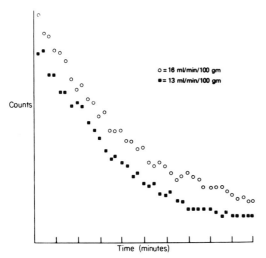

FIGURE 5–4. Computer-generated time/activity curves (non-log) for bilateral dorsal foot injection (transmetatarsal level) of ^{133}Xe in a normal subject. Notice the relatively rapid fall in radioactivity. (*From* Malone JM, Leal JM, Moore WS, et al: The "gold standard" for amputation level selection: Xenon-133 clearance. J Surg Res 30:449, 1981.)

at other amputation levels, such as toe, transmetatarsal, and Syme's amputation sites.[8] Later that same year, Malone and colleagues reported 137 lower extremity amputations

performed in 102 patients, who were tested prospectively with the xenon-133 clearance technique to determine appropriate amputation levels.[9] All 70 below-knee amputations with flow rates exceeding 2.2 ml/min/100 g tissue healed primarily. In addition, the use of the xenon-133 clearance technique allowed successful amputations at a lower level—including toe, transmetatarsal, and Syme's amputations and knee disarticulation—in the majority of patients who otherwise would have had a higher amputation on the basis of purely clinical grounds.

Other independent investigators have reported similar findings. Holloway and Burgess in 1978 reported that 19 of 22 amputations healed when flow rates were greater than 1.0 ml/min/100 g tissue.[11] Silberstein and coworkers in 1983 reported that 38 of 39 below-knee amputations healed primarily in the presence of flow rates greater than 2.4 ml/min/100 g tissue.[12] In contrast, only four of seven amputations healed if the flow rates were less than 2.4 ml/min/100 g tissue. Most recently, Harris and associates reported healing in 12 of 12 amputations when flow rates were greater than 1.0 ml/min/100 g tissue, in contrast to five of five wound failures when

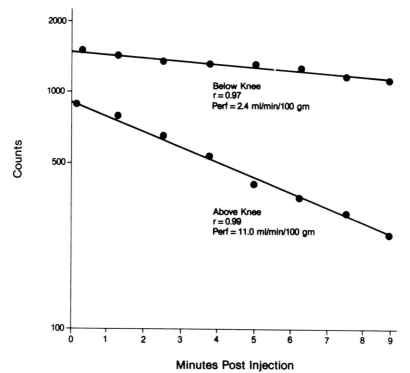

Minutes Post Injection

FIGURE 5–5. ^{133}Xe washout in a lower extremity with a gangrenous foot (log scale). Computer-generated time/ activity curves (log) for above-knee and below-knee amputation levels in the same leg. Xenon skin blood flow values are calculated at 6 minutes after injection. (*From* Malone JM, Leal JM, Moore WS, et al: The "gold standard" for amputation level selection: Xenon-133 clearance. J Surg Res 30:449, 1981.)

flow rates were less than 1.0 ml/min/100 g tissue.[13] Although the authors will perform a below-knee amputation in the presence of flow rates of 2.0 to 2.6 ml/min/100 g tissue, the best objective cut-off point for successful prediction of primary healing remains 2.4 ml/min/100 g tissue.[8, 9, 12] Overall, this criterion accurately predicts successful healing in over 95% of reported cases.[4, 5, 7, 9–12, 14]

DISCUSSION

One of the major difficulties of the xenon-133 clearance technique is the limited availability of the xenon-133 isotope.[1] The manufacturer of the isotopes no longer supplies xenon-133 dissolved in saline for injection. Xenon-133 is now available commercially only in the gas form. Although the injectable form can be purchased locally by the nuclear medicine departments, many medical centers do not have this technique available. Furthermore, the test is highly technician dependent, and its reliability is influenced by the technician's skill. All of these problems were borne out in a recent study in which Malone and associates prospectively compared xenon-133 clearance and transcutaneous oxygen pressure determinations.[15] In this study, because of a large overlap in test results, xenon-133 blood flow did not reliably predict proper amputation levels. The widely variable test results were due to all of the factors mentioned previously.

Other investigators, particularly in Europe, have used other radioisotopes and a variation of the clearance technique because of several theoretical issues. Xenon-133, being a lipophilic substance, is trapped in the subcutaneous fat and therefore may not be cleared entirely by the circulating capillary bed.[16] To overcome this theoretical problem, Holstein and coworkers used technetium-99–pertechnetate, sodium iodine-131, or iodine-131–antipyrine in the presence of external pressure.[16–18] These investigators reported skin perfusion pressure rather than capillary blood flow. The skin perfusion pressure is defined as the external counterpressure that is just sufficient to stop the washout of an intradermal deposit of radioactive isotope. These investigators reported that 60 of 62 amputations healed when skin perfusion pressure was greater than 30 mmHg. In

contrast, only six of 13 amputations healed if the pressure was between 20 and 30 mmHg, and only one of nine amputations healed if the perfusion pressure was less than 20 mmHg. These results are similar to those achieved by Moore and Malone and colleagues using the xenon-133 clearance technique.[7–9]

SUMMARY

Despite some theoretical disadvantages of the isotope and the general unavailability of its injectable form, the xenon-133 clearance technique for measuring skin blood flow has proved an accurate means of determining proper amputation levels. Flow rates greater than 2.4 ml/min/100 g tissue accurately predict amputation healing in over 95% of reported cases. Elective lower extremity amputation should not be performed in the absence of objective testing, such as the xenon-133 clearance technique.

REFERENCES

1. Malone JM, Goldstone J: Lower extremity amputation. In Moore WS (ed): Vascular Surgery: A Comprehensive Review, 2nd Ed. Orlando, Grune & Stratton, 1986, pp 1139–1210.
2. Moore WS: Amputation level determination. In Rutherford RB (ed): Vascular Surgery, 2nd Ed. Philadelphia, WB Saunders Co, 1984, pp 1479–1483.
3. Kety S: Measurement of regional circulation by local clearance of radioactive sodium. Am Heart J 38:321, 1949.
4. Kostuik JP, Wood D, Hornby R, et al: Measurement of skin blood flow in peripheral vascular disease by epicutaneous application of xenon-133. J Bone Joint Surg 58:833, 1964.
5. Serjrsen P: Blood flow in cutaneous tissue in man studied by washout of radioactive xenon. Circ Res 25:215, 1969.
6. Lassen NA, Lindbjerg J, Munck O: Measurement of blood flow through skeletal muscle by intramuscular injection of xenon-133. Lancet 1:686, 1964.
7. Moore WS: Determination of amputation level. Measurement of skin blood flow with xenon Xe 133. Arch Surg 107:798, 1973.
8. Moore WS, Henry RE, Malone JM, et al: Prospective use of xenon Xe 133 clearance for amputation level selection. Arch Surg 116:86, 1981.
9. Malone JM, Leal JM, Moore WS, et al: The "gold standard" for amputation level selection: Xenon-133 clearance. J Surg Res 30:449, 1981.
10. Roon AJ, Moore WS, Goldstone J: Below-knee amputation: A modern approach. Am J Surg 134:153, 1977.

11. Holloway GA Jr, Burgess EM: Cutaneous blood flow and its relation to healing of below knee amputation. Surg Gynecol Obstet 146:750, 1978.
12. Silberstein EB, Thomas S, Cline J, et al: Predictive value of intracutaneous xenon clearance for healing of amputation and cutaneous ulcer sites. Radiology 147:227, 1983.
13. Harris JP, McLaughlin AF, Quinn RS, et al: Skin blood flow measurements with xenon-133 to predict healing of lower extremity amputations. Aust NZ J Surg 1987, in press.
14. Daly MJ, Henry RE: Quantitative measurement of skin perfusion with xenon-133. J Nucl Med 21:156, 1980.
15. Malone JM, Anderson GG, Lalka SG, et al: A prospective comparison of noninvasive techniques for amputation level selection. Am J Surg 154:179, 1987.
16. Holstein P, Lund P, Larsen B, Schomacker T: Skin perfusion pressure required to stop isotope washout: Methodological considerations and normal values on the legs. Scand J Clin Lab Invest 37:649, 1977.
17. Holstein P: Level selection in leg amputation for arterial occlusive disease. Acta Orthop Scand 53:821, 1982.
18. Holstein P, Trap-Jensen J, Bagger H, et al: Skin perfusion pressure measured by isotope washout in legs with arterial occlusive disease. Clin Physiol 3:313, 1983.

6

Amputation Level Selection by Transcutaneous Oxygen Pressure Determination

Rodney A. White, M.D.
Stanley R. Klein, M.D.

Optimal therapy for the patient with severe peripheral vascular disease who is not a candidate for reconstruction relies on determining the most distal amputation level that will heal. The importance of making an accurate preoperative assessment is emphasized by the excessive morbidity and mortality that are associated with breakdown of ischemic tissues after vascular reconstruction and amputation.[1] Arteriography remains the standard for determining the distribution of arterial lesions, but this invasive procedure does not quantitate local tissue perfusion. Noninvasive techniques, including Doppler segmental pressure measurement,[2] pulse volume recording (PVR),[3] and quantitative flow velocity determination,[4] reflect primarily the hemodynamics of the extremity. Xenon-133 clearance has been shown to accurately quantitate skin blood flow and predict healing but is minimally invasive and requires operator expertise and facilities that are not available in many hospitals.[5] Transcutaneous oximetry is a noninvasive technique that requires minimal operator time and expertise, is per-

formed with low-cost instruments, and accurately reflects local tissue perfusion and oxygenation. This method has been used to assess peripheral arterial occlusive disease[6–16] and to monitor the status of patients with replanted limbs[17] and those who are critically ill.[18, 19]

METHODOLOGY OF TRANSCUTANEOUS OXIMETRY

Transcutaneous oxygen sensors are placed at the desired sites, which are shaved, if necessary, and wiped with an alcohol pad. The selected areas should not be directly over superficial veins or ischemic lesions. The selection of flat or slightly convex areas provides reliable sensor contact when a minimal amount of contact gel, recommended by the manufacturer, is used. Leads are taped to the leg approximately 1 inch proximal to the sensor or are held in place by an adhesive ring. A two-point gas calibration of the electrode is performed before and after each study to ensure accurate data. If there is significant discrepancy in the electrode drift, the instrument is recalibrated. The electrode requires approximately 15 to 20 minutes to equilibrate before transcutaneous oxygen pressure (PTC_{O_2}) values can be recorded. Minor variations in this procedure may be found with instruments from different manufacturers, but the procedure is uniformly easy to perform. Differences in performance among the various units available are discussed in a subsequent section.

PHYSIOLOGY OF TRANSCUTANEOUS OXYGEN PERFUSION

Transcutaneous oximetry is performed with a heated Clark polorographic oxygen electrode to measure oxygen diffusion to the skin surface from the dermal capillaries. Heating of the skin to 44° C changes the lipid structure of the stratum corneum, increasing the rate of oxygen diffusion; decreases oxygen solubility; shifts the oxygen-hemoglobin dissociation curve to the right; and dilates the capillaries.[20] Heating the skin increases PTC_{O_2} and compensates for the oxygen diffusion gradient between the capillaries and the electrode and for oxygen consumption by dermal and epidermal cells. PTC_{O_2} values have been shown to approximate arterial oxygen pressure (Pa_{O_2}) values closely in both neonates and adults when blood flow is normal. When blood flow is reduced, PTC_{O_2} is correlated with oxygen delivery: the product of oxygen content and flow.[21] Experimentally, PTC_{O_2} measured with the patient breathing room air decreases nonlinearly in relation to flow, with a marked drop occurring below 20% of baseline flow. PTC_{O_2} measured at increased fractional inspired oxygen (FI_{O_2}) is dependent primarily on Pa_{O_2} at flow rates greater than 50% of baseline. With reduction in flow below 25% of baseline, PTC_{O_2} is dependent solely on flow and is not augmented by increasing Pa_{O_2}.[22]

PTC_{O_2} values have been shown to be affected by ambient temperature, change of the extremity's position,[6, 23, 24] stress induced by transient ischemia or exercise,[10, 11, 14, 25] and changes in FI_{O_2}.[22, 26] For these reasons, tests should be performed at the same room temperature and with the patient at rest in the supine position, breathing room air, to assure reproducibility of results and make comparative studies. Changes in position, stress, or percentage of inspired oxygen are being evaluated to increase the discriminatory capability of PTC_{O_2} values and show some promise, particularly in the evaluation and classification of the degree of peripheral vascular disease.[10, 11, 26] Determination of the true benefit of these maneuvers in enhancing diagnostic accuracy awaits further investigation.

SELECTION OF AMPUTATION LEVEL

Selection of amputation level is an appealing application for transcutaneous oximetry, as tissue oxygenation is the primary determinant of the potential for wound healing. Secondary factors such as infection can be controlled if the tissue oxygen supply is adequate. Several studies have examined the value of PTC_{O_2} as a predictor for healing at the chosen amputation level and are summarized in Table 6–1 and in the following discussion. Most of the studies concur as to the PTC_{O_2} value necessary for healing, and there is uniformity of its predictive capability within a particular institution, as each has an established methodology for use with the available instrumentation. The methods for acquiring measurements are simple and comparable among the studies, and variations in the absolute values are attributed to differences in the quantitative characteristics of the different instruments used.

In 1982, three studies were published that described preliminary results using PTC_{O_2} to determine the level for successful amputation. A group of 17 patients with foot ulcers, minor and major amputations, and ischemic ulcers that healed following reconstructive procedures were studied by the authors' group at the Harbor-UCLA Medical Center.[27] Patients with PTC_{O_2} values greater than 44 mmHg healed, whereas those with values less than 40 mmHg did not. In the authors' study, the PTC_{O_2} values offered a distinct advantage in predictive value over Doppler pressure measurements, PVR, pulse reappearance time, and angiography.

Table 6–1. SUMMARY OF STUDIES USING $P_{TC_{O_2}}$ TO SELECT AMPUTATION LEVEL

Reference	No. of Patients	Level of Amputation	$P_{TC_{O_2}}$ of Successful Amputations (mmHg)	$P_{TC_{O_2}}$ of Failed Amputations (mmHg)
White et al[27]	17	Toe, transmetatarsal, BK, AK, hip disarticulation	> 44*	< 40
Franzeck et al[6]	35	Foot, transmetatarsal, ray, ankle, BK, AK	36.5 ± 17.5†	0–3
Burgess et al[28]	37	BK	42 ± 11‡ (26–72)	16 ± 15 (0–36)
Dowd et al[7]	24	Toe, transmetatarsal, BK, AK	> 40‡ (40–74)	< 40 (0–40)
Mastapha et al[8]	14	BK	52.9 ± 13.1‡ (39–53)	28.4 ± 8.0 (19–36)
Ratliff et al[29]	34	BK	42.3 ± 15.6§ (8–72)	23.2 ± 11 (10–35)
	33	AK	53.3 ± 14	28.3 ± 14
Katsamouris et al[30]	37	Transmetatarsal, BK	54 ± 9§ (37–76)	7 ± 3
Cina et al[9]	29	Toe, transmetatarsal, BK, AK	> 38§	< 38

BK = below-knee, AK = above-knee.
*Measured with a Tecomette, Novametrix Medical Systems, Inc, Wallingford, Connecticut.
†Measured with a Transoxode, Hellige-Drager, FRG, manufactured in the USA by Litton Medical Electronics.
‡Measured with a Radiometer TCM 1, The London Company, Denmark.
§Measured with a Roche Model 5302, Roche Medical Electronics, Switzerland.

Franzeck and associates evaluated the healing of 35 patients who had foot, transmetatarsal, ray, ankle, below-knee, and above-knee amputations.[6] The mean $P_{TC_{O_2}}$ value from 26 patients with primary healing was 36.5 ± 17.5 mmHg, whereas six patients with failed amputations had $P_{TC_{O_2}}$ values between 0 and 3 mmHg. An additional three patients had delayed healing, with $P_{TC_{O_2}}$ values between 10 and 32 mmHg. The researchers concluded that values greater than 20 mmHg indicate good healing potential.

Burgess and colleagues reported their series of 37 patients having below-knee amputations.[28] Thirty of the amputations with $P_{TC_{O_2}}$ values of 42 ± 11 mmHg (a range of 26 to 72) healed, and seven amputations with $P_{TC_{O_2}}$ values of 16 ± 15 mmHg (a range of 0 to 36) failed. Fifteen patients with $P_{TC_{O_2}}$ values of 40 mmHg or more had no delay in healing, whereas 17 of 19 patients with values greater than 0 but less than 40 mmHg healed. Three patients with values of 0 required reamputation above the knee.

Several subsequent studies have been published regarding the use of $P_{TC_{O_2}}$ to determine amputation level. Dowd and coworkers studied 24 patients with $P_{TC_{O_2}}$ values measured at the level of toe, midtarsal, below-knee, and above-knee amputations and found that those with values less than 40 mmHg (a range of 0 to 40) failed to heal

irrespective of the level, whereas those patients with $P_{TC_{O_2}}$ values greater than 40 mmHg (a range of 40 to 74) all healed.[7] Mastapha and associates reported that nine of 14 patients had successful below-knee amputations, with $P_{TC_{O_2}}$ values of 52.9 ± 13.1 mmHg (a range of 39 to 53), and that five patients who had failed amputations requiring revisions had values of 28.4 ± 8.0 mmHg (a range of 19 to 36).[8] They concluded that $P_{TC_{O_2}}$ values of 40 mmHg or more indicate adquate perfusion for successful amputation; with values of 35 mmHg, there is some doubt as to the viability of the skin; and when lower values are recorded, it appears unlikely that amputation will be successful.

Ratliff and colleagues studied 62 below-knee and above-knee amputations and found that the mean below-knee $P_{TC_{O_2}}$ value was 42.3 ± 15.6 mmHg (a range of 8 to 72) in healed and 23.2 ± 11 mmHg (a range of 10 to 35) in failed below-knee amputations.[29] All below-knee amputations with $P_{TC_{O_2}}$ values above 35 mmHg healed; however, there were some amputations with values less than 35 mmHg that healed. All failed below-knee amputations had a below-knee $P_{TC_{O_2}}$ of 35 mmHg or less. The mean above-knee $P_{TC_{O_2}}$ value was 53.3 ± 14 mmHg in healed above-knee amputations and 28.3 ± 14 mmHg in those that failed.

Katsamouris and associates studied 37 patients with forefoot and below-knee amputations and found that successful amputations had PTC_{O_2} values of 50 ± 8 mmHg over the anterior calf, whereas failed procedures had values of 22 ± 16 mmHg.[30] This group also measured posterior calf PTC_{O_2} values and found them to enhance the discriminating ability of transcutaneous oximetry, with successful amputations having values of 54 ± 9 mmHg (a range of 37 to 76), and failed procedures, 7 ± 3 mmHg (a range of 3 to 10). Cina and coworkers further characterized this group's experience by describing PTC_{O_2} values in 29 patients who had toe, transmetatarsal, below-knee, and above-knee amputations.[9] Healing of amputations occurred when PTC_{O_2} values were equal to or greater than 38 mmHg, and failure to heal in the absence of infection was associated with PTC_{O_2} values less than 38 mmHg. This was true even in diabetic patients, in whom tests based on hemodynamic function are less reliable.

ATTEMPTS TO IMPROVE THE SPECIFICITY OF PTC_{O_2} DETERMINATIONS

Several investigators have tried to improve the specificity of PTC_{O_2} values beyond an individual reading at the proposed site in determining the amputation level. Harward and associates performed a blind prospective study of 119 amputations (39 forefoot, 57 below-knee, and 23 above-knee) to compare PTC_{O_2} values before and 10 minutes after inhalation of 100% oxygen as predictors of healing.[26] On the basis of preliminary studies in their institution, PTC_{O_2} values greater than 10 mmHg or an increase greater than 10 mmHg after oxygen inhalation was considered to predict a successful outcome, whereas failures were predicted when the initial PTC_{O_2} value was less than 10 mmHg and the increase after oxygen inhalation did not exceed the 10 mmHg level. Amputation level was determined by the operating surgeon on clinical criteria alone, without knowledge of the laboratory data. Results were then tabulated by retrospective analysis of operative outcome and preoperative tests. At the below-knee amputation level, the test was 95% sensitive, 100% specific, and 95% accurate; at the above-knee level, 100% sensitive, 100%

specific, and 100% accurate; at the transmetatarsal level, 80% sensitive, 0% specific, and 57% accurate; and at the toe level, 83% sensitive, 60% specific, and 61% accurate. From these results, it is apparent that the test was a good predictor of above- and below-knee healing but was not successful at the forefoot level. The results of studies from this group show promise for increasing the capability of PTC_{O_2} to discriminate those patients who have above- or below-knee PTC_{O_2} values less than 35 to 40 mmHg (the values that have been found by most other groups to predict delayed or failed healing) but who have a high likelihood for healing amputations. These results have not yet been duplicated by independent investigators. In general, the finding by this group that PTC_{O_2} values of 10 mmHg or more predict healing is significantly lower than that demonstrated by other groups, and the reason for this discrepancy is not apparent. One possible explanation is that this group is the only one using the Oxymonitor (Litton Medical Electronics), although this is speculative, as there has been no controlled comparison of the accuracy or absolute oxygen tension values obtained from the different instruments that are available.

Additional attempts to increase the discriminatory capability of PTC_{O_2} determinations include making a ratio of extremity to chest (i.e., central) values[8–10, 24, 30] and observing PTC_{O_2} changes induced by positional change,[6, 23, 24] exercise,[10, 14] or temporary ischemia.[11, 25] Extremity-to-chest ratios have been shown to increase the discrimination between groups in predicting successful level of amputation. The difference between patients whose amputations heal and those whose fail is statistically significant for both absolute transcutaneous oxygen tension values and transcutaneous oxygen tension ratios, and it is not clear that the PTC_{O_2} ratio is helpful in evaluating the disease, since tissue metabolism is probably related to the absolute value of oxygen tension and not to a normalized value.[9] Additional studies are required before a conclusion can be made regarding the improved predictive ability of these additional maneuvers.

SUMMARY

On the basis of cumulative experience, PTC_{O_2} value has been uniformly shown to be an accurate predictor of the potential for wound healing and successful amputation level. $P_{TC_{O_2}}$ determination has been shown to be superior to hemodynamic modalities and is not limited by underlying diseases, particularly diabetes. Although there is some variation among institutions in the absolute values reported to be required for healing, each group has shown a minimal learning curve and a high, reproducible accuracy once they have become familiar with the instrumentation.

The advantages over other available methods for quantitating local circulatory adequacy are that $P_{TC_{O_2}}$ determination

1. Can be used in 96 to 98% of all patients
2. Is inexpensive, is completely noninvasive, and requires minimal operator training
3. Can be used to make quantitative, serial assessments at multiple levels
4. Is not limited in extremities with absent pulses, absent Doppler signals, noncompressible vessels, or painful lesions
5. Is rapidly responsive to changes in local circulatory status, such as those induced by position
6. Provides a physiological correlate for and has the potential to increase the accuracy of other modalities

In the authors' institution, $P_{TC_{O_2}}$ values of 40 mmHg are used to predict the successful outcome of amputations. Values of less than 40 mmHg suggest an unsuccessful outcome, unless revascularization can be combined with the amputation to increase oxygenation. Limbs with persistently low $P_{TC_{O_2}}$ ($<$ 30 mmHg) have a high probability of amputation failure, and selection of a more proximal level is called for in high-risk patients.

REFERENCES

1. Blaisdell WF, Steele M, Allen R: Management of acute lower extremity arterial ischemia due to embolism and thrombosis. Surgery 84:822, 1978.
2. Barnes RW, Shank CW, Slaymaker EE: An index of healing in below knee amputations: Leg blood pressure by Doppler ultrasound. Surgery 79:13, 1976.
3. Raines JK, Darling C, Buth J, et al: Vascular laboratory criteria for the management of peripheral vascular disease of the lower extremities. Surgery 79:21, 1976.
4. Dilley RB, Fronek A: Quantitative velocity measurements in arterial disease of the lower extremity. *In* Bernstein EF (ed): Noninvasive Diagnostic Techniques in Vascular Disease. St Louis, CV Mosby Co, 1978, p 294.
5. Moore WS: Determination of amputation level. Measurement of skin blood flow with xenon Xe 133. Arch Surg 107:798, 1973.
6. Franzeck UK, Talke P, Bernstein EF, et al: Transcutaneous PO_2 measurements in health and peripheral arterial occlusive disease. Surgery 91:156, 1982.
7. Dowd GSE, Linge K, Bentley G: Measurement of transcutaneous oxygen pressure in normal and ischemic skin. J Bone Joint Surg 65:79, 1983.
8. Mustapha NM, Redhead RG, Jain SK, Wielogorski JW: Transcutaneous partial oxygen pressure assessment of the ischemic lower limb. Surg Obstet Gynecol 156:582, 1983.
9. Cina C, Katsamouris A, Megerman J, et al: Utility of transcutaneous oxygen tension measurements in peripheral arterial occlusive disease. J Vasc Surg 1:362, 1984.
10. Hauser CJ, Shoemaker WM: Use of a transcutaneous PO_2 regional perfusion index in peripheral vascular disease. Ann Surg 197:337, 1983.
11. Kram HB, White RA, Tabrisky J, et al: Transcutaneous oxygen recovery and toe pulse reappearance time in the assessment of peripheral vascular disease. Circulation 72:1022, 1985.
12. Wyss CR, Matsen FA, Simmons CW, Burgess EM: Transcutaneous oxygen tension measurements on limbs of diabetic and non-diabetic patients with peripheral vascular disease. Surgery 95:339, 1984
13. Clyne CAC, Ryan J, Webster JHH, Chant ADB: Oxygen tension on the skin of ischemic legs. Am J Surg 143:315, 1982.
14. Byrne P, Provan JL, Ameli FM, Jones DP: The use of transcutaneous oxygen tension measurements in the diagnosis of peripheral vascular insufficiency. Ann Surg 200:159, 1984.
15. Tonnesen KH: Transcutaneous oxgyen tension in imminent foot gangrene. Acta Anaesthesiol Scand 68:107, 1978.
16. Hauser CJ, Klein SR, Mehringer CM, et al: Superiority of transcutaneous oximetry in noninvasive vascular diagnosis in patients with diabetes. Arch Surg 119:690, 1984.
17. Matsen FA, Bach AW, Wyss CR, Simmons CW: Transcutaneous PO_2: A potential monitor of the status of replanted limb parts. Plast Reconstr Surg 65:732, 1980.
18. Tremper KK, Shoemaker WM: Transcutaneous oxygen monitoring of critically ill adults, with and without low flow shock. Crit Care Med 9:706, 1981.
19. Kram HB: Noninvasive tissue oxygen monitoring in surgical and critical care medicine. Surg Clin North Am 65:1005, 1985.
20. Lubbers DW: Theoretic basis of the transcutaneous blood gas measurements. Crit Care Med 9:721, 1981.
21. Tremper KK, Waxman K, Shoemaker WM: Effect of hypoxia and shock on transcutaneous PO_2 values in dogs. Crit Care Med 7:526, 1979.
22. Moosa HH, Makaroun MS, Steed, DL, Webster MW: $TcPO_2$ values in limb ischemia: Effects of blood flow and arterial oxygen tension. Proceedings of the Association for Academic Surgery Meeting, Cincinnati, November 10–13, 1985, p 109.
23. Matsen FA, Wyss CR, Pedegana LR, et al: Transcutaneous oxygen tension measurement in peripheral vascular disease. Surg Gynecol Obstet 150:525, 1980.
24. Hauser CJ, Appel PA, Shoemaker WM: Pathophysiologic classification of peripheral vascular disease

by positional changes in regional transcutaneous oxygen tension. Surgery 95:689, 1984.

25. Kram HB, Appel PL, White RA, Shoemaker WM: Assessment of peripheral vascular disease by post occlusive transcutaneous oxygen recovery time. J Vasc Surg 1:628, 1984.

26. Harward TR, Volny J, Golbranson F, et al: Oxygen inhalation-induced transcutaneous PO_2 changes as a predictor of amputation level. J Vasc Surg 2:220, 1985.

27. White RA, Nolan L, Harley D, et al: Noninvasive evaluation of peripheral vascular disease using transcutaneous oxygen tension. Am J Surg 144:68, 1982.

28. Burgess EM, Matsen FA, Wyss CR, Simmons CW: Segmental transcutaneous measurements of PO_2 in patients requiring below the knee amputation for peripheral vascular insufficiency. J Bone Joint Surg 64:378, 1982.

29. Ratliff DA, Clyne CAC, Chant ADB, Webster JHH: Prediction of amputation wound healing: The role of transcutaneous PO_2 assessment. Br J Surg 71:219, 1984.

30. Katsamouris A, Brewster DC, Megerman J, et al: Transcutaneous oxygen tension in selection of amputation level. Am J Surg 147:510, 1984.

7

Amputation Level Selection by Skin Fluorescence

David G. Silverman, M.D.*

Since 1882, when Paul Ehrlich used the dye to study fluid in the anterior chamber of the eye, fluorescein's major role in clinical medicine has been for ophthalmologic studies such as retinal angiography. Although employed more than 40 years ago as an indicator of skin and bowel perfusion, fluorescein did not enjoy widespread use in these areas. However, more recent efforts to preserve compromised tissue with conservative amputation, revascularization, microvascular surgery, and vasoactive therapy have often required a sensitive indicator of the microcirculation. Fluorescein has been found to be well suited for such use in the skin and viscera, where it assesses perfusion and helps predict viability with high sensitivity and accuracy.[1-10]

After systemic administration, fluorescein is distributed throughout the circulation. During this phase, its passage through the retinal vessels may be documented by retinal angiography. Staining patterns in the skin

are assessed 10 to 20 minutes later—after the small fluorescein molecules have diffused into the pericapillary interstitium—by visual inspection, fluorescent photography, or fluorometry. Illumination by ultraviolet or blue light excites fluorescein's outermost electron, with maximum excitation at approximately 490 nm. Return to the original energy state is characterized by emission of yellow-green fluorescence, with maximum emission in the range of 515 to 520 nm.[11, 12] Several filter combinations have been proposed to delineate well-perfused areas from ischemic nonviable regions, which do not stain and simply reflect the excitation light. The excitation filter should be specific for wavelengths below 500 nm, whereas the emission filter should transmit only those above 510 nm. Narrowband interference filters appear to provide the clearest discrimination. For photography, it generally is advisable to use a rapid shutter speed that is synchronized with a powerful flash. This maximizes the fluorescent signal, minimizes the effect of ambient light, and permits the camera to be hand-held (Table 7-1).[11-17]

The fluorescein test is well suited for evaluating the hypoperfused limb undergoing amputative surgery. Assessment of tissue

*Many of the studies reported were funded by a Veterans Administration Career Development Award and Veterans Administration Rehabilitative Research and Development Award 150.

Table 7–1. FLUORESCENT PHOTOGRAPHY: FILTERS, CAMERAS, AND FILM

	Excitation Filters	Emission Filters	Camera & Film	References
In Darkened Room	W47B Blue plexiglass SE40* or PTR blue* PTR blue*	W4 W8 SB50* or W15 Edmund 520*	f2 to f5.6, 64 ASA film f5.6 to f11, 200 ASA film f8, 200 ASA film unspecified	Valencia et al,[12] Welch,[13] Myers & Donovan,[14] Myers et al[16]
	Kodak 18A glass	W15 or W12	unspecified	
In Normal Room Light	SE40, W47B, or plexiglass #2114 or PTR blue	W15, W2A, W8, W4, or SB50	f8, 64 ASA film, or faster shutter speed (1/125 sec)	Myers,[15] Myers et al,[16] Myers[17]
	W47	W12	f8, 400 ASA film processed at 1600	
"Instant" Prints	SE40	W15, consider adding neutral density filter	Polaroid SX70 camera modified to attain f 8, 1/90 sec, 150 or 600 ASA film. Also can modify Polaroid 680 or attach Polaroid "back" to a 35 mm camera.	Myers,[15] Myers et al[16]

*Interference filter.

W = Wratten series (Eastman Kodak Co, Rochester, New York), SE = Spectrotech Excitation (Spectrotech Inc, Lincoln, Massachusetts), SB = Spectrotech Barrier, blue plexiglass #2114 (Rohm and Haas, Dallas, Texas), PTR (PTR Optics Corp, Waltham, Massachusetts), Edmund 520 (Edmund Scientific Co, Barrington, New Jersey).

staining after systemic fluorescein administration is specific for nutritive blood flow[4, 5] and can determine skin perfusion to widespread areas of the leg. Intraoperative assessment of a newly created amputation flap is analogous to that for skin flaps in other regions, where intraoperative fluorescence assessment consistently has provided highly reliable predictions of ultimate flap viability.[1–3] However, the difficult task for the fluorescein test or any of its counterparts is to predict preoperatively whether a given site will be able to heal a subsequent insult such as amputative surgery. Despite the changes that occur because of the operative procedure, most surgeons want the test's information preoperatively. The traditional fluorescein test, visual inspection under ultraviolet illumination (Table 7–2), has proved to be valuable in this setting. As will be discussed later, quantification of tissue fluorescence by fluorometry may be the best available means for documenting critical variations in the perfusion of the hypoperfused limb.

fluorescein distribution corresponded to viable and nonviable ischemic limbs.[6] A line of demarcation was most clearly evident at sites of vascular occlusion due to acute embolization.

Table 7–2. TRADITIONAL FLUORESCEIN TEST FOR PREOPERATIVE ASSESSMENT OF SKIN PERFUSION

Preinjection: Have patient assume comfortable position (preferably semi-Fowler's) on stretcher. Establish intravenous route in hand or forearm.

Injection: Administer sodium fluorescein 10–40 mg/kg (10–20 mg/kg in light- or 20–40 mg/kg in dark-skinned subject) via intravenous cannula. A physician should be available at the time of injection. Slow injection diminishes the likelihood of a reaction to the dye.

Postinjection: Turn lights off and scan limb under ultraviolet light with or without yellow glasses,[6] or photograph with a blue flash and a green emission filter.

Interpretation: Assess perfusion according to staining patterns.

Staining Pattern	Probable Perfusion
Homogeneous green	Adequate
Fine reticular	Borderline/adequate
Patchy	Borderline/poor*
Mostly blue	Critical hypoperfusion
Solid blue	No flow

*Particularly worrisome if nonfluorescent regions are greater than 1 cm in diameter.

PIONEERING STUDIES

More than 40 years ago, Lange and Boyd reported that the time course and extent of

Fluorescein permitted us to establish exactly the level of blood supply to the skin. . . . There is a sharp line of demarcation where normal fluorescence stops. . . . In two patients with acute embolism we were able to demonstrate that the embolus had not led to complete vascular occlusion. . . . Since the tips of all toes were fluorescent, we were sure that gangrene would not occur; the subsequent clinical course bore out our contention.*

In long-standing arteriosclerosis, Lange and Boyd noted two main patterns of altered perfusion secondary to arterial occlusion.[6] The most common was in the setting of generalized atherosclerosis, which was characterized by diffuse hypofluorescence and, perhaps, scattered fluorescent islands.

. . . there is a generalized marked decrease in fluorescence of both limbs with the appearance of an entirely nonfluorescent distal gangrenous area. Usually there is no hyperfluorescent ring surrounding the gangrenous tissue to indicate "walling off"; rather there is a definite trend toward further spread of the gangrene. The ulcers showed no fluorescence of their base which indicated complete ischemia. This type of condition offers an extremely poor prognosis, and an amputation must be performed at a high level. Low amputations lead to poorly healing stumps. . . .*

Less common, but more distinct, was localized hypofluorescence due to local occlusion.

The ulcer may or may not show a few fluorescent capillaries. The surrounding tissue is extremely hyperfluorescent, with increased capillary permeability. . . .The general fluorescence of the leg is normal or only slightly depressed. . . . This does not preclude the appearance of a gangrenous spot with the same picture of demarcation within a short time in another area. . . . Patients with this type of arteriosclerotic gangrene do well with local debridement and self demarcation. . . . In six cases we could predict that gangrene would probably occur in a certain spot on the foot within a short time, for this area of skin showed no, or markedly diminished, fluorescence.*

To maximize the fluorescent signal in the extremity under study, other investigators administered the dye directly into the femoral artery. Groin-to-leg circulation times and patterns of fluorescence provided valuable information, particularly in light-skinned subjects. The value of this approach was demonstrated by Lowry and associates in an elderly diabetic with dry gangrene of his left third toe.[18]

The fluorescein test revealed circulation times of six seconds to the knee and 14 seconds to the toes, and a staining pattern which showed excellent fluorescence of the leg and foot to the base of the involved toe. This information suggested that local amputation should heal and a wedge-shaped ray amputation was performed and healed primarily.[18]

Unfortunately, there are not always distinct demarcations of perfusion in the arteriosclerotic limb, a feature that has complicated all means of perfusion assessment. With respect to the traditional fluorescein test, this lack of distinct demarcations has contributed to staining patterns that are difficult to interpret, especially in dark-skinned subjects. Although homogeneous fluorescence and complete absence of staining are readily identifiable, it may be difficult to interpret the intermediate perfusion patterns that typify the arteriosclerotic limb. Attempts to modify the technique, although potentially beneficial, have tended to compromise its simplicity. This certainly is the case for intra-arterial injection. It has been reported that making scratches or wheals along the extremity facilitates visualization of fluorescent staining,[19, 20] but this approach also has attracted few converts.

In contrast to the subjective and somewhat invasive (see "Fluorescein Safety") fluorescein test, measurement of segmental limb pressures by Doppler ultrasound apparently constituted a highly reliable, noninvasive means for amputation site determination. Such was the case when more proximal amputations (below- and above-knee) were routinely performed; thus, the fluorescein test was rarely employed.

RENEWAL OF INTEREST

More recently, the reliability of segmental limb pressure measurements has been challenged by reports that they often fail to predict skin necrosis in the contexts of diabetic calcification and distal amputative sur-

*From Lange K, Boyd LJ: Use of fluorescein method in establishment of diagnosis and prognosis of peripheral vascular diseases. Arch Int Med 74:175, 1944. Copyright 1944, American Medical Association.

gery. In 1978, it was proposed that a monitor of skin perfusion would significantly decrease morbidity and save millions of dollars annually in the care of the amputee.[21] No technique has proved to be ideal in this regard, prompting a "second look" at fluorescein.

The intravascular phase of fluorescein distribution has been assessed with capillary angiography (in a manner comparable to that used for retinal angiography).[8, 22] Tanzer and Horne microscopically analyzed fluorescein angiograms at one minute after bolus injection.[8] Without knowledge of the fluorescein findings, the surgeon's choice of amputation level was too distal in nine of 27 amputations; assessment of fluorescein staining patterns predicted five of these nine amputation failures. However, interpretation of fluorescein patterns incorrectly predicted necrosis of three amputations that eventually healed by prolonged secondary healing.

In Sweden, Lund has introduced a sophisticated means for dynamic monitoring of fluorescein appearance and filling times to the sole and for densitometric analysis of sole staining.[23, 24] Patterns of perfusion are delineated by bolus injection of dye into a patient who becomes vasodilated by drinking alcohol and lying in a heat box. This technique has provided clear documentation of changes in perfusion after vasoactive therapy; however, assessment restricted to the sole provides limited information as to the optimum site of amputation.

Visual and fluorometric assessments of skin staining after dye distribution also have been applied successfully. Such assessments have been shown to be specific for nutritive perfusion in animal models.[4, 5, 32] They do not necessitate rapid documentation within seconds of bolus injection of dye. Thus, they facilitate evaluation of widespread regions. In addition, although such assessments traditionally have been performed after bolus injection, they can be performed after a slower means of administration and thereby be associated with a lesser incidence of adverse effects (see "Fluorescein Safety"). McFarland, Lawrence, and colleagues compared fluorescent staining (as outlined in Table 7–2) and segmental Doppler pressures in 30 patients with lower extremity ischemic lesions.[9, 25] Healing of an amputation was predicted if the proposed amputation site became fluorescent or if the segmental pressure was greater than 50 mmHg. Each amputation was performed at the most distal site compatible with function at which either criterion was met. Segmental blood pressures were accurate and useful in only 47% of cases. They predicted the outcome of digital ischemia with only 45% usefulness and accuracy (5/11 patients); in four cases, there was critical ischemia even in the presence of normal ankle Doppler pressures. In contrast, fluorescein studies were accurate in 91% of the cases of digital ischemia and 80% overall—the 20% failure was attributed to infection or deep tissue necrosis, consistent with the test's specificity for skin, not muscle, blood flow. These authors concluded:

> . . . skin fluorescence appeared to be more reliable and had several advantages over the more commonly used blood pressure method. First, it gave an accurate assessment of digital or forefoot ischemia. Second, it proved useful when stiff arteries made blood pressure measurements unreliable. And, finally, it frequently predicted that a more distal site of amputation would heal than the blood pressure method, thus preserving tissue that can be very valuable during a patient's rehabilitation.[9]

QUANTITATIVE FLUORESCENCE ASSESSMENT

Despite their encouraging findings, advocates of the fluorescein test noted that visual assessment of dye distribution is not without its limitations. More than 40 years ago, it became evident to Lange and associates that quantification of fluorescence would overcome many of the limitations of the fluorescein test.[6, 26]

> . . . if there is doubt exactly where fluorescence ends, the dermofluorometer provides a solution, for an increase in fluorescein skin units after the injection always indicates the presence of some circulation. This alone, however, did not determine whether the area should be included in the amputation. Only when the values are two-thirds of the lowest normal may one safely refrain from amputation.[26]

However, in its original form, dermofluorometry did not gain widespread acceptance, primarily because it required strapping a bulky electrical device to the area under study.[27] The advent of fiberoptic light guides, matched interference filters, and highly sensitive photomultiplier tubes has permitted design of a fiberoptic fluorometer (Fig. 7–1)

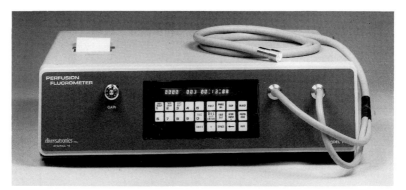

FIGURE 7–1. Fiberoptic fluorometer. A branched fiberoptic light guide transmits blue excitation light to, and emitted fluorescence from, the tissue under study. The gain control permits adjustment of the photomultiplier tube output, which is displayed on the light-emitting diode and recorded by the printer. The keyboard is used for microprocessor analysis of the data and permits information storage in a permanent memory. (*Courtesy of* Diversatronics, Inc, Broomall, Pennsylvania.)

that overcomes the limitations of the 1940 prototype.

The 1980s have seen a plethora of studies suggesting that fluorometry is superior to the more traditional means of fluorescence assessment (Table 7–3). The fluorometer's increased sensitivity has enabled more precise determination of skin and bowel survival in laboratory and clinical settings. The technique has been shown to delineate nutritive blood flow in compromised tissue with the precision of radiolabeled microspheres.[32] In contrast, techniques such as thermometry and laser Doppler flowmetry may be influenced by nonnutritive arteriovenous shunt flow. In comparative studies, fluorometry was found to be more sensitive and specific for

gradations in perfusion than laser Doppler flowmetry.[37–39] In addition, the fluorescein test does not require local skin warming, which may alter local perfusion and limit the speed at which a test such as transcutaneous oximetry can be performed at multiple sites.

Several studies have indicated that fluorometry is a very good technique for predicting healing of a proposed amputation site.[6, 33, 40–42] Hundreds of reading sites may be outlined on each subject to provide multiple study sites at each potential amputation level (Fig. 7–2). Most commonly, the dye fluorescence (DF) value of each study site is expressed as a percentage of the DF in a well-perfused reference region: the dye fluorescence index, or DFI (Table 7–4). As will be described later, other means of analysis have been recommended.

In a series of 86 amputations in which fluorometry was performed preoperatively but did not influence the surgeon's decision, it appeared that inclusion of fluorometric findings would have significantly improved amputation outcome.[33] The relative fluorescence (DFI) of healing sites averaged 79%, whereas those that failed had a mean DFI of 27%. Fluorometric predictions remained accurate at each amputation level, including distal sites (Table 7–5). Fluorometry's clear discrimination was maintained in diabetic patients, in whom the DFI of healing and nonhealing sites averaged 81% and 25%, respectively, and in the presence of varied skin pigmentation (Fig. 7–3). Overall, discriminant analysis provided an optimum DFI cutoff of 40%. This identified a critical amount of perfusion, as all but two of the failed amputations had DFI values below 40%. Out-

Table 7–3. ADVANTAGES OF FLUOROMETRY OVER THE TRADITIONAL FLUORESCEIN TEST

Visual Inspection	Fluorometry
Subjective interpretation "All or none"	Quantitative measurement Delineates gradations[28–31] with precision of radiolabeled microspheres[32]
Detects 10^{-6} g/ml fluorescein in water	Detects 10^{-10} g/ml[28]
Dosage in range of 10–40 mg/kg	2–8 mg/kg, thus less side effects[3, 33]
Difficult to assess in black skin	More accurate in black skin[33–35]
Single assessment of dye uptake	Documents uptake and elimination; this may identify extravasation[30, 35, 36] and negate effect of pigmentation[34, 35]
Not repeatable for 24 hours	Repeatable within minutes[29]

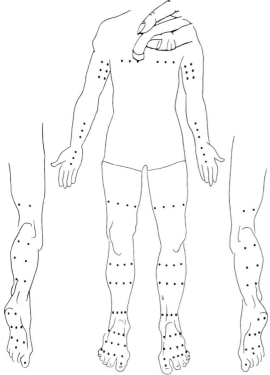

FIGURE 7–2. Sample fluorometric grid pattern, with fiberoptic light guide on chest.

Table 7–4. ESTABLISHED PROTOCOL FOR FLUOROMETRIC EVALUATION* OF SITES FOR LOWER LIMB AMPUTATION

Preinjection: Demarcate fluorometric study sites with a nontoxic marker. Allow fluorometer to warm–up for 20 minutes, and adjust it so that it records a value of zero when the photomultiplier tube is shielded from incoming light. Obtain preinjection background readings by gently placing the fiberoptic light guide on each study and reference site for 2–3 seconds. Record photomultiplier tube output, or transmit data to an interfaced microprocessor by depressing a foot pedal.

Injection: Dilute fluorescein 4–8 mg/kg to 20 ml with saline 0.9%; administer dye via peripheral intravenous route over a 2–3 minute interval. A physician should be available at the time of injection.

Postinjection: Record fluorometric readings at 10–20 minutes after injection. Obtain "postdye" dye fluorescence (DF) value by subtracting preinjection background reading from each postinjection reading (accomplished automatically by microprocessor). Extra points can be monitored even if preinjection background readings have not been recorded at these sites; background values can be approximated from those of neighboring sites of comparable pigmentation.

Analysis: Determine dye fluorescence index (DFI) by comparing DF value of study site to that of the appropriate reference site.

$$DFI = (DF \text{ of study site/DF of reference}) \times 100$$

*Proposed modifications with respect to dye administration and normalization for pigmentation are described in the text and outlined in Table 7–7.

Modified from Silverman DG, Roberts A, Reilly CA, et al: Fluorometric quantification of low-dose fluorescein delivery to predict amputation healing. Surgery 101:335, 1987.

side of the narrow "transitional zone" of DFI values between 38 and 42%, the cutoff predicted amputation success accurately in 74 of 75 cases (except at sites of cellulitis and edema). This attests to the precision of fluorometric determinations; however, one should predict cautiously when DFI values lie near or within the transitional range. Certainty is limited by the questionable fate of tissues with marginal perfusion (a condition that plagues every means of preoperative evaluation) and by the fact that DFI values are themselves subject to variation.[28, 29]

In the same report,[33] it was noted that fluorometry did not predict success accurately in 12 other cases in which an amputation was performed in the presence of cellulitis or edema. This finding was consistent with that reported by Lange and Boyd.[6] This inaccuracy may be attributed, in part, to poor healing of amputations in such settings regardless of the means of preoperative assessment and to the finding that fluorescence may be distorted if there is endothelial damage and subsequent dye extravasation;[30, 35, 36, 43] the latter will be addressed later in this chapter when new means of fluorometric analysis are discussed.

Table 7–5. PREOPERATIVE FLUOROMETRIC INDICES* AND ULTIMATE AMPUTATION SITE HEALING

	No. of Patients	DFI (mean ± SD)
All Levels		
Healing	62	79.1 ± 37
Failing	24	26.9 ± 14
All Distal Amputations		
Healing	23	62.5 ± 19
Failing	21	25.5 ± 12
Diabetic Patients		
Healing	41	80.8 ± 41
Failing	20	25.0 ± 12
Dark-skinned Patients		
Healing	35	75.6 ± 36
Failing	21	25.4 ± 14

*Fluorescence expressed as a percentage of well-perfused reference area with the dye fluorescence index (DFI).

From Silverman DG, Roberts A, Reilly CA, et al: Fluorometric quantification of low-dose fluorescein delivery to predict amputation healing. Surgery 101:335, 1987.

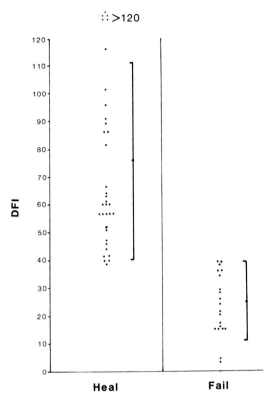

FIGURE 7–3. Fluorometry in dark-skinned patients. A distinct separation is shown between healing and failing amputation sites. (*From* Silverman DG, Roberts A, Reilly CA, et al: Fluorometric quantification of low-dose fluorescein delivery to predict amputation healing. Surgery 101:335, 1987.)

In a more recent prospective study of 137 cases without cellulitis and edema, fluorometric predictions based on the aforementioned cutoffs were made preoperatively, and the surgeon was given the option of incorporating the data into the selection of an amputation level. The previously established cutoffs proved to be accurate in 112 cases, inconclusive in 11 (a DFI between 38 and 42%), and inaccurate in 14.[41]

These clinical trials demonstrated the importance of documenting fluorescence at multiple sites along a potential amputation level. Regional variations in perfusion may make the mean DFI misleading. Actually, this illustrates a potential advantage of the fluorescein test in that the test can delineate perfusion throughout the potential amputation flap before, during, and after the operation.

The advent of fluorometry has improved the ability to evaluate and optimize therapeutic interventions designed to increase tissue perfusion. However, it should be noted that expanded applications of fluorometry and other clinical means of assessment in arteriosclerotic extremities have been restricted primarily by two factors. First, there is no nonradioactive "gold standard" with which to readily assess a technique such as fluorometry in the clinical setting (except ultimate viability). Second, it has been difficult to simulate in the laboratory the chronic effects of arteriosclerosis on the human extremity. Thus, clinicians can only extrapolate from laboratory findings, and determination of clinical significance awaits clinical trials.

Fluorometric assessments of changes in perfusion after creation of an interpolated flap[44–46] and a surgical delaying procedure[47] may prove to be relevant to the ischemic limb. They demonstrate that it is possible to identify when a compromised tissue should be able to tolerate a subsequent surgical insult such as pedicle severance or flap creation (as would be the case during amputative surgery). Furthermore, they may lead to ways of improving ulcer or amputation site perfusion and certainly have established means of documenting such changes.

Fluorometry's repeatability (consistent results have been obtained after four successive dye injections at 15-minute intervals[29]) has also permitted monitoring of the effects of vasoactive drug therapy and sympathectomy.[6, 43, 48–52] The value of fluorometry in the assessment of vasoactive therapy has been illustrated by a series of studied evaluating the local erythematous response after topical application of a prostaglandin E_2 analog. Fluorometry documented significant increases in dye delivery and elimination at sites of drug application on healthy volunteers, indicating that the erythema represented an increase in nutritive perfusion.[48]

The ability of fluorometry to document interruption and restitution of perfusion in island and free flaps[3, 43, 51, 53–55] and replanted digits[56] has led to the application of the technique to the ischemic extremity undergoing vascular reconstruction or angioplasty. Fluorometry has been performed before and after the therapeutic procedure, and the improvement in the DFI of the desired skin region, or lack thereof, has correlated highly with clinical outcome (Table 7–6). That the change in fluorescence of the study area did indeed represent an increase in perfusion via the reconstituted vessel was supported by a study in rabbits, which confirmed that limb

Table 7–6. PERCENT CHANGE IN DFI COMPARED WITH CLINICAL COURSE AFTER VASCULAR RECONSTRUCTION OR ANGIOPLASTY

	Treated Leg % Change (SD)	Untreated Leg % Change (SD)
Leg Pain		
Relieved in treated leg (n = 11)	+87 (106)	+5 (11)
Not relieved in treated leg (n = 6)	−27 (9)	0 (99)
Ischemic Wound		
Healed (n = 8)	+73 (110)	−3 (7)
Not healed (n = 7)	−20 (20)	0 (28)

In 20 patients with ischemic leg pain or an ischemic wound, fluorometry was performed before and after attempted recanalization. The relative fluorescence (DFI) of the relevant vascular territories were compared before and after treatment, and values were expressed as mean change and standard deviation (in parentheses). Discriminant analysis provided a DFI increase of 11% as the optimum cutoff. Values above this cutoff accurately documented clinical improvement in 16 of 17 cases of leg pain and 15 of 17 cases of ischemic ulceration (unpublished data). Care was taken not to perform measurements at sites of cellulitis or edema, as readings at such sites may have been distorted; even so, there was high variability among subjects. It is anticipated that recent modifications of dye administration and fluorometric analysis will improve test consistency (see text).

fluorescence correlates highly with distal aortic flow.[57]

Thus, fluorometry appears to be well suited for the assessment of nutritive blood flow in the extremity with compromised perfusion. However, there are two aspects of the fluorescein test in the evaluation of the potential amputee that must be addressed: re-

liability, especially in dark-skinned individuals, and safety of dye administration. In multicolored pigs, Brousseau and colleagues noted that the DFI of flap regions with comparable fates varied by less than 4% when referenced to comparably pigmented areas.[34] In that setting, the well-perfused reference area was adjacent to or contralateral to the study area. Clinicians are hampered, somewhat, in evaluating the patient with occlusive arterial disease, since remote reference sites on the upper extremity or chest are generally used. This has led to a search for a "color-independent" fluorescein test, even though the basic technique has proved to be highly reliable in experienced hands.[33, 40, 41]

The influence of pigmentation may be virtually eliminated if one analyzes the time course of fluorescein distribution or elimination (Fig. 7–4). Such parameters are not dependent on an absolute measurement of fluorescence at a single point in time and thus are independent of site-to-site variations in fluorescence that result from noncirculatory factors such as skin pigmentation.[34, 35] The author first accomplished this by analysis of dye elimination. As the tissues accumulate fluorescein and blood levels decline, the blood-tissue gradient reverses, and fluorescein is eliminated from tissues in proportion to their perfusion.[58, 59] Analysis of dye elimination after delivery to the ischemic limb and reference region enabled Hurford and Silverman to clarify accurately all cases in which uptake (DFI) at a given site was not definitive.[60] Failure of wound healing was predicted if, by the time the fluorescence of the reference area had returned to preinjection

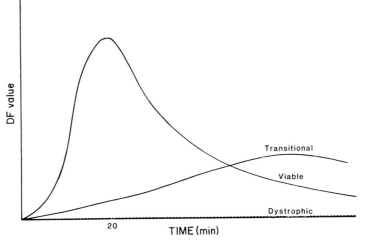

FIGURE 7–4. Idealized uptake and elimination of fluorescein in well-perfused (Viable), moderately perfused (Transitional), and nonperfused (Dystrophic) regions of a pedicle skin flap.

values, the equivocal site still retained more than 50% of its 20-minute fluorescent reading. The value of elimination lies not only in its being independent of skin pigmentation, but also in its being more indicative of an intact microvasculature than is delivery alone. Damaged endothelium, as seen after intestinal strangulation[30, 36] or prolonged vascular compromise and injury,[43] may allow some leakage of dye even if perfusion is not sufficient for effective elimination.

Unfortunately, a limiting feature of elimination analysis is that it requires documentation of skin fluorescence for as long as 2 to 6 hours after dye administration. Therefore, despite the excellent results that had been reported with assessment of elimination,[60] in subsequent clinical trials, only a single measure of dye delivery at 10 to 20 minutes after dye administration was documented.[33, 40, 41] To achieve a stronger fluorescent signal, the maximal dosage of dye was increased from 4 to 8 mg/kg. As noted earlier, this has achieved excellent results (see Table 7–5), but there are situations in which the DFI alone is not definitive and a color-independent measurement would be helpful.

A less time-consuming means of dynamic assessment can be achieved with analysis of fluorescein delivery. As noted by previous investigators, dye appearance time may prove to be valuable in this setting. Generally, the arm-to-calf circulation time is twice that for the arm-to-lip time, which averages approximately 17 seconds. In the context of arteriosclerosis, arm-to-calf times may be two to six times normal, and further prolongation may be noted in the circulation time to the foot and toes.[6, 18, 42, 61] Unfortunately, such measurements have not been practical at multiple sites. Visual assessment of dye appearance times entails bolus injection of a relatively large dose of dye. This increases the likelihood of patient reaction to dye administration (see "Fluorescein Safety") and compromises repeated assessments. In addition, measurement of appearance times at multiple sites has been difficult with Lange's original ("bulky") fluorometer or Lund's tripod-based camera. Alternatively, the flexible light guide used for fiberoptic fluorometry has permitted rapid scanning of multiple sites. This has been used to document perfusion of flap regions[29] and to delineate vascular territories in conjoined twins (in whom there was a relative delay in dye delivery to the twin remote from the site of injection).[62]

The kinetics of dye delivery may be monitored in far less time than is required for dye elimination. Retrospective analysis of data previously obtained after intravenous fluorescein injection[29] indicates that the time to peak fluorescence can accurately distinguish between well-perfused and poorly perfused regions of rat pedicle flaps. Although the fluorescence of reference areas and viable flap sections peaked in 16.0 ± 4.5 minutes and 34.2 ± 13 minutes, respectively, that of dying sections failed to peak during the 200-minute study period. Such serial monitoring of fluorescence at close time intervals after a single injection of dye is practical for the small animal skin flaps and at a limited number of sites in the clinical setting;[63] however, the brief period of uptake after rapid intravenous administration does not allow the analysis of uptake kinetics at the multiple sites evaluated in arteriosclerotic limbs.

This limitation may be overcome by slower administration of dye. Oral ingestion and slow continuous intravenous infusion each provide the time interval required for efficient accumulation of data to monitor uptake kinetics. Laboratory studies have confirmed the reliability of fluorometry after these routes of administration.[35, 64] The time to peak fluorescence after oral administration of dye clearly delineated gradations in pedicle flap perfusion (Fig. 7–5), and it remained consistent at sites of varied pigmentation on multicolored dogs[35] and in a dark-skinned member of the author's research group who drank the fluorescein preparation (Fig. 7–6).

To obviate the need for serial assessments of dye uptake or elimination, investigations have been undertaken to determine whether a single determination after dye injection could be analyzed in a way that minimizes distortion by skin pigmentation.[35] It appears that melanin has a similar effect on background and postdye values. Thus, by noting the relative background readings of light and dark regions, one can approximate the relative effects of pigmentation on postdye values. The ratio of the preinjection background value of the light site to that of the dark site provides a normalization factor by which to multiply the postdye value of the darker site. Normalized postdye values of darker canine skin were within 10% of the values of lighter sites. Likewise, after dye administration, the mean proportional increase in fluorescence at darker sites also was within 10% of that for lighter sites.[35] Retrospective application

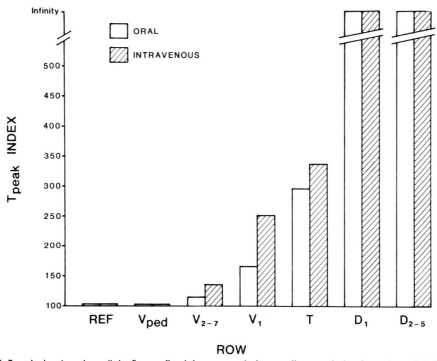

FIGURE 7–5. T_{peak} Index in rat pedicle flaps after intravenous (retrospective analysis of previous data[29]) and oral[64] administration of dye. As the distance from the pedicle increases, the relative time it takes for the dye to get there increases. This is indicated by a relative increase in the time to peak fluorescence (T_{peak}) of more distal sites, as expressed by the T_{peak} Index = [(T_{peak} of study site)/T_{peak} of reference area) × (100)]. After administration by either route, there is a significant difference between the values in the last viable row (V_1) and those in the first critically ischemic row (termed D_1 because it is the first row destined to become dystrophic).

FIGURE 7–6. Graph of dye fluorescence (DF) vs time in two regions of a healthy dark-skinned volunteer after oral ingestion of fluorescein. The outer forearm was much darker (background value of 40, compared with a value of 85 at the inner forearm—after the fluorometer was appropriately zeroed[35]) and therefore transmitted less fluorescence. However, the difference in skin color did not significantly affect the kinetics of dye delivery. This was evidenced by a T_{peak} of 53.5 ± 2.6 and 57.5 ± 3.8 minutes at dark and light arm sites, respectively, and 53.8 ± 10.5 minutes overall. Likewise, the values for the slope of the uptake phase were 4.77 ± 0.02 and 4.65 ± 0.41 per hour for the respective arm sites and was 4.46 ± 0.45 per hour for the 60 study sites overall.

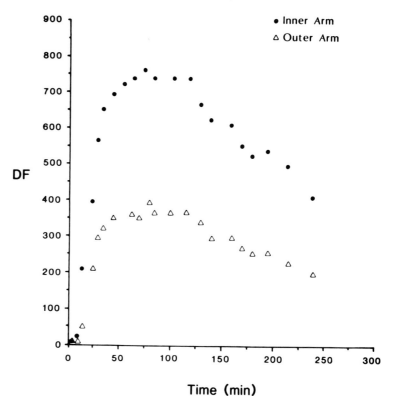

of this means of analysis to the data in Figure 7–6 provides a normalization factor of 2.1 (85/40, after appropriate zeroing of the machine[35]). The uncorrected DFI of the dark site compared with that of the light site at 50 minutes after dye ingestion would have been approximately 50% (350/700 × 100). The normalized DFI would be 105% (50% × 2.1), indicating comparable perfusion. Likewise, the proportional increases at both sites were similar (350/40 vs 700/85). The realization that such "simple" means of analysis can permit accurate determination of fluorescein delivery after low doses of dye—regardless of skin pigmentation—should significantly improve assessment of skin perfusion in the patient with an ischemic limb.

FLUORESCEIN SAFETY

A study of 200 dye administrations (4 to 8 mg/kg injected over 2 to 3 minutes) for fluorometry in awake subjects suggests that the test is safe.[33] There were no major reactions noted and no significant changes in vital signs. Four subjects experienced nausea upon infusion; two of them evidenced mild urticaria and pruritus, which responded promptly to diphenhydramine (Benadryl). The remaining 196 injections (98%) were associated with no adverse effects. In an additional 30 subjects undergoing fluorometry for intraoperative flap assessment during reconstructive head and neck surgery, there were no adverse effects.[3] Because of the relatively low doses of dye used for fluorometry, there was no skin discoloration, dysuria, or photophobia; however, the urine and occasionally the sclera were stained for up to 24 hours after injection. These findings were similar to those noted by Lange and Boyd in over 1000 patients who received 100 to 200 mg rapidly and then the remainder of a dose of 6.5 mg/kg slowly over 90 seconds.[6] Eleven of their patients vomited but evidenced no other untoward reactions.

Despite the apparent safety of this technique, the author still limits injection for fluorometry to settings in which trained personnel and resuscitative supplies are available. A review of the literature indicates that the incidence of minor effects from dye injection generally is higher than the aforementioned experience and that there is a risk, albeit rare, of cardiovascular and respiratory dysfunction. After rapid bolus injection of dye for retinal angiography, minor reactions (nausea, vomiting, pruritus, and urticaria) have been reported in 5 to 25% of patients.[65–67] More significant systemic reactions have also been noted.[68–72] In contrast to the stable blood pressure reported with low-dose fluorescein for fluorometry,[3, 33] Buchanan and Levine[68] reported a 20 mmHg or more decrease in systolic blood pressure in 32% of patients receiving rapid injection of the higher dose traditionally used for intraoperative visual inspection. Occasionally, severe angioedema, respiratory obstruction, hypotension, and cardiovascular collapse have been noted.[69–71] A recent international survey of 260 ophthalmologic clinics noted the incidence of "serious accidents" to be 1 in 18,020 and that of fatalities to be 1 in 49,557.[72]

In most cases, side effects suggest a non–hapten-mediated (anaphylactoid, not anaphylactic) release of histamine in sensitive individuals, as may be the case for radiopaque dyes and certain anesthetic agents.[73–75] After fluorescein injection, there is a positive correlation between the rise in plasma histamine concentration and the onset of nausea and urticaria.[65, 66] Such an anaphylactoid response is amenable to antihistamine prophylaxis and therapy. It appears to be dose related; thus, a low dose of dye is preferable. Traditionally, doses of 10 to 20 and 20 to 40 mg/kg have been used in light-skinned and dark-skinned subjects, respectively. The fluorometer's matched interference filters and highly sensitive photomultiplier tube provide clear discrimination after only 2 to 8 mg/kg. This certainly has contributed to the lesser incidence of nausea, vomiting, urticaria, and pruritus with fluorometry and to the reported absence of blood pressure changes or other major systemic effects.[33] Interestingly, in Buchanan and Levine's subjects in whom high-dose fluorescein elicited a significant decline in blood pressure, administration of a lower dose on a subsequent occasion resulted in a much less pronounced effect.[68]

Slow infusion or oral administration of dye should further minimize peak plasma levels and associated histamine release while permitting adequate tissue staining. The author's initial trial with bolus injection of a low dose (4 to 8 mg/kg) elicited nausea in three of 40 patients (7.5%). Administration of this dose over a 2- to 3-minute interval is associated with only a 2% incidence.[33] Slow continuous

Table 7–7. PROPOSED CLINICAL PROTOCOL WITH CONTINUOUS INTRAVENOUS INFUSION OF DYE*

Preparation & Preadministration: Calibrate and zero fluorometer. Demarcate study and reference (ref) sites. Obtain background (bckgd) values.

Dye Administration: Begin continuous infusion of fluorescein 0.25 mg/kg/min. Monitor reference areas to determine when dye fluorescence (DF) has increased to 2–3 times bckgd value (15–20 minutes).

Postinfusion:

A) If T_{peak} is to be monitored, obtain set of DF readings upon discontinuing the infusion and at 5-minute intervals until desired patterns are evident.

B) For static assessment of delivery, obtain set of readings at approximately 5 minutes after infusion, and determine dye fluorescence index (DFI), Normalized DFI (if varied pigmentation), or Proportional Increase (PI) at each site.

DFI = (DF of study site/DF of ref) × 100

Normalized DFI =
(DFI) × (Bckgd of lighter site/Bckgd of darker site)

PI =
(DF of study site/Bckgd of study site)

(When the PI of the study site is expressed as a percentage of the PI of the reference site, the comparative PI is equivalent to the normalized DFI, since they take the same factors into account.)

C) Monitor at later time intervals if dye leakage across damaged endothelium is suspected.[35]

*This protocol can be adapted to monitor fluorescein delivery or elimination after oral dye administration.

infusion (0.25 mg/kg/min for 20 minutes) further tapers the rise in plasma levels and offers the added advantage of permitting cessation of dye delivery at any time. Oral administration, generally considered the most convenient, safe, and economical route of drug administration,[76] with the least frequent and mildest allergic reactions,[77] also may provide a practical alternative. Reports have noted that oral administration of fluorescein for ophthalmologic studies has been well tolerated and is safe.[78–82] However, except for the requisite needle injection, continuous intravenous infusion may prove to be better suited for fluorescein delivery, as it permits titration of dye administration and cessation of dye delivery at any time.

SUMMARY

It is evident that a measure of skin perfusion is essential for optimal management of the potential amputee. Fluorescein fills this role. Using visual assessment of staining and, more recently, fluorescent photography and fluorometric quantification of dye delivery, several investigators have recommended application of fluorescence assessment to the ischemic limb. Sensitive means of quantifying fluorescence have improved the precision of the test and have enabled such critical issues as patient safety and the influence of skin pigmentation to be addressed. It is now possible to control for differing skin pigmentation and monitor uptake kinetics after continuous intravenous infusion or oral ingestion of dye (Table 7–7).

In conclusion, it is somewhat humbling to note the conclusions of Lange and Boyd in 1944[6] on the potential value of the fluorescein test.

In general, the test seems to have distinct advantages over methods formerly employed, since it gives a direct insight into nutrition of the tissues in peripheral vascular diseases. It is necessary, however, for a complete survey of the functional capacity of the vessels of the limb to perform the usual tests, such as determinations of cutaneous temperature and oscillometric studies, in order to obtain as complete a picture as possible.*

*From Lange K, Boyd LJ: Use of fluorescein method in establishment of diagnosis and prognosis of peripheral vascular diseases. Arch Int Med 74:175, 1944. Copyright 1944, American Medical Association.

REFERENCES

1. Myers MB, Brock D, Cohn I: Prevention of skin sloughs after radical mastectomy by the use of a vital dye to delineate devascularized skin. Ann Surg 173:920, 1971.
2. McCraw JB, Myers B, Shanklin KD: The value of fluorescein in predicting the viability of arterialized flaps. Plast Reconstr Surg 60:710, 1977.
3. Weisman RA, Pransky S, Silverman DG, et al: Clinical evaluation of flap perfusion by fiberoptic fluorometry. Ann Otol Rhinol Laryngol 94:226, 1985.
4. Prather A, Blackburn JP, Williams TR, Lynn JA: Evaluation of tests for predicting the viability of axial pattern skin flaps in the pig. Plast Reconstr Surg 63:250, 1979.
5. Reinisch JF: The pathophysiology of skin flap circulation—the delay phenomenon. Plast Reconstr Surg 54:585, 1974.
6. Lange K, Boyd LJ: Use of fluorescein method in establishment of diagnosis and prognosis of peripheral vascular diseases. Arch Int Med 74:175, 1944.
7. Sloan GM, Sasaki GH: Noninvasive monitoring of tissue viability. Clin Plast Surg 12:185, 1985.
8. Tanzer TL, Horne JG: The assessment of skin

viability using fluorescein angiography prior to amputation. J Bone Joint Surg 64:880, 1982.

9. McFarland DC, Lawrence PF: Skin fluorescence, a method to predict amputation site healing. J Surg Res 32:410, 1982.

10. Buckley GB, Zuidema GD, Hamilton SR, et al: Intraoperative determination of small intestinal viability following ischemic injury. Ann Surg 193:628, 1981.

11. DeLori F, Ben-Sira I, Trempe C: Fluorescein angiography with an optimized filler combination. Am J Ophthalmol 82:559, 1976.

12. Valencia S, Schmekl RH, Wacholty WF, Myers B: Absorption and emission spectra of fluorescein in man. Plast Reconstr Surg 79:667, 1987.

13. Welch J: The photography of fluorescein. Plast Reconstr Surg 69:990, 1982.

14. Myers B, Donovan W: An evaluation of eight methods of using fluorescein to predict the viability of skin flaps in the pig. Plast Reconstr Surg 75:245, 1985.

15. Myers B: Personal communications with respect to different filter combinations, 1983–1984.

16. Myers B, Guber M, Donovan W: The fluorescence camera—how to use fluorescein dye in a normally illuminated room—even in black patients. Ann Plast Surg 10:248, 1983.

17. Myers B: How to photograph fluorescein in a normally illuminated room. Plast Reconstr Surg 67:809, 1981.

18. Lowry K, Kirkpatrick JF, Thoroughman JC: Evaluation of peripheral vascular disease using intraarterial fluorescein. Am Surg 30:35, 1964.

19. Neller JL, Schmidt ER: Wheal-fluorescence. A new method of evaluating peripheral vascular diseases. Ann Surg 121:328, 1945.

20. Asokan R, Caffee HH: The fluorescein test in darkskinned patients. Plast Reconstr Surg 66:766, 1980.

21. Malone JM, Moore WS, Gladstone J, Malone SJ: Therapeutic and economic impact of a modern amputation program. Ann Surg 189:798, 1978.

22. Bollinger A: Function of the precapillary vessels in peripheral vascular disease. J Cardiovasc Pharmacol 3:S147, 1985.

23. Lund F: Fluorescein angiography of the skin in diagnosis, prognosis and evaluation of therapy in peripheral arterial disease. Bibl Anat 16:257, 1976.

24. Lund F: Can a clinical effect of pyridinocarbamate be objectively assessed in advanced peripheral atherosclerosis? *In* Carlson LA, Paoletti R, Sirtori CR, Weber G (eds): International Conference on Atherosclerosis. New York, Raven Press, 1978, pp 679–687.

25. Lawrence PF, McFarland DC, Seeger JM, Lowry SF: Evaluation of extremity ischemia by skin fluorescence. Surg Forum 31:349, 1980.

26. Lange K, Krewer SE: The dermofluorometer. J Lab Clin Med 28:1746, 1943.

27. Lange K: Personal communication, 1980.

28. Silverman DG, LaRossa DD, Barlow CH, et al: Quantification of tissue fluorescein delivery and prediction of flap viability with the fiberoptic dermofluorometer. Plast Reconstr Surg 66:545, 1980.

29. Silverman DG, Norton KJ, Brousseau DA: Serial fluorometric documentation of fluorescein dye delivery. Surgery 97:185, 1985.

30. Silverman DG, Hurford WE, Cooper H, et al: Quantification of fluorescein distribution to strangulated rat ileum. J Surg Res 34:179, 1983.

31. Graham BH, Walton RL, Elings VB, Lewis FR: Surface quantification of injected fluorescein as a prediction of flap viability. Plast Reconstr Surg 71:826, 1983.

32. Klein SG, Hansell JR, Brousseau DA, Silverman DG: Fluorescein and microsphere distribution to ischemic skin and bowel. Surg Forum 36:542, 1985.

33. Silverman DG, Roberts A, Reilly CA, et al: Fluorometric quantification of low-dose fluorescein delivery to predict amputation healing. Surgery 101:335, 1987.

34. Brousseau DA, Klein SK, Weinstock BS, Silverman DG: Fluorometric assessment of perfusion in multicolored skin. Surg Forum 34:641, 1983.

35. Silverman DG, Ostrander L, Lee BY, et al: Monitoring delivery of fluorescein dye independent of skin pigmentation. Submitted.

36. Carter MS, Fantini GA, Sammartano RJ, et al: Qualitative and quantitative fluorescein fluorescence for determining intestinal viability. Am J Surg 147:117, 1984.

37. Chasse WR, Min YG, Silverman DG, Brousseau DA: Assessment of pedicle flap viability by fluorometry and laser Doppler. Surg Forum 34:579, 1983.

38. Cummings CW, Trachy RE, Richardson MA, Patterson HC: Prognostication of myocutaneous flap viability using laser Doppler flowmetry and fluorescein microfluorometry. Otolaryngol Head Neck Surg 92:559, 1984.

39. Silverman DG, Weinstock BS, Brousseau DA, et al: Comparative assessment of blood flow to canine island flaps. Arch Otolaryngol 111:677, 1985.

40. Silverman DG, Rubin SM, Reilly CA, et al: Fluorometric prediction of successful amputation level in the ischemic extremity. J Rehabil Res Dev 22:29, 1985.

41. Roberts AB, Reilly CA, Bakshi KR, et al: Fiberoptic fluorometry as a useful adjunct in determining lower extremity amputation level. Submitted.

42. Perbeck L, Sevastik B, Sonnenfeld T: The transcapillary exchange of sodium fluorescein in ischaemic limbs measured by fluorescein flowmetry. Clin Physiol 7:95, 1987.

43. Douglas B, Weinberg H, Song Y, Silverman DG: Improved flap tolerance to warm ischemia after ibuprofen. Plast Reconstr Surg 79:366, 1987.

44. Gatti J, LaRossa D, Brousseau DA, Silverman DG: Assessment of neovascularization and timing of flap division. Plast Reconstr Surg 73:396, 1984.

45. Semashko D, Song Y, Silverman DG, Weinberg H: Ischemic induction of neovascularization: A study by fluorometric analysis. Microsurgery 6:244, 1985.

46. Brousseau DA, Klein SG, Norton KJ, Silverman DG: Monitoring flap neovascularization by fiberoptic fluorometry. Surg Forum 38:561, 1987.

47. Norton KJ, Brousseau DA, Silverman DG: Documentation of delay in bilateral thoracoabdominal flaps. Arch Otolaryngol 110:660, 1984.

48. Silverman DG, Brousseau DA, Engelman K: Fluorometric documentation of increased cutaneous blood flow after topical application of a PGE_2 analog in man. Prostaglandins 33:627, 1987.

49. Brousseau DA, Clark NL, Rubin SM, et al: Tolerance to warm ischemia after topical nitroglycerin and a PGE_2 analog. Surg Forum 36:591, 1985.

50. Norton KJ, Brousseau DA, Silverman DG: Improved flap survival with a new topical vasodilator. Surg Forum 35:585, 1984.

51. Silverman DG, Brousseau DA, Norton KJ, et al:

The effects of a topical PGE$_2$ analog on global flap ischemia. Submitted.

52. Gatti JE, Silverman DG, Brousseau DA, LaRossa D: Intravenous nitroglycerin as a means of improving ischemic tissue hemodynamics and survival. Ann Plast Surg 16:521, 1986.

53. Vidas MC, Weisman RA, Silverman DG: Serial fluorometric assessment of experimental neurovascular island flaps. Arch Otolaryngol 109:457, 1983.

54. Denneny J, Weisman RA, Silverman DG: Monitoring of free flap perfusion by serial fluorometry. Otolaryngol Head Neck Surg 91:372, 1983.

55. Weinberg H, Song Y, Silverman DG, et al: Vascular island flap tolerance to warm ischemia: An analysis by perfusion fluorometry. Plast Reconstr Surg 73:949, 1984.

56. Graham BH, Gordon L, Alpert BS, et al: Serial quantitative skin surface fluorescence: A new method for postoperative monitoring of vascular perfusion in revascularized digits. J Hand Surg 10:226, 1985.

57. Bongard FS, Upton RA, Elings VB, Lewis FR: Digital cutaneous fluorometry: Correlation between blood flow and fluorescence. J Vasc Surg 1:635, 1984.

58. Silverman DG, Cedrone FA, Hurford WE, et al: Monitoring tissue elimination of fluorescein with the perfusion fluorometer: A new method to assess capillary blood flow. Surgery 90:409, 1981.

59. Silverman DG, Denneny J, Brousseau DA, Weisman RA: Continuous monitoring of flap perfusion by fiberoptic fluorometry. Surg Forum 33:559, 1982.

60. Hurford WE, Silverman DG: Evaluation of ischemic extremities by quantitative fluorescence assessment. Surg Forum 33:442, 1982.

61. Lange K, Boyd LJ: The use of fluorescein to determine the adequacy of the circulation. Med Clin North Am 26:943, 1942.

62. Ross AJ III, O'Neill JA Jr, Silverman DG, et al: A new technique for evaluating cutaneous vascularity in complicated conjoined twins. J Pediatr Surg 20:743, 1985.

63. Gatti JE, LaRossa D, Silverman DG, Hartford CE: Evaluation of the burn wound by perfusion fluorometry. J Trauma 23:202, 1983.

64. Silverman DG, Kim DJ, Brousseau DA, et al: Fluorometric assessment of skin perfusion after oral fluorescein. Surgery 103:221, 1988.

65. Arroyave CM, Wolbers R, Ellis PP: Plasma complement and histamine changes after intravenous administration of sodium fluorescein. Am J Ophthalmol 87:474, 1979.

66. Ellis PP, Schoenberger M, Rendi MA: Antihista-

mines as prophylaxis against side reactions to intravenous fluorescein. Trans Am Ophthalmol Soc 78:190, 1980.

67. Chazan BI, Balodimos MC, Konez L: Untoward effects of fluorescein angiography. Ann Ophthalmol 3:42, 1971.

68. Buchanan RT, Levine NS: Blood pressure drop as a result of fluorescein injection. Plast Reconstr Surg 70:363, 1982.

69. Stein MR, Parker CW: Reactions following intravenous fluorescein. Am J Ophthalmol 72:861, 1971.

70. Cunningham EE, Balu V: Cardiac arrest following fluorescein angiography. JAMA 242:2431, 1979.

71. LaPiana F, Penner R: Anaphylactoid reaction to intravenously administered fluorescein. Arch Ophthalmol 79:161, 1968.

72. Zografos L: International survey on the incidence of severe or fatal complications which may occur during fluorescein angiography. J Fr Ophtalmol 6:495, 1983.

73. Lorenze W, Doernicke A: Histamine release in clinical conditions. Mt Sinai J Med 45:357, 1978.

74. Lieberman P, Siegle RL, Taylor WW Jr: Anaphylactoid reactions to iodinated contrast material. J Allergy Clin Immunol 62:174, 1978.

75. Roscow CE, Moss J, Philbin DM, Savarese JJ: Histamine release during morphine and fentanyl anesthesia. Anesthesiology 56:93, 1982.

76. Mayer SE, Melmon KL, Gilman AG: The dynamics of drug absorption, distribution and elimination. *In* Gilman AG, Goodman LS, Gilman A (eds): The Pharmacological Basis of Therapeutics. New York, MacMillan, 1980, pp 1–27.

77. Orange RR, Donsky GJ: Anaphylaxis. *In* Middleton E Jr, Reed CE, Ellis EF (eds): Allergy Principles and Practice. St Louis, CV Mosby Co, 1978, pp 563–573.

78. Araie M, Sawa M, Nagataki S, Mishima S: Aqueous humor dynamics in man as studied by oral fluorescein. Jpn J Ophthalmol 24:346, 1980.

79. Sawa M, Sakanishi Y, Shimizu H: Fluorophotometric study of anterior segment barrier function after extracapsular cataract extraction and posterior chamber intraocular lens implantation. Am J Ophthalmol 97:197, 1984.

80. Palestine AG, Brubaker RF: Pharmacokinetics of fluorescein in the vitreous. Invest Ophthalmol Vis Sci 21:542, 1981.

81. Kelley JS, Kincaid M, Hoover RE, McBeth C: Retinal fluorograms using oral fluorescein. Ophthalmology 87:805, 1980.

82. Kelley JS, Kincaid M: Retinal fluorography using oral fluorescein. Arch Ophthalmol 97:2331, 1979.

8

Amputation Level Selection by Laser Doppler Flowmetry

G. Allen Holloway, Jr., M.D.

The general principles of amputation level selection have been addressed in a previous chapter. To assist in this level selection, a quantitative measurement is needed to tell the surgeon whether or not an amputation, or for that matter an ulcer, can be expected to heal. It would be a significant advantage if the time required for healing could also be determined.

A number of methods have been suggested for this purpose, several of which are addressed in this book. These range from the most basic, clinical judgment to various newer noninvasive methods. However, the basic need is for a method that will show whether there is an adequate environment for cells in the skin to survive and replicate, covering any defects in the skin surface. This method should assess all areas of skin that might be at risk. Additionally, it would be advantageous if this method could take into account changes that might occur with time as well as the effects that wound care or surgical technique might superimpose. Needless to say, such a method does not exist at present, and it is highly unlikely that there will ever be one that satisfies all of these needs. A biochemical sensor that assesses energy or substrate production in the affected area is a

more realistic goal but does not currently exist.

Laser Doppler flowmetry is a method that provides a continuous quantitative measurement of microcirculatory perfusion from a volume of approximately 1 mm^3 of skin or other exposed organ; as the bearer of nutrients to and waste products from the skin, capillary perfusion provides perhaps the closest assessment of intracellular biochemical activity as is possible at this time. The method is similar to that commonly used in radar or ultrasonography in that flow measurement is based on the Doppler frequency shift induced by moving objects; however, it uses laser light instead of the lower frequency wave energy of ultrasound and radar systems.

THEORETICAL PRINCIPLES

The Doppler principle was first described by Christian Doppler in 1842 and is best exemplified by the decrease in the pitch of a train whistle as it passes a railroad crossing. Sound that is emitted from a moving object is shifted in frequency in proportion to the velocity of the object. The sound waves are compressed as the object moves toward an observer, resulting in a higher frequency, whereas they are spread farther apart when an object moves away from an observer, thus producing a lower frequency. If the waves are emitted from the observer rather than from the object, the frequency is shifted both going to and coming from the object, and the shift in frequency is doubled. If this shift in frequency is known, the velocity of the object can be calculated.

The laser Doppler flowmeter uses light waves instead of sound waves.[1] Monochromatic, coherent laser light—usually from a helium-neon laser, owing to its lower cost—illuminates the skin, or other surface, being examined. Some of the light is backscattered from the nonmoving skin tissues and some absorbed. A lesser part is backscattered from moving red blood cells in the microcirculation and shifted in frequency in proportion to their relative velocity. The volume from which the scattered light is obtained, the sample volume, is about 1 mm³. The shifted and nonshifted backscattered light mix together on the surface of a photodetector, where they beat or heterodyne. The output from the photodetector is the difference between the two frequencies, the Doppler frequency. Because red blood cells are moving at many different angles and velocities, a spectrum of Doppler-shifted frequencies is

obtained. The first moment of the power spectrum of the Doppler-shifted frequencies, a single number that represents the spectrum, is derived through a mathematical algorithm. This number has been shown empirically to compare favorably and vary linearly with values obtained by other methods measuring skin blood flow.[2, 3]

INSTRUMENTATION

Several laser Doppler instruments are now available commercially. A 2 mW helium-neon laser has been the standard light source, but solid-state laser diodes are beginning to be used. The light is directed through optical connectors into small optical fibers that lead the light to and from the surface of the skin. The optical fibers usually terminate in a simple probe of which there may be several different interchangeable types. The return optical fiber is coupled to a photodiode, the electrical output from which enters the signal processor system where the power spectrum algorithm is applied. Output of the system is usually to a meter or strip chart recorder. These instruments are portable and, with advances in electronics, are becoming smaller all the time. Figure 8–1 is an example of such a system.

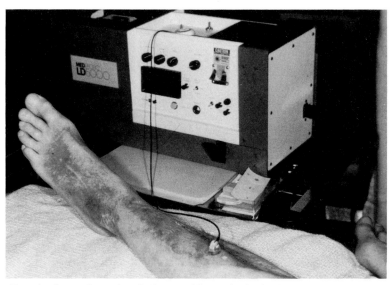

FIGURE 8–1. Laser Doppler flowmeter system being used to evaluate skin blood flow in the lower leg of a patient with ischemic vascular disease.

CALIBRATION

Because of the anatomic complexity of the microcirculation in the skin, in terms of both light scattering and red blood cell flow, it has not been possible to develop an analytical model against which to test these flowmetry systems. There is also no "gold standard," absolute or empirical, for measurement of microcirculatory flow or perfusion; thus, the laser Doppler system has been "calibrated" by comparing its values with those derived from other methods, such as radioisotope clearance or plethysmography. Initially, skin circulation was compared with xenon-133 clearance, showing a good correlation.[2, 3] Calibration has subsequently been done in other organ systems, including the kidney[4] and gastrointestinal tract,[5, 6] also with good correlation. The correlation is never exact, however, no matter what organ system is studied, as the other methods examine different sample volumes and physical parameters, e.g., isotope clearance in the xenon-133 method with a sample volume of roughly 1 cm^3 and volume change with plethysmography from a volume the size of the tissue contained in the plethysmograph.

METHODOLOGY AND TECHNIQUES IN SKIN

Although the laser Doppler system has been used in most organ systems in the body, the greater part of the studies have been performed in skin. Techniques in skin have included measurement of resting microcirculatory blood flow and flow after perturbation or stress. As the metabolic needs of skin are small, baseline resting flow to supply these needs is also low and may well be the same in patients with vascular disease as in normal adults. However, if a stimulus is applied, flow in the normal adults will increase, whereas in patients with occlusive vascular disease, flow will tend not to increase or may even fall in response. Several different stimuli to increase flow have been used. Transient vascular occlusion with a blood pressure cuff at the ankle or knee has been tried, and the degree and duration of the subsequent hyperemic response, examined. Some investigators have looked at the response to local heating. This has typically involved making a baseline measurement, heating the skin to 44° C for 10 minutes with a transcutaneous PO_2 heater probe or similar system, and repeating the laser Doppler measurement.

Yet another measurement has been that of skin occlusion pressure, in which a blood pressure cuff is inflated to suprasystolic levels and blood flow monitored over the desired skin area. The cuff is then gradually deflated until the return of flow is seen with the laser Doppler. The pressure at which flow first returns has been called the skin perfusion pressure.

REVIEW OF EXPERIENCE IN AMPUTATION LEVEL SELECTION

The use of laser Doppler flowmetry in ischemic and diabetic limbs has occurred only recently. The author first published results in 1983[7] and has been followed by others. This initial experience was with 16 patients, eight diabetic and eight nondiabetic, undergoing 20 amputations. The protocol involved examining perfusion at the dorsum of the foot and below and above the knee both under resting conditions and after heating for 10 minutes at 44° C. All 14 of the below- and above-knee amputations (BKAs and AKAs) healed primarily, whereas reamputation was required in the ray, transmetatarsal, and two Syme's amputations. Resting flow was about the same as in normals in both nonhealing foot and healing below- and above-knee amputations. However, the healing amputations showed a significant rise in flow with heating, although less than in the normals, whereas in the nonhealing amputations, flow increased minimally and to a level less than one third of that seen in normals.

Pabst and Castronuovo[8] examined eight normal controls, ten moderately ischemic patients with claudication, and ten very ischemic patients with rest pain, ulcers, or gangrene. Resting skin blood flow, reactive hyperemia after 2 minutes of occlusion, and skin perfusion pressure were measured. The latter was obtained by placing a blood pressure cuff over the laser Doppler probe, inflating the cuff to a suprasystolic pressure, and gradually deflating it until flow signals were first recorded. Reactive hyperemia was indicated by the percentage increase from resting to maximal flow after occlusion. Measurements were taken on the ventral great toe, in the dorsal metatarsal area, and lateral to the tibia, 10 cm below the inferior patellar margin. Resting blood flow was significantly less in the toes, but not at the other levels, in patients as compared with normals. Skin perfusion pressure showed a significant difference between normals, moderately ischemic, and very ischemic patients at both the transmetatarsal and toe levels but not below the knee. However, reactive hyperemia revealed significant differences between all of the groups at all three levels. The investigators concluded that the laser Doppler technique using reactive hyperemia and skin perfusion pressure showed good potential as an adjunct in the prediction of healing, particularly in the more distal areas that provide the greatest challenge at present.

Karanfilian and associates[9] looked at 20 limbs in ten normal subjects and contrasted them with 12 limbs in nine patients with severe peripheral vascular disease (PVD): the study examined baseline skin blood flow and reactive hyperemia after 3 minutes of thigh occlusion. Baseline flow was found to be significantly greater in normals in the great toe, as was the pulse wave amplitude at the same location. The differences were more clearly seen after reactive hyperemia, in which the peak blood flow decreased and the time to peak flow significantly increased in the PVD patients. In a subsequent paper,[10] they compared both laser Doppler flowmetry and transcutaneous PO_2 (PTC_{O_2}) in the distal foot of 59 limbs in 48 patients with advanced PVD. Diabetes was present in 63%, and there were 20 transmetatarsal or digital amputations. Baseline skin blood flow, pulse wave amplitude, and ankle/brachial pressure indices were measured. They defined criteria for successful healing of these distal amputations as including a PTC_{O_2} of more than 10 mmHg, laser Doppler skin blood flow of more than 40 mV, and an ankle systolic pressure of more than 30 mmHg. With these criteria, the outcome was correctly predicted in 95% of amputations on the basis of the PTC_{O_2} alone, in 87% on the basis of the laser Doppler alone, but in only 52% if the sole criterion was ankle pressure. These represent the combined results in both diabetic and nondiabetic patients, with healing in diabetics being only 46% as compared with 68% in nondiabetics.

Fairs and colleagues[11] examined a series of 14 patients requiring BKA or AKA for vascular disease and a control group with no evidence of ischemia. PTC_{O_2} and laser Doppler measurements were obtained at 13 cm below the knee joint when the patient was in the rest state and after 5 minutes of heating at 43° C. In each case, there were significant differences between the normals and the vascular patients with both the PTC_{O_2} and heated laser Doppler measurements, and the PTC_{O_2} and laser Doppler flowmetry methods correlated quite well.

A brief preliminary laser Doppler study was reported by Kvernebo and coworkers;[12, 13] they showed that in patients with claudication who demonstrate a fall in resting segmental blood pressure from the distal thigh to the ankle, occlusion of the thigh just proximal to the patella results in a prolonged time to peak hyperemia after release. They thought that this might be a useful noninvasive parameter of vascular resistance in the leg and foot and could be used to assess vascular insufficiency.

Moneta and associates[14] looked at a related area, the relation of cutaneous vasomotion to the success or failure of angioplasty for limb salvage. Twenty-five patients were studied, with 15 successes and ten failures. Vasomotion was detected as regular cyclic variations in the laser Doppler output signal. In the successes, perfusion increased significantly, whereas it fell in the failures. Vasomotion was present in seven of eight patients with predilation ankle pressures of more than 80 mmHg but in only one of 11 with pressures less than 80 mmHg. Vasomotion appeared in all of six patients whose pressures after balloon angioplasty increased to more than 80 mmHg and disappeared in the two whose pressures fell to less than 80 mmHg.

In a somewhat different yet related area, Rayman and colleagues[15] used laser Doppler flowmetry to investigate the reflex changes in capillary perfusion in diabetics, both with and without neuropathy, as compared with normals. When the limb was placed in a dependent position, flow fell far less in subjects with neuropathy than in normals, which was thought to be compatible with a loss of sympathetic control. This may help to shed light on the problems with healing and amputation level selection in this group of patients.

The results of these studies indicate that laser Doppler flowmetry is beginning to be used at a number of institutions in the quantitative evaluation of amputation levels. On the basis of the ongoing work of investigators at other institutions, it appears that laser Doppler flowmetry is able to provide similar information on level selection and healing success as PTC_{O_2} below and above the knee. This is in the range of a 90 to 95% prediction of healing success, a level that will be hard to improve much further, as the intangibles, such as the effects of anesthesia, surgical technique, and postoperative management, do not enter into the measurement. There is opinion and initial evidence that the laser Doppler measurement may be of particular value in the foot in which PTC_{O_2} cannot be employed owing to irregular surfaces or is inaccurate because of inadequate diffusion through the thick epidermis on the sole of the foot. The laser Doppler method can be used on any of these surfaces, including the toes, as has been indicated in several of the references cited before, and there are anecdotal reports of a number of other instances in which it has proved of value. Awaited are further basic and clinical reports allowing for greater standardization of the method and additional cases that will permit determination of critical flow levels that are compatible with healing in the 90 to 95% range.

REFERENCES

1. Holloway GA Jr: Laser Doppler estimation of skin blood flow. *In* Rolfe P (ed): Noninvasive Physiological Measurements, Vol 2. London, Academic Press, 1983, pp 219–249.
2. Stern MD, Lappe DL, Bowen PF, et al: Continuous measurement of tissue blood flow by laser-Doppler spectroscopy. Am J Physiol 232:H441, 1977.
3. Holloway GA Jr: Cutaneous blood flow responses to injection trauma measured by laser Doppler velocimetry. J Invest Dermatol 74:1, 1980.
4. Stern MD, Bowen PD, Parma R, et al: Measurement of renal cortical and medullary blood flow by laser-Doppler spectroscopy in the rat. Am J Physiol 236:F80, 1979.
5. Feld AD, Fondacaro JD, Holloway GA Jr: Laser Doppler velocimetry: A new technique for the measurement of intestinal mucosal blood flow. Gastrointest Endosc 30:225, 1984.
6. Shepherd AP, Riedel GL: Mucosal blood flow in the intestine measured by laser Doppler anemometry. Fed Proc 41:1743, 1982.
7. Holloway GA Jr, Burgess EM: Preliminary experiences with laser Doppler velocimetry for the determination of amputation levels. Prosthet Orthot Int 7:63, 1983.
8. Pabst TS, Castronuovo JJ, Jackson SD, et al: Evaluation of the ischemic limb by pressure and flow measurements of the skin microcirculation as determined by laser Doppler velocimetry. Curr Surg 42:29, 1985.
9. Karanfilian RG, Lynch TG, Lee BC, et al: The assessment of skin blood flow in peripheral vascular disease by laser Doppler velocimetry. Am Surg 50:641, 1984.
10. Karanfilian RG, Lynch TG, Zirul VT, et al: The value of laser Doppler velocimetry and transcutaneous oxygen tension determination in predicting healing of ischemic forefoot ulcerations and amputations in diabetic and nondiabetic patients. J Vasc Surg 4:511, 1986.
11. Fairs SLE, Ham RO, Conway BA: Laser Doppler flowmetry in lower limb amputation level selection. Int J Microcirc Clin Exp 5:206, 1986.
12. Kvernebo K, Stranden E, Slagsvold CE: Reactive hyperemia in healthy controls and in patients with atherosclerosis evaluated with laser Doppler flowmetry. Int J Microcirc Clin Exp 3:450, 1984.
13. Kvernebo K, Bay K, Melby E: Laser Doppler flux reappearance time (FRT)—a parameter of peripheral resistance in the ischemic limb? Int J Microcirc Clin Exp 5:205, 1986.
14. Moneta G, Schneider E, Jager K, Bollinger A: Erythrocyte flux and the vasomotion of cutaneous arteriolar autoregulation in patients before and after transluminal angioplasty. Personal communication, 1986.
15. Rayman G, Hassan A, Tooke JE Jr: Blood flow in the skin of the foot related to posture in diabetes mellitus. Br Med J 292:87, 1986.

9

Amputation Level Selection by Skin Temperature Measurement

Frank L. Golbranson, M.D.

The functional superiority of below-knee over more proximal level amputations has initiated a trend toward more distal level amputations in patients with peripheral vascular disease. Although patients with more distal level amputations most often have shorter rehabilitation times and improved function, failures occur because of inadequate vascularity to support healing at the lower levels.[6] The determination of amputation levels in patients with ischemia or gangrene of the lower extremity secondary to peripheral vascular disease has been based on a number of clinical criteria, including skin nutrition, pulses, skin temperature by palpation, skin color, skin bleeding in surgery, angiography, and noninvasive techniques such as segmental blood pressure measurement.[1–3, 8] None of these techniques have been consistently reliable in predicting skin healing, however. Angiography and segmental blood pressure measurements have been criticized because they measure the status of larger arteries and arterioles and not that of the skin capillaries, which are impor-

tant in skin healing. Ideally, a method that directly or indirectly measures the skin blood flow at the selected level of amputation would provide a more reliable guide to selecting the most distal level compatible with healing.

In 1959, Peacock[4, 5] correlated cutaneous temperature and skin blood flow as measured by venous occlusion plethysmography and showed the effect of changes in local temperature on skin blood flow. Stirrat and associates[7] reported on the use of skin monitoring in following-up patients with replanted digits. They found skin temperature measurement a simple, noninvasive, and inexpensive technique for indirectly assessing changes in skin perfusion. In view of these correlations between skin temperature and skin blood flow, a prospective study exploring the role of skin temperature determination in predicting wound healing of peripheral vascular disease patients undergoing amputations distal to the knee joint was undertaken at the University of California, San Diego, Medical Center and the Veterans Administration Hospital, La Jolla.

MATERIALS AND METHODS

From January 1978 to September 1981, 30 amputations in 26 patients were performed for advanced end-stage lower extremity ischemia at the University of California, San Diego, Medical Center and the Veterans' Administration Hospital, La Jolla. There were 21 men and five women. Seventeen patients had diabetes mellitus. The indications for operation were gangrene in 21 patients, ischemia with infections in five, and ischemic pain in four. All patients had preoperative angiograms and blood viscosity and segmental pressure studies. Amputations were done at the toe level in three patients and at the transmetatarsal level in two; Syme's amputations were performed in five patients, and below-knee amputations, in 20. An immediate postoperative rigid dressing was used for all except the toe and transmetatarsal level amputations. Skin temperature studies were done on all patients in the following manner. Patients were studied in hospital rooms in which the temperature ranged from 22.7 to 28° C. Air movement was negligible. The patients were placed in a supine position, and the extremity to be examined was exposed for 15 minutes. Clothing consisted of hospital attire. Recordings were made using the Teletthermometer, USI series 400, model 46 PVC.* The patients lay on their beds with the involved extremity exposed to the hip region. A thermistor probe was used to record skin temperature over the anterior aspect of the lower extremity at 2-inch intervals starting at the toes and extending proximally to just above the patella. Readings were taken after the movement of the recording needle ceased. Ambient room temperatures were recorded at the time of examination.

RESULTS

Results were recorded as healed or failed. Failures, by definition, required revision or reamputation at a more proximal level. Of 30 amputations, 25 healed (83%), and five failed (16%). Of 14 residual limbs with skin temperatures above 32° C, 14 healed (100%).

*Yellow Springs Instrument Company, Yellow Springs, Ohio.

Of 14 residual limbs with skin temperatures between 30.5 and 32° C, 11 healed (78%), and three failed (22%). Two residual limbs had skin temperatures below 30.5° C, and both failed (100%).

The difference between ambient room temperature and skin temperature at the amputation level was determined for all patients. Patients with skin temperatures 5° C greater than the ambient temperature had primary wound healing, with one exception (Table 9–1). Patient MC had a 4.8° C difference but had healing of his below-knee amputation in 3½ weeks. Patients with less than a 5° C difference between the amputation level and the ambient temperature had failed amputations, with one exception (Table 9–1). Patient MA had a 5.1° C temperature difference but failed to heal his transmetatarsal amputation.

The mean difference between the ambient and skin temperatures for residual limbs with primary wound healing was 7.0° C. The mean difference in temperature for the failed residual limbs was 3.9° C. The difference in skin temperature for the two groups was statistically significant (p<0.001).

Lower extremity amputations for ischemic disease are performed in an attempt to preserve the maximum extremity length compatible with skin healing. The use of multiple diagnostic methods to determine the amputation level compatible with healing suggests the difficulty in predicting accurately the healing rate of selected amputation levels in ischemic disease.

The evaluation of extremity skin temperature by palpation, although useful, does not offer the accuracy needed to select specific amputation levels. The author is not aware of any published report using a skin temperature recording as a criterion for amputation level determination.

Between 1978 and 1981, the study demonstrated a direct correlation between skin temperature and skin healing. In 26 patients who had below-knee amputations for ischemic disease, all amputation levels with skin temperature readings above 32° C healed. All amputation levels with skin temperature readings below 30.5° C failed to heal. Amputation levels with skin temperatures between 30.5 and 32° C were associated with some healed wounds and some failures. If the difference between the skin temperature and the room temperature was less than

Table 9–1. AMPUTATION HEALING PREDICTED BY SKIN TEMPERATURE

Patient	Diagnosis	Skin Temperature (° C)	Room Temperature (° C)	Healing	Time of Healing (weeks)	Amputating Procedure
1 NW	Ischemia, infection	31.0	26.0	Healed	2	BKA
2 MC	Gangrene	30.8	24.2	Healed	2	BKA
3 CW	Ischemia, infection	31.6	26.0	Healed	2	BKA
4 WR	Ischemia, infection	33.0	25.0	Healed	3	5th ray resection
5 ME	Gangrene	32.2	27.4	Healed	3½	BKA
6 NE	Gangrene	31.3	23.4	Healed	3	Syme's
7 RC	Gangrene	33.6	26.0	Healed	2	TMA
8 AC	Gangrene	31.3	25.2	Healed	4	5th toe resection
9 MA	Gangrene	30.1	25.0	Failed		TMA
		31.5	23.0	Healed	4	Syme's
10 GC	Ischemic pain	30.8	26.0	Failed		Syme's
		33.2	26.0	Healed	2	BKA
11 SR	Ischemia, infection	31.8	25.2	Healed	2	BKA
12 SM	Gangrene	31.0	24.5	Healed	3	BKA
13 MR	Ischemia, infection	34.5	26.3	Healed	4	5th ray resection
14 LG	Ischemia, infection	33.4	27.3	Healed	3	BKA
15 JP	Gangrene	31.2	24.4	Healed	6	BKA
16 DO	Gangrene	32.2	26.0	Healed	2	BKA
17 KJ	Gangrene	31.2	25.0	Healed	3	BKA
18 RW	Gangrene	32.0	27.5	Failed		Syme's
		32.5	27.5	Healed	4	BKA
19 LP	Ischemic pain	37.8	28.0	Healed	2	BKA
20 IH	Gangrene	32.9	25.8	Healed	3	BKA
21 GF	Gangrene	34.6	28.0	Healed	2	BKA
22 NE	Gangrene	33.0	25.4	Healed	2	BKA
23 MC	Gangrene	32.8	23.4	Healed	2	BKA
24 CG	Gangrene	31.3	26.6	Failed		Syme's
		32.3	26.8	Healed	2	BKA
25 BM	Gangrene	31.5	22.7	Healed	3	BKA
26 LP	Gangrene	28.0	27.5	Failed		BKA

BKA = below-knee amputation, TMA = transmetatarsal amputation.

5° C, the amputation generally failed. Conversely, if the difference was greater than 5° C, the amputation healed. Although the number of patients studied was not large, the preliminary data suggest that the use of skin temperature measurements is a helpful indicator in the preoperative determination of amputation level in patients with peripheral vascular disease.

During the period January 1984 to December 1985, thermistor readings made on 21 patients were compared with transcutaneous oxygen pressure (PTC_{O_2}) readings, and the success or failure of the predictions of residual limb healing at a selected level were determined by the end results, a healed or nonhealed residual limb.

Patients' ages ranged from 41 to 83 years; 19 patients were diabetics; all patients were male. Amputations were done for infection in 12 and for ischemia in nine. Preoperative

vascular work-ups included segmental limb pressures, blood flow velocities, and PTC_{O_2} determinations. In addition, all patients had preoperative thermistor studies done by the intern or resident at the bedside.

After studying 486 patients in the vascular laboratory, the author's conclusion is that chances for primary or secondary healing are very poor if

1. PTC_{O_2} values at rest are 5 mmHg or less.
2. There is no increase in the PTC_{O_2} level at the end of a 10-minute exposure to 100% O_2.

DISCUSSION

PTC_{O_2} predicted healing accurately in 16 (76%) of 21 patients (Table 9–2). Of the five incorrect predictions, four predicted suc-

Table 9–2. AMPUTATION HEALING PREDICTED BY $P_{TC_{O_2}}$

Patient	Diagnosis	Skin Temperature (°C)	$P_{TC_{O_2}}$ (mmHg) Before O_2	After O_2	Time of Healing (weeks)	Amputating Procedure
1 CB	Ischemia	32	33	75	Failed	BKA
	Ischemia	32.4	6	31	4	AKA
2 JS	Infection	30.7	18	118	2	BKA
3 CR	Infection	32	1	106	6	Great toe amputation
4 CH	Ischemia, renal insufficiency	30.8	27	62	Failed	BKA
5 ES	Ischemia	33.3	47	114	2	BKA
6 EO	Infection	31.6	5	28	3	BKA
7 HH	Infection	32.5	9	42	7	2nd ray resection
8 JH	Infection	30.8	42	90	Failed	3rd ray resection
9 WC	Infection	29	15	44	Failed	5th ray resection
10 RH		32.5	62	113	2	AKA
11 RC	Ischemia	31.8	13	83	3	BKA
		30.5	39	62	3	BKA
12 BG	Infection	33.5	0	67.5	2	Syme's
13 BD	Infection	32.2	49	122	6	3rd ray resection
14 PR	Infection	32.4	5	27	7	5th ray resection
15 PC	Infection	31.8	31	53	5	TKA
16 CC	Ischemia	32	0	17	3	AKA
17 PR	Ischemia	32.1	0	0		AKA
18 ST	Ischemia	31.7	0	39	2	TKA
19 RY	Infection	30.7	40	154	2	BKA
20 DM	Ischemia	32.1	8	23	2	BKA
21 BL	Ischemia	31.7	12	41	3	BKA

BKA = below-knee amputation, AKA = above-knee amputation, TKA = transmetatarsal amputation.

cesses were failures, and one predicted failure was successful.

The thermistor technique predicted healing accurately in 18 (85%) of 21 patients. Of the three incorrect predictions, all of the predicted successes were failures.

The technique of using the thermistor has changed gradually as the author's philosophy has changed: readings should be taken at potential below-knee amputation sites over the *anterior* aspect of the leg for conventional anteroposterior flaps and *medially* and *laterally* if sagittal flaps are planned. At ankle level, measurements are taken over the anterior ankle joint and at the plantar aspect of the heel pad. *Anterior* readings in planned above-knee levels are considered adequate.

The "bottom line" determination of *skin bleeding* at surgery supercedes all other evaluations.

SUMMARY

Skin temperature determination with a thermistor is a useful procedure in the preoperative assessment of patients undergoing lower extremity amputation for peripheral vascular disease. The technique is simple, noninvasive, and can be done in a standard hospital room with the use of a relatively inexpensive thermistor apparatus.

REFERENCES

1. Baddelery RM, Fulford JC: The use of arteriography in conservative amputations for lesions of the feet in diabetes mellitus. Br J Surg 51:658, 1964.
2. Barnes RW, Shanik GD, Slaymaker EE: An index of healing in below-knee amputation: Leg blood pressure by Doppler ultrasound. Surgery 79:13, 1976.
3. Golbranson F, Yu E, Gelberman R: The use of skin temperature determinations in lower extremity amputation level selection. Foot Ankle 3:170, 1982.
4. Peacock JH: A comparative study of the digital cutaneous temperatures and hand blood flows in the normal hand, primary Raynaud's disease and primary acrocyanosis. Clin Sci 18:25, 1959.
5. Peacock JH: The effect of changes in local temperature on the blood flows of the normal hand, primary Raynaud's disease and primary acrocyanosis. Clin Sci 19:505, 1960.
6. Romano RL, Burgess EM: Level selection in lower extremity amputations. Clin Orthop 74:177, 1971.
7. Stirrat CR, Seaker AV, Urbaniak JR, Bright DS: Temperature monitoring in digital replantation. J Hand Surg 3:342, 1978.
8. Warren R, Kihn RB: A survey of lower extremity amputations for ischemia. Surgery 63:107, 1968.

10

Anesthesia Considerations for the Amputation Patient

Joseph A. Gallo, Jr., M.D.
Burnell R. Brown, Jr., M.D., Ph.D.

The three leading causes of lower extremity amputations are diabetes, arteriosclerosis, and trauma. In this chapter, these three clinical situations are discussed with particular reference to intraoperative medical management and institution of appropriate anesthetic drugs and techniques. Similar to other aspects of medicine, anesthesia selection can never be dogmatic. Rather, it depends on those elusive phenomena known as clinical judgment and experience. Anesthetic sequence is determined by the following concerns, in order of importance: (1) providing the greatest patient safety, (2) rendering the surgery as easy to perform as possible, and (3) honoring the patient's preference. Following are some considerations that modify anesthesia selection and perspectives on how to determine what is best for the patient.

THE INSULIN-DEPENDENT DIABETIC

The insulin-dependent diabetic (Type I diabetes) often presents to the surgeon with lower extremity gangrene or infection requiring amputation at various levels. There is incontrovertible evidence that surgical mortality in diabetic patients remains higher than in nondiabetic individuals.[51] The three leading causes of perioperative mortality in patients with this endocrinopathy, in order of frequency, are infection, complications of the accelerated atherosclerosis common to diabetics, and renal failure. Evidence is mounting that close control of glucose levels in insulin-dependent diabetics can ameliorate morbidity at least for long-term complications.[8] It must be emphasized that although it appears logical, lowering the perioperative complications of diabetes by ensuring ubiquitously normal glucose levels has not been definitely proved. Certainly short-term moderate hyperglycemia does not produce long-lasting problems for the diabetic. Nonetheless, good control improves platelet and white cell function and increases red cell survival. Since infection plays such a major role in increasing surgical morbidity and mortality, it would seem prudent, in view of such salutary short-term effects, to control blood sugar as much as possible. There is no question that ketoacidosis represents a risk in diabetics with uncontrolled glucose levels and can be avoided by proper and thoughtful preparation.

Preoperative Assessment

Care of the diabetic before anesthesia and surgery can be a critical factor in the final outcome of the surgical procedure.[43] The two major areas for preoperative assessment are the current metabolic status of the individual and the chronic effects of the endocrinopathy on other systems, primarily the cardiovascular, urinary, and nervous systems.

Control of infection is paramount in these individuals. Although total control of infection may not be possible before definitive surgery, appropriate antibiotics should be administered as well ahead of the contemplated operation as possible. Reduction of bacterial activity is a definite catalyst in gaining metabolic control. In addition to the treatment of obvious extremity infection, the possibility of a less obvious infection, such as in the urinary tract, should be investigated through appropriate urinalysis and other diagnostic procedures. The astute clinician should also remember that if the patient has renal function impairment, significant dosage modifications of certain antibiotics (synthetic penicillins, aminoglycosides, cephalosporins, tetracyclines) may be required.[32] The aminoglycosides can potentiate the effects of curariform drugs used during anesthesia.

Chronic complications of diabetes can lead to acute problems perioperatively. Thus, pathological factors should be assessed as much as time permits. The patient's general level of fitness can easily be evaluated by means of questions regarding exercise tolerance. Cardiovascular problems and problems associated with atherosclerosis should receive careful attention from the physician. In one study of 100 diabetic patients operated on for lower extremity disease, 63% had cardiac disease, 44% peripheral vascular disease, and 24% cerebrovascular problems.[1] The difficulties presented by atherosclerosis of the cardiovascular and cerebral systems are detailed later in this chapter, as they are pathophysiologically identical for clinical purposes to nondiabetic atherosclerotic problems. In addition to the history and physical examination, electrocardiograms, chest X-ray films,

and pulmonary function studies may be indicated to rule out or document the degree of myocardial ischemia, myocardial conduction abnormalities, and cardiorespiratory reserve. The presence of congestive heart failure, even if insidious, is a grave prognostic sign and should be aggressively treated before all but the most extreme emergency surgical procedures.[16] Many patients with cardiac problems take β-adrenergic receptor blockers. It must be remembered that these drugs interact with insulin to slow the recovery time from hypoglycemia. Severe bradycardia and an increase in diastolic pressure have been observed in patients taking beta-blockers who have episodes of hypoglycemia.[27] Thus, the margin for error in insulin dose is far less in diabetics taking concomitant beta-blockers. Potent inhalational anesthetics can further enhance the action of the beta-blockers on the mechanical performance of the myocardium.

Neurologic complications of diabetes can present real problems insofar as anesthetic management is concerned. Autonomic nervous system neuropathy can cause serious vasomotor instability. This is particularly manifest during anesthesia, as both potent general inhalation anesthetics and regional anesthetics further reduce activity of the sympathetic nervous system. Cardiac arrest has been reported secondary to this interaction.[33] Motor neuropathy also can be present and lead to problems. For example, evaluation of pharmacologically induced myoneural blockade may be difficult. The anesthesiologist must take care that the nerve stimulator, used to assess the degree of myoneural block, is placed on uninvolved muscle if possible.

Another concern that frequently arises is the unanswered question of exacerbation of peripheral neuropathy by use of regional anesthesia, e.g., spinal, epidural, or peripheral nerve block. For most circumstances, regional anesthesia may well be the anesthesia of choice in the diabetic. It prevents stress, produces marked improvement in peripheral blood flow owing to sympathetic nervous system blockade, and has the salient advantage that verbal contact can be maintained with the patient so that reports of symptoms (e.g., chest pain, shortness of breath, central nervous system changes due to hypoglycemia) can be directly reported to and observed by the anesthesiologist. This problem, exacerbation of peripheral neuropathy by regional anesthesia, is more theoretic than real. There has been no scientific study demonstrating a worsening of diabetic neuropathy by spinal anesthesia. Perhaps a logical case can be made for avoidance of epinephrine-containing local anesthetic solutions in the diabetic, although again this is more clinical folklore than a proven point. Large doses of epinephrine can potentiate glucose intolerance, and if the catecholamine is used to bathe nerves, neuropathic vascular insufficiency could theoretically result.

Another anesthesia problem that is a consequence of the autonomic neuropathy seen in some diabetics is gastric atony. Diabetics in these circumstances can be prone to slower gastrointestinal transit times. This will amplify the often lethal complications of gastric aspiration on induction of or emergence from general anesthesia. This potential problem is circumvented to a certain degree by use of regional anesthesia and should give weight to the use of this technique in lower extremity surgical procedures. Metoclopramide in intravenous doses of approximately 10 mg in adults can stimulate peristaltic activity and diminish the threat of aspiration if administered 45 to 60 minutes before induction of anesthesia. However, this does not totally solve the problem of aspiration hazard.

Renal disease has been mentioned in relation to prolongation of the antibiotics' effects. It must be remembered that the pharmacodynamics and pharmacokinetics of many therapeutic and anesthetic drugs and adjuvants can be significantly prolonged and amplified with diabetic nephropathy. Diminished renal function may produce extra concerns about fluid management and may thus necessitate more sophisticated monitoring techniques, such as pulmonary artery catheterization.

The Decompensated Diabetic

The decompensated diabetic is defined as one who is (1) hypoglycemic, (2) hyperglycemic with ketoacidosis, or (3) hyperglycemic with hyperosmolar coma. Obviously patients in these categories have special risks and must be zealously prepared for surgery. Hypoglycemia and hypoglycemic tendencies are generally easily treated with glucose, either as a single injection of 50% dextrose intravenously or as a 10% dextrose intravenous drip. Note should be made of whether a beta-blocker may be producing exaggerated hypoglycemic responses to insulin. Stress can delay the distribution of subcutaneously administered insulin, leading to late hypoglycemic effects. It is quite difficult to diagnose hypoglycemia by clinical signs when the patient is under general anesthesia. This is another of the salient reasons for the strong support given to the use of regional anesthesia techniques for lower extremity surgery in the diabetic. If general anesthesia is mandated, it is imperative to check blood glucose levels often intraoperatively and be alert for the rather protean features of hypoglycemia seen during this technique. Such features include otherwise unexplained changes in heart rate, blood pressure, and other autonomic activities (pupil size, sweating). However, there is nothing of specific diagnostic value during even severe degrees of hypoglycemia in the anesthetized state.

Patients with hyperglycemia and ketoacidosis often require urgent or emergency surgery.[29] Ketoacidosis is almost universally accompanied by fluid and electrolyte losses that must be replaced before surgery. Treatment should be aggressive and include administration of sufficient volumes of saline-containing solutions and employment of large-dose intravenous insulin or continuous low-dose insulin infusion.[48] Sodium bicarbonate may be required to raise blood pH during the management of diabetic ketoacidosis. It must be remembered that if such acidotic patients are given bicarbonate, the cerebrospinal fluid may become more acidotic, with consequent clinical deterioration. Arterial blood gas samplings are usually necessary under such circumstances to ensure that the Pa_{CO_2} is kept low to militate against the cerebrospinal fluid changes. Clearance of ketones from the urine has been used as a sign surgery may safely proceed.

Hyperglycemic hyperosmolar coma is produced by osmolality increases and dehydration secondary to very high serum glucose levels. Blood glucose may exceed 1000 mg/dl, and osmolality may range as high as 360 mOsm/kg. Because of dehydration, the results of serum electrolyte determinations may be inaccurate. Such states are medical and surgical emergencies, and affected patients require intensive therapy and monitoring before surgery. Initial treatment is usually intravenous insulin and hypotonic electrolyte solutions. Glucose solutions are added as the blood sugar decreases with the increases in fluids and insulin. The therapeutic aim is restitution of serum osmolality to 310 mOsm/kg or below. This can generally be accomplished in 4 to 6 hours with aggressive therapy. In hyperosmolar hyperglycemic coma, the mortality rate is high. If at all possible, surgery and anesthesia should be forestalled until the patient's condition is stable.

Preoperative and Intraoperative Management of Glucose

Historically, serum glucose levels in the diabetic patient undergoing elective surgery were managed by one of the following regimens.

Withholding All Insulin the Morning of Surgery

The rationale for this seemingly irrational procedure was the aforementioned difficulty in adequately diagnosing hypoglycemia during general anesthesia. The proponents of this nihilistic technique held that hyperglycemia, even with its attendant problems of electrolyte and osmolality disturbances and diuresis, was a lesser evil than hypoglycemia and brain damage.[13] This concept is somewhat antedeluvian by current standards of practice and is now rarely used. In the average diabetic, mean increases in glucose concentrations under this regimen approximate 22 mg/dl/h.

Administration of a Partial Dose of Long-Acting Insulin Before Surgery (One Third to One Half Usual Daily Dose)

Although several years ago this empirical regimen was subscribed to by many adherents, there is little concrete evidence to justify its use. In fact, it may be detrimental. Since the latency period of isophane (NPH) insulin is 2 to 4 hours (Table 10–1) and peak action is not until 8 to 12 hours, a morning dose can theoretically produce, and actually has

Table 10–1. TIME COURSE OF INSULIN PREPARATIONS

	Time to Onset (hours)	Duration of Action (hours)
Crystalline zinc insulin	1–2	8
Lente insulin	2	24
NPH insulin	2	24
Ultralente insulin	7	36

produced, delayed hypoglycemia.[49] Since the effect of NPH insulin persists in the patient when monitoring is least (after the recovery room period), unrecognized hypoglycemia can be quite dangerous.

Continuous or Intermittent Insulin Therapy in the Perioperative Period

Use of either a continuous drip or syringe pump infusion of regular insulin or intermittent boluses of regular insulin coupled with a continuous drip of 5% dextrose in water is now considered by most interested investigators as the preferable technique for the perioperative management of the diabetic surgical patient. Several protocols have been suggested. All withhold the usual dose of long-acting insulin the morning of surgery, and all require frequent (e.g., every 30 minutes) estimates of blood glucose during anesthesia and in the recovery room. One group advocates infusion of 2 units/h of regular insulin.[45] Another regimen recommends 50 ml/h 5% dextrose solution "piggybacked" with an infusion pump delivering insulin at a fixed rate. The hourly insulin requirements in units of regular (crystalline) insulin are determined by dividing the current plasma glucose level by 100 (e.g., a blood glucose of 380 mg/dl requires 3.8 units of regular insulin in the next hour).[30]

A more empiric and simpler, but nonetheless successful, regimen consists of withholding long-acting insulin the morning of surgery and administering 2 ml/kg/h glucose as 5% dextrose (100 mg/kg/h). Insulin, regular crystalline, is given in 1 to 2 units/h for blood glucose levels exceeding 250 mg/dl. Extra glucose is given when blood glucose levels fall below 150 mg/dl.[31]

Regardless of the technique employed, constant monitoring of blood glucose and occasionally of blood ketones is required. It must also be kept in mind that the insulin molecule tends to "stick" to glass and plastic intravenous tubing. Therefore, injection or infusion close to the intravenous catheter site is preferable. Again, Table 10–1 demonstrates that serum levels of intravenously administered insulin do not peak immediately. Thus, at least 2 to 3 hours of careful observation are necessary after the last dose of insulin.

Selection of Anesthetic Technique for Amputation in the Diabetic

There is no one anesthetic technique that can be advocated over any other in the insulin-requiring diabetic scheduled for lower extremity amputation. Certainly, however, regional anesthetic techniques have many theoretic advantages over general anesthesia, as described earlier in this chapter. Regional anesthesia sites and indications are described.

Ankle Block

This technique is applicable for digital amputation or even for a transmetatarsal amputation. There is basically no physiological change produced with this procedure, and it must be advocated as an excellent method of anesthesia for the high-risk patient. Injections are probably contraindicated if infection and edema have spread to the ankle area. Although there are theoretic objections against this block in the presence of vascular occlusion or infection, experience does not contraindicate its use. Local anesthetics, such as lidocaine, actually increase blood supply by producing vasodilation as long as injected volumes are not sufficiently large to produce mechanical vascular occlusion. Local anesthetics are also bacteriocidal. In the last 10 years at the University of Arizona Hospitals, 125 ankle blocks have been performed for toe amputations, without complication.

Sciatic-Femoral Nerve Block

This block is applicable for lower extremity surgical procedures below the knee only. It is probably underused. Similar to ankle block, it produces few physiological disturbances. The disadvantage of the sciatic-femoral block is the high failure rate in the hands of anes-thesiologists who use the technique infrequently.

Epidural (Peridural) Block

This is a highly useful anesthetic technique for lower extremity amputations. When a catheter is inserted into the peridural space, pain relief after amputation can be maintained for several days. The resulting profound sympathetic blockade may be of therapeutic value for the ischemic limb. Often used local anesthetics are bupivacaine and lidocaine, the former having a duration of neural blockade some 2 to 3 times that of the latter.

Spinal (Subarachnoid) Block

This is a highly preferable technique and, with epidurals, must be considered as almost the procedure of choice in the diabetic requiring lower extremity surgery. Speculative contraindications concerning exacerbations of diabetic neuropathy have no basis in actual experimental fact. It must be kept in mind that the peripheral sympathetic blockade produced by both epidural and spinal block is a two-edged sword. The good aspect is obviously that more blood is shunted into an ischemic extremity. Problems can arise, however, with subsequent hypotension. Usually this constitutes little hazard and can be adequately and safely treated with fluids or vasopressors such as ephedrine or phenylephrine.

General Anesthesia

Although there appear to be greater numbers of advocates of regional techniques for diabetic patients undergoing lower extremity amputation, general anesthesia can be a safe alternative. Monitoring may be increased if general anesthesia is selected, since this technique, unlike regional nerve block, has nonselective effects on organ systems. There is no one general anesthetic or combination of anesthetics and adjuvants that can be considered superior. Selection is generally predicated on the pathophysiological condition of the patient, closely coupled with the experiences of the anesthesiologist. It is far wiser with the emergency-complicated diabetic for anesthesiologists to use techniques in which they are skilled and confident rather than new ones based on arcane pharmacological innuendo. If the patient has a full stomach or gastric atony, a rapid sequence induction with an assistant providing a Sellick's maneuver (cricoid pressure) is necessary. Most potent inhalation anesthetics have a tendency to inhibit the uptake of glucose by peripheral tissues. This pharmacological action is more academic than hazardous but can keep glucose levels fairly high. This effect has been termed the anti-insulin phenomenon of general anesthetics.

ATHEROSCLEROTIC DISEASE

The patient with atherosclerotic peripheral vascular disease who requires lower extremity amputation presents the anesthesiologist with many complex problems. The primary consideration is, of course, the safety and general well being of the patient. As many as 50% of these patients present with hypertension on hospital admission, regardless of whether or not they are taking antihypertensive medication.[11] Additionally, many have a history of myocardial infarction or symptoms of significant coronary artery disease.[7] It is also common for these patients to have atherosclerotic involvement of their cerebrovasculature, constituting an additional anesthetic risk.[10] All of these factors and many others provide a true anesthetic challenge.

In order to deliver optimal anesthetic care, the anesthesiologist must be well versed in all aspects of pre-, intra-, and postoperative care. Rather than outline the anesthetic considerations appropriate for all surgical patients, the next several pages will describe those aspects of anesthetic care that specifically apply to the patient with atherosclerotic vascular disease. As a general rule, all of these patients should be managed with the assumpton that they have significant coronary artery disease. The incidence of coronary artery disease in this patient population is high even without symptoms or electrocardiographic changes. Thus, it is essential to review those factors crucial in determining the myocardial oxygen supply/demand balance. Subsequently, the criteria for anesthetic risk classification, preoperative evaluation, determinants of the choices for intraoperative monitoring, and anesthetic and pharmacologic management of these patients will be discussed.

Determinants of Myocardial Oxygen Homeostasis

There have been several attempts, by different investigators, to assist the clinician in estimation of myocardial oxygen consumption. Measures such as the tension-time index or rate-pressure product have been forwarded.[35, 37] The latter has been found, by the authors, to be too imprecise to provide a clinically predictable index of myocardial homeostasis. The tension-time index is a reproducible index of myocardial oxygen consumption; it is estimated by multiplying the mean root aortic pressure (when the aortic valve is open) by the time, per minute, the valve is open. This time is calculated by determining the time between the valve opening (upstroke of the pressure wave) and closing (dicrotic notch). The index at which oxygen demand exceeds supply varies among patients, depending on coronary anatomy and hemodynamics, and the tension-time index is often difficult to calculate and use clinically. However, the clinician may play an important role in balancing myocardial oxygen supply and demand by regulating those determinants that can be controlled and influenced clinically.

Determinants of Myocardial Oxygen Supply

Myocardial oxygen supply depends primarily on two factors, coronary blood flow and the oxygen delivery capability of the blood perfusing the coronary arteries. As can be seen in Table 10–2, there are several determinants of each of these two primary variables. Each determinant will be briefly discussed in order to further elucidate its role in this process.

Table 10–2. DETERMINANTS OF MYOCARDIAL OXYGEN SUPPLY

Coronary Blood Flow
  Diastolic aortic blood pressure
  Heart rate
  Preload
  Coronary vascular resistance
Oxygen Delivery
  Oxygen saturation
  Hematocrit and 2,3-DPG levels
  Pa_{CO_2}, pH, temperature

Coronary Blood Flow

Normal coronary blood flow is approximately 225 ml/min or 0.7 to 0.8 ml/g heart muscle.[20] This is equivalent to about 4 to 5% of the normal resting cardiac output.[20] It is evident that there is a phasic alteration of coronary blood flow in relation to systole and diastole, with the majority of the flow occurring during diastole and very little flow taking place during systole.[20] This phasic change in coronary blood flow is much more pronounced in the left ventricle than in the right. The reason or this discrepancy between the right and left ventricles is because the left ventricle generates much higher intramyocardial pressures during systole and compresses the coronary vasculature to a much greater extent.[20] However, in cases of right ventricular failure, pressures within the right ventricle will increase, and it will become more like the left ventricle in relation to the phasic changes in coronary blood flow.[25] Additional determinants of myocardial blood flow include diastolic aortic blood pressure, heart rate, preload, and coronary vascular resistance.

Diastolic Blood Pressure. Normal coronary perfusion pressure is equal to diastolic aortic blood pressure minus left ventricular end-diastolic pressure (LVEDP). Hence, the amount of coronary blood flow is closely linked to diastolic pressure, particularly in light of the fact that most flow occurs during diastole. In most patients, this is not a crucial point, since their diastolic blood pressure is adequate to provide sufficient coronary flow. However, if coronary artery disease is superimposed, a fall in diastolic pressure—as occurs with vasodilator therapy, aortic insufficiency, or induction of a regional or general anesthetic—may precipitate myocardial ischemia. Thus, optimal management of these patients with coronary artery disease includes maintaining diastolic blood pressure at or near the patient's baseline. An additional factor making this crucial is that in coronary artery disease, the perfusion pressure is not dependent on the diastolic pressure; rather, it is the pressure in the coronary artery distal to the obstructive atherosclerotic plaque that is significantly lower than the actual aortic diastolic blood pressure.

Heart Rate. The duration of the diastolic portion of the cardiac cycle is critical to the adequacy of myocardial blood supply. As heart rate increases, the duration of diastole decreases, and there is a decrease in diastolic cycle length as a percentage of total cardiac cycle time.[4] Thus, tachycardia produces a decrease in myocardial oxygen supply and should be assiduously avoided in patients with coronary artery disease.

Preload. Coronary perfusion pressure is partially dependent on the end-diastolic volume of the ventricle. Thus, preload should be preserved at adequate levels to maintain normal cardiac output. Overdistention of the ventricle by high filling pressures is to be avoided. A patient who presents with congestive heart failure and elevated filling pressures needs aggressive therapy.

Coronary Vascular Resistance. Blood flow through the coronary vessels is regulated by the vascular response to the local nutritional needs of cardiac muscle.[22, 36] However, the coronary vasculature in the ischemic myocardium may already be maximally dilated distal to the lesion and almost entirely dependent on perfusion pressure, with autoregulation playing little or no role in control of blood flow.[6] Cardiac wall tension during diastole may also contribute to changes in coronary vascular resistance due to alterations in intramyocardial pressure on coronary arteries, produced by varying ventricular end-diastolic volumes.[5]

Oxygen Delivery

All too often, the clinician views myocardial oxygen supply only in terms of coronary blood flow. Little or no consideration is given to the quality of the delivered hemoglobin in its ability to adequately supply the myocardium with oxygen. In the normal resting state, 65 to 70% of the oxygen in arterial blood is removed by the heart from the coronary circulation.[20] It is important that the delivered blood have a sufficient quantity of oxygen and possess the ability to deliver it to myocardial tissue. This fact also emphasizes why increases in myocardial oxygen demand are met primarily with increases in coronary blood flow. When increases in flow are not possible, ischemia occurs.

Oxygen Saturation. Since such a high percentage of the oxygen is extracted from the blood by the myocardium, to produce optimal oxygen delivery, the arterial hemoglobin should be maintained at over a 90% saturation whenever possible. This may be an important factor in the case of the patient with chronic obstructive pulmonary disease

(COPD) in whom it is not always possible to achieve a high arterial oxygen saturation. In patients who smoke, oxygen delivery may be further impaired owing to the carboxyhemoglobin content of their blood.

Hematocrit and 2,3-DPG Levels. Anemic patients obviously have less oxygen carried to the myocardium compared with patients with normal hemoglobin concentrations, regardless of saturation. In addition, if levels of 2,3-diphosphoglycerate (2,3-DPG) are low, the blood will be less able to deliver the oxygen it is carrying to the tissues. Normally, the authors attempt to maintain the hematocrit around 30% in these patients.

Pa$_{CO_2}$, pH, and Temperature. Also related to the oxygen-hemoglobin dissociation curve and delivery of oxygen at the tissue level are Pa$_{CO_2}$, pH, and temperature. Hypocarbia, alkalosis, and hypothermia will all adversely effect unloading of oxygen to the tissues.

By and large, all of the factors discussed previously with regard to oxygen delivery normally play little role in myocardial oxygen supply compared with coronary bood flow. However, in the critically ill or borderline patient, fine tuning these variables may make the difference in the eventual outcome of the patient. This is particularly true in the patient who has suffered massive blood loss or has received multiple transfusions.

Determinants of Myocardial Oxygen Demand

Myocardial oxygen demand depends primarily on four factors: afterload (defined as mean aortic pressure or impedance to left ventricular ejection), heart rate, preload, and contractility (Table 10–3). Similar to supply, myocardial oxygen demand must be aggressively controlled to maintain an optimal oxygen supply/demand balance. It is also interesting that heart rate and preload are important in determining demand, just as they were in regulating supply.

Afterload (Impedance to Left Ventricular Ejection)

Sarnoff and associates in 1958 showed that if the pressure against which the heart pumped doubled, oxygen consumption also doubled.[37] This increase in consumption is partially offset by the supply/demand ratio,

Table 10–3. DETERMINANTS OF MYOCARDIAL OXYGEN DEMAND

Afterload (mean aortic pressure)
Heart rate
Preload (diastolic volume)
Contractility

since an increase in pressure will also increase supply. However, it is evident that an afterload increase is not well tolerated in a patient with a borderline ischemic myocardium. Hence, hypertension must be controlled.

Heart Rate

Myocardial oxygen consumption per beat remains constant over a very wide range of heart rates.[28] However, if the number of beats per minute increases, the oxygen demand per minute increases. This is particularly detrimental to the patient with coronary artery disease, since an increase in heart rate will decrease myocardial oxygen supply by decreasing coronary blood flow.

Preload

Using the same experimental design, Sarnoff and associates also showed that doubling preload increased oxygen consumption by 8%.[37] This increase is substantially less than those seen with changes in afterload. Thus, volume loading is better tolerated by the myocardium than systemic pressure increases. The increase is primarily due to the change in the tension the heart must generate secondary to the enlarged radius of the ventricular chamber from the increased preload. The relationship is described by the law of Laplace (T = P × r2h, where T = tension, P = pressure, r = radius, and h = thickness).

Contractility

Contractility is said to increase when the rate of active contraction or force developed during active contraction is increased while extrinsic factors (muscle loading or length) remain the same.[20] Sonnenblick and colleagues in 1965 found that myocardial oxygen consumption increased with positive inotropic stimulation.[41] Contractility may be increased by such perturbations as digoxin, epinephrine, isoproterenol, increased heart rate, and sympathetic stimulation. The increase in oxygen demand produced by an

Table 10–4. METHODS OF IMPROVING MYOCARDIAL OXYGEN SUPPLY

Maintain diastolic aortic blood pressure at or near the patient's baseline.

Maintain a low normal heart rate, particularly in patients with coronary artery disease (i.e., consider use of beta-blockers).

Preserve adequate preload in order to maintain normal cardiac output while avoiding fluid overload and increases in ventricular wall tension.

Treatment of coronary vasospasm (i.e., use of calcium channel blockers).

Improve arterial oxygenation by treating underlying pulmonary pathological condition.

Improve oxygen carrying capacity of blood with iron or blood transfusions (i.e., maintain a hematocrit of 30–35%).

Avoid states such as hypocarbia, hypothermia, alkalosis, or decreased levels of 2,3-DPG.

Treat arrhythmias that may decrease coronary blood flow.

increased contractile state is partially offset with respect to the oxygen supply/demand ratio by an increase in myocardial oxygen supply.

It is clearly evident that there are multiple variables and interactions that determine optimal myocardial oxygen homeostasis. Even more evident is the fact that the clinician must be well versed in these interactions if the cardiovascular stability of the patient is to be maintained. Tables 10–4 and 10–5 summarize the important therapeutic goals. Dilemmas in therapy occur, evident for example in the treatment of congestive heart failure, in which nitrates, other vasodilators, diuretics, and possibly positive inotropic drugs are administered. The first three therapeutic interventions are aimed at decreasing ventricular volume and wall tension, all of which increase supply and decrease demand; however, the latter intervention improves myocardial performance, which may in turn improve the congestive heart failure, increase myocardial oxygen supply, *and* to a greater extent increase myocardial oxygen demand. Obviously, the clinician must weigh the ben-

Table 10–5. METHODS OF DECREASING MYOCARDIAL OXYGEN DEMAND

Aggressive treatment of increased afterload (hypertension).

Maintain the heart rate at or below the patient's baseline (i.e., avoid tachycardia).

Aggressive treatment of congestive heart failure.

Avoid *unnecessary* increases in contractility (i.e., avoid inotropic drugs and sympathetic stimulation).

efits and risks of each therapeutic maneuver while monitoring the patient's progress and response to each intervention. Knowledge of cardiac physiology is the mainstay in the care of these patients and underlies the anesthesiologist's preoperative evaluation.

Preoperative Evaluation

A thorough preoperative evaluation is critical if the anesthesiologist is to adequately care for the patient. Table 10–6 outlines the many aspects integral to an appropriate preoperative assessment.

Assessment of Risk Factors

There have been many attempts to categorize patients by preoperative risk factors so that the clinician can reliably predict the eventual outcome. Although results have been variable, two classifications that are referred to often in this patient population are the American Society of Anesthesiologists (ASA) classification (Table 10–7) and the New York Heart Association Functional Class (Table 10–8). The New York Heart Association classification is the more appropriate in predicting outcome. Goldman and coworkers proposed a Cardiac Risk Index score to be used for patients undergoing surgery with a history of coronary artery disease.[16] Of particular importance in their classification was the increased perioperative risk associated with a myocardial infarction 6 months before surgery; evidence on physical examination of myocardial dysfunction, such as S_3 gallop or jugular venous distention (JVD); or the presence of arrhythmia. Even so, this classification has been found to be too unwieldy and unpredictable to find widespread clinical use; however, a specific and totally reliable predictor of patient outcome for this population has yet to be determined. Despite such short-

Table 10–6. THE PREOPERATIVE EVALUATION

Assessment of risk factors
Evaluation of the myocardial oxygen supply/demand state
History, physical examination, laboratory data, chest X-ray, EKG, stress testing data, cardiac catheterization data
Preoperative drug therapy
Preoperative interview
Preoperative cardiology consultation

Table 10–7. AMERICAN SOCIETY OF ANESTHESIOLOGISTS (ASA) PATIENT CLASSIFICATION

Class 1:   The patient has no organic, physiological, biochemical, or psychiatric disturbance. The pathological process for which the operation is to be performed is localized and does not entail a systemic disturbance.

Class 2:   The patient has mild to moderate systemic disturbance caused either by the condition to be treated surgically or by other pathophysiological processes.

Class 3:   The patient has severe systemic disturbance or disease from whatever cause, even though it may not be possible to define the degree of disability with finality.

Class 4:   The patient has severe systemic disorders that are already life threatening—not always correctable by operation.

Class 5:   The moribund patient who has little chance of survival but is submitted to operation in desperation.

Emergency Operation (E): Any patient in one of the previous classes who is operated on as an emergency is considered to be in poorer physical condition than patients undergoing normal surgery.

Adapted from Dripps RD, Eckenhoff JE, Vandam LD: Preanesthetic consultation and choice of anesthesia. *In* Introduction to Anesthesia: The Principles of Safe Practice, 7th Ed. Philadelphia, WB Saunders Co, 1988.

comings, it is useful to classify patients with peripheral vascular disease using the ASA and New York guidelines. These classifications can estimate anesthetic risk relative to

Table 10–8. NEW YORK HEART ASSOCIATION FUNCTIONAL CLASS

Class I: Ordinary physical activity is well tolerated with normal hemodynamic parameters. Anesthesia and surgery are well tolerated.

Class II: Physical activity is mildly limited, with normal hemodynamic parameters at rest. Anesthesia and surgery are usually well tolerated with adequate monitoring and therapy.

Class III: Physical activity is moderately limited, with a normal cardiac output and abnormal hemodynamic parameters at rest. Anesthesia and surgery are tolerated with adequate monitoring and therapy.

Class IV: Physical activity is severely limited, with failure to maintain normal cardiac output at rest. Hemodynamic parameters are abnormal. Anesthesia and surgery are poorly tolerated even with appropriate therapy and management.

other patient populations so that the patient may be adequately informed of risks.

In addition to patient classification, there have also been several efforts to help identify those patients at risk for cardiovascular instability, perioperative myocardial infarction, or stroke. The patient with atherosclerotic peripheral vascular disease may be at risk for all of these complications. Thus, it is imperative that the anesthesiologist and surgeon be aware of the factors that predict these complications so that they may be avoided.

Foëx and Prys-Roberts in 1974 found that the absolute perioperative hemodynamic fluctuations are less in treated than in untreated patients with hypertension.[34] This was later confirmed by Goldman and Caldera.[15] Other studies have stressed the importance of this finding.[17] One such study looked at patients with a history of a myocardial infarction who were undergoing anesthesia and surgery; it found that wide swings in vital signs, such as a 30% lowering of systolic blood pressure for a period of greater than 10 minutes, was associated with a fivefold increase in cardiac related death from 3.2 to 15.2%.[17] One would also want to avoid large swings in vital signs in patients with known cerebrovascular disease. A marked fall in systemic pressure could result in a marked fall in cerebral perfusion pressure and blood flow, producing ischemic brain injury. Thus, it seems unwise to proceed with surgery when hypertension is poorly controlled, unless absolutely necessary.

Tarhan and associates have demonstrated an increase in the incidence of perioperative myocardial infarction if surgery occurs within 6 months of a previous myocardial infarction;[46] Table 10–9 summarizes their findings. They also found that 33% of the periopera-

Table 10–9. THE INCIDENCE OF PERIOPERATIVE MYOCARDIAL INFARCTION (MI)

History	Incidence (%) of Perioperative MI
No previous MI	0.13
MI in the past	6.6
MI within the last 3 months	37
MI within 3–6 months	16
MI more than 6 months before surgical procedure	4–5

Based on data from Tarhan S, Moffitt EA, Taylor WF, et al: Myocardial infarction after general anesthesia. JAMA 220:1451, 1972.

tive myocardial infarctions occurred on the third postoperative day and carried a mortality rate of 54%, with 80% of the deaths occurring within 48 hours. It was postulated that the third postoperative day also carried an increased incidence of infection, sepsis, atelectasis, and activity, all of which may increase the patient's oxygen demand.[46] It was postulated that this oxygen demand could be the cause of the high incidence of perioperative myocardial infarctions at that time. These findings suggest that every effort should be made to delay anesthesia and surgery until 6 months after a myocardial infarction.

Many other factors have been associated with an increased incidence of perioperative myocardial infarctions.[17, 46] One of these is a history of a transmural versus subendocardial myocardial infarction, with the transmural variety carrying on increased risk.[3] This, however, has not been substantiated by other studies. A myocardial infarction complicated by arrhythmias or congestive heart failure is also associated with greater risk.[17] Furthermore, it has been found in one study, but not yet substantiated, that the longer the operative procedure, the greater the risk of a perioperative myocardial infarction.[39] The severity and location of the surgical procedure have been directly associated with increased perioperative risk, particularly with procedures on the thorax and upper abdomen.[16]

All in all, what does this mean? Is this information needed? Does the classification of risk factors change the care the patient receives? The latter question is the key to why such information is important in care. Classification allows the anesthesiologist to identify patients at increased risk and thereby adjust the degree of monitoring and anesthetic technique. It also lends support to postponing elective surgery until a more propitious date, if necessary.

Evaluation of the Myocardial Oxygen Supply/Demand State

Those factors important in the determination of myocardial oxygen homeostasis have already been reviewed. During preoperative evaluation of the patient, the anesthesiologist must assess whether therapeutic intervention could improve the supply/demand ratio. As previously stated, congestive heart failure, arrhythmias, hypertension, anemia, abnormal pulmonary function, and similar conditions may all adversely affect this balance. Thus, clinicians must improve what they can. If no improvements are possible, prior knowledge of an individual patient's preoperative state allows better intraoperative care.

Examination of the Patient

The examination is an integral part of a total evaluation. The anesthesiologist should use the following step-by-step approach, which emphasizes those points pertinent to the patient population under discussion.

History. Patients about to undergo anesthesia and surgery should have their recent and distant medical history reviewed by the anesthesiologist in charge of the case. Of particular importance is the patient's prior anesthetic experiences, and in the case of patients with atherosclerotic peripheral vascular disease, any history of hypertension, ischemic heart disease, or cerebrovascular insufficiency should be noted. The frequency and severity of symptoms should be noted, and the adequacy of treatment should be assessed, particularly in relation to the patient's exercise tolerance. In addition, any associated disease states such as pulmonary or renal insufficiency should be thoroughly discussed, and a preoperative consultation should be obtained in the appropriate circumstance. One should also evaluate the cause and course of all previous hospitalizations.

Physical Examination. A complete physical examination is required on all patients; particular attention should be paid to the cardiac and pulmonary systems. Physical findings of cardiomegaly, rales, gallop, pedal edema, bronchospasm, and similar conditions may dictate a more in-depth patient profile, with further testing necessary before surgery can proceed (e.g., stress test, pulmonary function tests). Evidence of cerebrovascular disease, such as the presence of carotid bruit, should be sought. If disease is suspected, further investigation is warranted to document severity. This procedure should impress upon the anesthesiologist the importance of maintaining cerebral perfusion pressure during the surgical procedure. Whenever possible, abnormalities noted on physical examination, such as hypertension, congestive heart failure, and pulmonary dysfunction, should be treated before surgery.

Laboratory Data. The laboratory examinations in this patient group should stress determinations of serum potassium, blood urea nitrogen (BUN), creatinine, hematocrit, clotting factors, and liver function. These measures are frequently abnormal in this patient population owing to medications or associated disease states. Abnormal findings may suggest therapeutic intervention or further laboratory examination. They may also influence the type of anesthesia used and the type of monitoring required by the anesthesiologist.

Potassium depletion is particularly common owing to the frequency with which diuretics are administered to this patient group for therapy of hypertension or congestive heart failure.[9, 16, 26] When patients receive chronic diuretics and suffer urinary potassium loss without adequate potassium repletion, severe total body potassium depletion can occur.[38] When this situation is present, there exists a high likelihood of arrhythmias with even small changes in serum potassium intraoperatively.[26, 38] Thus, all but emergency surgery should be postponed, and potassium replacement should be given orally over several days. This is especially true in states of chronic potassium depletion in which the serum potassium level is less than 3.0 mEq/l. In this situation, it is dangerous to consider rapid intravenous potassium administration owing to the arrhythmogenic potential of this therapy during the ensuing anesthesia.[52] This arrhythmogenic potential is created by the imbalance of the intra-/extracellular potassium ratio produced by this therapy, which simulates acute hyperkalemia. When oral potassium therapy is not possible, one should follow the treatment guidelines in Table 10–10.[42] Last, a serum potassium level greater than 4.0 mEq/l is preferred by the authors when patients are taking digoxin preoperatively.

Chest Radiograph. A multitude of information may be obtained from the chest radiograph. This is especially true for the functional state of the heart and lungs. Evidence of cardiac injury or dysfunction, such as pulmonary edema, vascular redistribution, valvular calcifications, cardiomegaly, or pleural effusion, can be observed. Additionally, evidence of pulmonary pathological conditions may be evident, such as emphysematous changes, atelectasis, and infiltrates.

Table 10–10. GUIDELINES FOR INTRAVENOUS POTASSIUM REPLACEMENT

1. Give up to but no more than 20 mEq/h of K^+ intravenously. The amount of intravenous solution necessary depends on whether it is being administered via a central or peripheral vein. Peripherally, a concentration of greater than 40 mEq/l should be avoided, and when given centrally, a concentration of greater than 100 mEq K^+/l should be avoided.
2. Administer no more than 240 mEq K^+/24 h.
3. Continuously montior the EKG for T-wave and QRS-complex alterations, as well as rate and rhythm disturbances.
4. Frequently measure (every 4 hours) plasma electrolyte concentrations.
5. Allow at least 13 hours for repletion of minimal to moderate K^+ depletion (2.8–3.2 mEq/l) and at least 24 to 48 hours for greater total body K^+ depletion.

Modified by permission from Clark NJ, Stanley TH: Anesthesia for vascular surgery. *In* Miller RD (ed): Anesthesia, 2nd Ed. New York, Churchill Livingstone, 1986.

Electrocardiogram. A systematic approach to the electrocardiogram is essential so that no information is lost in its interpretation. One should look for evidence of arrhythmias, heart block, and ischemia. One should be particularly aggressive in addressing those abnormal findings that may be improved or resolved preoperatively to enhance the myocardial oxygen supply/demand balance. Patients with right bundle branch block (RBBB) and left anterior or left posterior hemiblock with or without a prolonged P-R interval may be at increased risk of developing complete heart block. In addition, if planning to place a pulmonary artery catheter in a patient with left bundle branch block (LBBB), the clinician must always bear in mind that there is a 5% incidence of producing an RBBB during placement of the catheter, and pacing equipment should be close at hand.[47]

Additional Data Pertaining to the Cardiovascular System. For the most part, additional data on the cardiovascular status of the patient will not be available. The information obtained can be invaluable to the physicians caring for the patient, but if it is not available, one must determine from the rest of the historical, physical, and laboratory findings whether these data should be pursued. Additional data include results of noninvasive carotid artery studies in order to estimate carotid patency, exercise stress testing to examine myocardial reserve, or cardiac catheterization, which will determine the extent of coronary and myocardial disease.

Noninvasive studies of the carotids may dictate surgical intervention or, at the very least, impress upon the anesthesiologist the importance of maintaining adequate cerebral perfusion pressure during the surgical procedure and may lead to surgical intervention in the future.

If stress testing data are available, one should note at what heart rate and blood pressure ischemia occurred and in what lead of the electrocardiogram ST segment changes first occurred. This may indicate the myocardial reserve of the patient and defines which lead of the electrocardiogram to monitor intraoperatively.

Cardiac catheterization data in the critical or borderline patient could prove to be invaluable information. In the severely ill patient, it may be appropriate to obtain a cardiac catheterization preoperatively when indicated, since the morbidity and mortality of this procedure is so low compared with the potential benefit of the desired information.[40] If catheterization data are available, one should note the degree and significance of the coronary lesions present (particularly disease of the left main coronary artery), left ventricular end-diastolic pressure, ejection fraction, and myocardial wall motion abnormalities. Occlusion of the left main coronary artery of greater than 50% indicates a large part of coronary perfusion is extremely dependent on perfusion pressure, and hypotension must be aggressively treated. An LVEDP of greater than 15 mmHg or an ejection fraction of less than 50% indicates marked myocardial dysfunction with minimal reserve and poor ventricular compliance. These patients poorly tolerate any stress or myocardial depression from anxiety, light anesthesia, or volatile anesthetics.

Chronic or Preoperative Drug Therapy

It is beyond the scope of this chapter to review the pharmacology of possible medications patients with atherosclerosis may be taking chronically; however, there exists a core of pertinent medications that will be briefly discussed.

Digoxin. Digoxin is used primarily in the treatment of congestive heart failure or in the control of ventricular response to supraventricular tachyarrhythmias. In the latter instance, digoxin is continued through the morning of surgery. In fact, the night before surgery, patients should be examined at rest and during exercise (ambulation or arm exercises) to determine whether they are receiving adequate amounts of the drug. If the ventricular response rises to over 100 beats/min with exercise, additional digoxin is administered preoperatively. The amount of digoxin administered is determined on an individual basis. Of critical importance is maintainance of normokalemia (a serum potassium [K^+] level of greater than 4.0 mEq/l) throughout the perioperative period. When digoxin is administered for reasons other than rate or rhythm control, it is continued up to the day of surgery, with the dose the morning of surgery being withheld. There has been some controversy as to whether a severely ill elderly patient should be given a prophylactic dose of digoxin before surgery.[14] It is the authors' belief that this practice is prudent only in patients with a history of congestive heart failure, nocturnal angina, or frequent supraventricular tachyarrhythmias.

Antihypertensives. A high percentage of this patient population will be hypertensive and may or may not be taking chronic antihypertensive medication.[11] All antihypertensive medication is continued up to the time of surgery and is withheld the morning of surgery. In the operating room, it is much easier to treat hypertension than hypotension or hypovolemia. Whenever discussing this class of medications, one must always caution the clinician about clonidine. Interruption of clonidine therapy has been reported to cause refractory rebound hypertension.[21] Thus, it should be reinstituted or replaced by other antihypertensive medication as soon as possible after surgery. In the same way, the clinician should be ready to reinstitute antihypertensive therapy as soon after surgery as is deemed feasible, since postoperative hypertension is a concern.

Beta-blockers. Beta-blockers are frequently administered to control myocardial ischemic episodes, arrhythmias, or hypertension. Beta-blockers are continued up to the time of surgery, including the day of surgery, using the normal daily dosage schedule. However, it is the practice of the authors to reduce the dose of beta-blockers administered the day of surgery if it is greater than 300 mg/day. In this situation, one half the normal dose is administered 6 hours before surgery. Additionally, if a patient is taking a long-acting beta-blocker, it is continued up to the day of surgery. On the morning of surgery, the long-acting preparation is withheld, and an appropriate dose of short-acting beta-blocker (e.g., propranolol) is administered. Both of these maneuvers aim to reduce intraoperative myocardial depression. Last, the adequacy of beta-blockade should be assessed during the preoperative visit. If blockade is judged to be inadequate, administration of additional medication is considered.

Nitrates. Nitrates are continued in the usual dose amount up to the time of surgery and are administered the morning of surgery. If the patient is normally receiving high doses of nitrates in order to control myocardial ischemic episodes, prophylactic intravenous nitroglycerin is given intraoperatively in doses of approximately 1 to 2 μg/kg/min or as necessary to control ischemia.

Calcium Channel Blockers. Calcium channel blockers, such as nifedipine and diltiazem, are administered the morning of surgery and are continued through the day of surgery. The authors have found little problem continuing them up to the time of surgery. However, if the patient is on extremely high doses, the dose is reduced the morning of surgery in an effort to reduce intraoperative vasodilation or myocardial depression.

Subacute Bacterial Endocarditis (SBE) Prophylaxis. Any patient with structural heart disease or a prosthetic valve should receive SBE prophylaxis. The reader is referred to an appropriate text for current recommendations.[2, 24]

Preoperative Interview

Besides the history and physical examination, the preoperative interview by the anesthesiologist plays several important roles. It helps establish a rapport between patient and anesthesiologist. It allows the anesthesiologist to assess adequately premedication requirements and appropriate anesthetic techniques. Additionally, the patient becomes adequately informed regarding the anesthetic risk and the rationale behind the chosen anesthetic technique. Most mportant, psychological reassurance is given to reduce patient anxiety. In point of fact, Egbert and associates showed that a reassuring preoperative interview alone was just as good as a preoperative interview with a sedative in reducing nervousness in a patient arriving in the operating room;[12] moreover, it was judged to be supe-

rior to premedication alone. For patients with atherosclerotic disease, a reassuring interview can make the difference between a calm patient and a patient with marked hypertension who complains of chest pain.

Once the interview has taken place and the patient has been well informed, with all questions answered, the anesthesiologist must decide on preoperative medication. The goal of premedication is to further reduce the anxiety of the patient being transported to the operating room, *not* to induce general anesthesia. Thus, the type and amount of premedication must be individualized for each patient. For procedures involving peripheral vascular surgery or amputation of a limb, the authors premedicate patients while keeping in mind that they are, for the most part, elderly, and often have decreased requirements for sedative medications, which may produce a prolonged effect extending into the postoperative period. A discussion of several common premedications follows.

Anticholinergics. Many anesthesiologists continue to use a drying agent, such as atropine, whenever a general anesthetic is used. The authors discourage such routine use but suggest that if a drying agent is thought to be necessary, glycopyrrolate be used in place of atropine, since tachycardia is reduced with it. In addition, glycopyrrolate has a quaternary ammonium structure that prevents blood-brain barrier penetration. Thus, it does not possess the central nervous system effects of atropine or scopolamine. Scopolamine is useful if the patient's trachea is to remain intubated postoperatively, owing to its sedative effects when used in conjunction with a narcotic premedication. However, for short surgical procedures, when the patient is expected to be awake at the end of the procedure, the degree of postoperative sedation produced by scopolamine is unacceptable, particularly in the elderly.

Tranquilizers. Tranquilizers, such as diazepam (Valium), used in low oral doses provide excellent sedative effects preoperatively. These are commonly used in peripheral vascular or amputation surgery. However, higher oral or intravenous doses of diazepam and other benzodiazepines may also produce unacceptable sedation postoperatively.

Narcotics. The only narcotic the authors routinely use in this patient population is morphine; meperidine (Demerol) is specifically avoided owing to its effects on heart rate, systemic vascular resistance, and the contractile state of the heart.[23, 44] Although the dose must be individualized, a patient with fairly well-preserved cardiac function and normal central nervous system activity will receive 0.1 mg/kg of morphine intramuscularly 1 hour before transport to the operating room. This is administered with an appropriate dose of an adjunctive agent, such as scopolamine, promethazine (Phenergan), or hydroxyzine (Vistaril), depending on the individual patient and the anesthetic management planned. The advantage of a narcotic is that its action may be reversed with naloxone if necessary.

Barbiturates. As a routine, the authors rarely use barbiturates as a premedication for these patients. Barbiturates produce unacceptable sedation and myocardial depression and are not reversible.

Although these are only some of the general considerations to be taken into account when an anesthesiologist premedicates a patient for amputation or peripheral vascular surgery, the reader should now be familiar with the rationale behind the premedication administered. If nothing else, it is crucial to remember that the interview is just as important as the premedication and that each premedication must be individualized for the particular needs of the patient.

Preoperative Cardiology Consultation

Very commonly, the amputee patient or the patient with peripheral vascular disease has limited physical activity; thus, it is difficult to assess exercise tolerance and myocardial reserve. The fact that often they are taking multiple medications presents a further dilemma. Up to 50% of patients with angina have a normal electrocardiogram. Thus, the purpose of a preoperative cardiology consultation is twofold.[50] First, it assists the anesthesiologist and surgeon in determining the extent of the myocardial pathology and what further work-up, if any, is indicated. Second, the cardiologist is best able to determine if the patient is in optimal condition medically and if not, what needs to be done. The preoperative consultation is *not* to tell the anesthesiologist to avoid hypoxia and hypotension nor is it suggested that the cardiologist dictate the type of monitoring and anesthesia used during the surgical procedure.

The preoperative consultation may be extended into other subspecialties of medicine. Whenever there is a question regarding the preoperative medical condition of a patient, the appropriate consultation should be obtained. In this way, optimal care may be delivered to the patient in the operating room.

Monitoring

The monitoring used during a surgical procedure should be appropriate for the medical condition of the patient, *not* the surgical procedure. Thus, the more critically ill the patient, the more numerous and the more invasive are the monitors. When placing monitoring catheters, the clinician should remember several key points. First, adequate premedication, either on the ward or once the patient arrives in the operating room, greatly facilitates monitoring line placement. It is difficult to deal with an uncooperative, anxious patient, who may be complaining of chest pain. One must also be careful to provide adequate local anesthesia with lidocaine without epinephrine. Many times, despite adequate premedication, insufficient use of local anesthetic causes the patient to complain bitterly of pain, become uncooperative, and remember vividly the poor care received in the operating room. In addition to administering adequate amounts of local anesthetic, the clinician must continuously communicate with the patient. This tends to allay anxiety further and helps avoid unnecessary movement. Last, when placing a central venous catheter, one should always try to reduce time in the head-down position. Not only is this position uncomfortable, but patients with minimal cardiac reserve cannot tolerate it for long periods, if at all. Therefore, it is the practice of the authors to prepare and drape patients before placing them in the Trendelenburg position. As soon as the guide wire has been inserted in the vessel, the patient is returned to the supine position.

Before discussing anesthetic management, one must consider the rationale for monitoring, which is particularly useful in these patients. Whenever selecting appropriate monitoring, one must weigh the risks and benefits of each procedure in order to decide whether to proceed with or forego its use.

Electrocardiogram

All patients undergoing an anesthetic and surgical procedure should receive electrocardiographic monitoring. If the patient has known coronary artery disease, the optimal situation is to monitor lead II (for inferior wall ischemia and arrhythmia detection) and lead V_5 (for detection of anterolateral ischemia) simultaneously.[18] However, this is not always possible, particularly with a three-lead electrocardiogram. In this situation, the authors use a modified lead V_5.[18] In order to accomplish this, the leads are placed in the following manner: right arm and left leg electrodes remain in their normal positions, and the left arm electrode is placed in the V_5 position.[19] Lead I is monitored to examine the modified V_5 lead, and lead II may still be used normally with this configuration.

Intra-arterial Pressure

The use of an intra-arterial catheter depends on the severity of the patient's medical condition and the surgical procedure proposed. In general, an arterial catheter would not be used for peripheral vascular procedures or amputations; however, if the patient has significant coronary artery disease, minimal cardiovascular reserve, severe uncontrolled hypertension, or significant cerebrovascular disease, intra-arterial monitoring is serously considered in order to monitor systemic blood pressure continuously. An arterial catheter may also be placed if the patient's medical condition warrants frequent blood sampling, as in pulmonary failure, which requires frequent measurement of arterial blood gases.

Central Venous Pressure

The primary reason a central venous pressure (CVP) catheter is placed in this patient group is for central venous drug administration. If the patient has significant myocardial disease, sufficient to warrant central monitoring, a pulmonary artery catheter should be placed.

Pulmonary Artery Pressure

The authors consider placement of a pulmonary artery catheter to be indicated in the following groups: patients with severe coronary artery disease, patients with known congestive heart failure who may require intraoperative positive inotropic drugs and vasodilators, patients who are hemodynamically unstable, and patients in respiratory failure or who have suspected pulmonary emboli.

Anesthetic Management

As stated in the introduction, the primary goal of the anesthesiologist is to ensure the safety and well being of the patient. A state of anesthesia must be achieved such that the patient is insensitive to pain; amnesic, in the case of general anesthesia; and hemodynamically stable. Amputation or peripheral vascular procedures can be performed with local, regional, or general anesthesia. No technique has been found to be superior to another with regard to the perioperative risk of myocardial infarction.[18]

Local Anesthesia

This technique is usually reserved only for the critically ill. The rationale is that the hemodynamic instability produced by regional or general anesthesia is avoided. However, when using local anesthesia, one must remain aware of the volume of anesthetic in order to prevent toxicity in either the cardiovascular or central nervous system. Obviously, the use of epinephrine is avoided, since these patients have severe peripheral vascular disease and many have coronary artery disease.

Regional Anesthesia

Regional anesthesia includes spinal and epidural anesthesia, two common, and possibly preferred, anesthetic techniques for lower extremity amputation. This type of anesthesia has several advantages: major hemodynamic instability is avoided owing to the low dermatome level of the nerve conduction block, continuous communication with the patient may be maintained so that cardiac or central nervous system symptoms may be detected immediately, and prolonged postoperative sedation owing to general anesthesia is avoided. The major problem with the use of a spinal or regional anesthetic in elderly patients is either nerve block persisting in the recovery room or hemodynamic instability produced by too high a level of anesthesia with sympathetic blockade. Thus, the anesthesiologist must carefully choose the agent and dose administered.

General Anesthesia

If the patient and the anesthesiologist have elected to proceed with general anesthesia, the anesthesiologist must decide if an inhalation, a nitrous-narcotic, or a high-dose narcotic technique is indicated. The latter technique produces the greatest cardiovascular stability, but the patient will require several hours of ventilation postoperatively. An inhalation technique is adequate for most patients, but in those with a poor myocardium, the vasodilatation and myocardial depression produced by the inhalation anesthetics are unacceptable. A nitrous-narcotic technique may provide more cardiovascular stability, but patients tend to have high sympathetic tone with this technique, which may not be tolerated well in patients with hypertension or an ischemic myocardium. Each technique has its risks and benefits, and the anesthesiologist must decide which is best suited to the patient and proceed accordingly.

Regardless of technique, the authors feel it is best to use a graded response technique for induction. In this way, the induction proceeds in a manner such that graded stimuli—oropharyngeal airway, Foley catheter, laryngotracheal spray—occur sequentially during induction in order to test the adequacy of the general anesthetic. In this way, the anesthesiologist is not faced with a hypertensive, tachycardiac patient on intubation or surgical stimulation. The anesthesiologist must also decide whether intubation is necessary in view of the stress and the cardiovascular responses to both intubation and extubation.

Last, all anesthetics, general or regional, can produce undesirable cardiovascular effects. All volatile anesthetics produce some degree of myocardial depression and systemic vasodilation. Regional anesthesia may produce hypotension secondary to loss of sympathetic tone, with resultant vasodilation. Even narcotic anesthesia may, if given too rapidly, produce hypotension secondary to bradycardia, histamine release, and loss of the patient's own sympathetic tone.[50] Addi-

tionally, most muscle relaxants have undesirable cardiovascular effects; however, newer muscle relaxants ostensibly devoid of significant cardiovascular effects, vecuronium and atracurium, have been introduced. To maintain coronary and cerebral perfusion pressures and cardiovascular stability, anesthesiologists must have at their disposal the ability to counteract these effects with vasoconstrictors or inotropic drugs. They must also be well versed in the intraoperative detection and therapy of myocardial ischemia and dysfunction. This is crucial if the outcome is to be favorable.

Postoperative Care

If surgical results are to improve, the extensive preoperative preparation and intraoperative care must be extended into the postoperative period. Remember, most perioperative myocardial infarctions occur on the third day after surgery.[46] Thus, in the appropriate patient, serial electrocardiograms, enzyme assays, and possible intensive care unit monitoring must be considered if ischemic events are to be detected and treated early. This type of care can and will reduce the overall morbidity and mortality. Consideration of continuous oxygen therapy in patients with borderline myocardial oxygen supply/demand balances or cerebrovascular insufficiency may also make a difference. Thus, it is imperative that the knowledge utilized in the preceding pages be extended into the postoperative period in order to offer the best possible care.

ANESTHESIA FOR TRAUMA OF THE LOWER EXTREMITY

Many cases of lower extremity trauma occur in adolescents and young adults—individuals who are generally in the peak of health. Anesthetic problems in such patients revolve about three major issues.

1. Associated injuries (e.g., subdural hematoma, pneumothorax, fat embolism from fractures)
2. Shock due to blood loss
3. Problems associated with a full stomach. The first problem, diagnosis and therapy

of the many associated injuries that may be initially unrecognized, is truly beyond the scope of this chapter. However, astute recognition and heightened awareness of potential problems in multiple trauma are important duties of the anesthesiologist.

Lower extremity injuries can, of course, lead to considerable loss of blood. It is difficult to estimate the amount of blood lost at the scene of the accident and en route to the hospital emergency room. Clinical signs are the best guidelines during definite operative procedures. Usually the short interval between trauma and surgery is not sufficient time to draw inferences from changes in hematocrit. Central venous pressure, blood pressure, color, pulse rate, and urinary output monitoring are necessarily integrated into the final decision for volume of blood required. Extensive third space loss can occur with trauma of the leg. Also, it should be remembered that shock per se due to blood loss causes alterations in skeletal muscle surface potential, favoring the intracellular movement of sodium ions and water. Thus, a crystalloid solution, usually in the form of Ringer's lactate, is often required in generous quantities in these patients; the high renal output obtained by administration of such solutions helps protect against development of renal failure after extensive skeletal muscle crush injuries.

The problem of the full stomach has been discussed earlier in this chapter in relation to the gastric atony seen in diabetes. Pain and trauma also act in a similar manner to delay gastric emptying.The anesthesiologist should therefore consider the lower extremity trauma victim as having a full stomach with all the attendant problems. Thus, if general anesthesia is required, a Sellick's maneuver with rapid sequence induction is mandatory, and certainly use of metoclopramide should be considered if time for effective intravenous administration of this drug (45 to 60 minutes) exists before surgery.

Selection of regional versus general anesthesia for the trauma victim depends on a host of circumstances. In general, if cardiovascular instability due to incomplete volume resuscitation is still present, general anesthesia may be considered first. However, if the patient is hemodynamically stable, regional anesthesia, such as a spinal, has advantages in the patient with a full stomach.

SUMMARY

To the neophyte in anesthesia, there is always a desire for a set pattern—a formula or recipe—of anesthesia specific for disease states. Such clear-cut anesthetic protocols do not exist in the real world. Selection of anesthesia and intraoperative management are variables that depend on an astronomic number of interactions. Such is the case with anesthesia for lower extremity amputation. Although a strong case has been made for the use of regional techniques with surgery of this type, this suggestion cannot be taken as absolute. Integration of the pathophysiological condition of the patient with the technical experience of the anesthesiologist remains the "safest way" of delivering optimal patient care.

REFERENCES

1. Alberti KGMM, Thomas OJB: The management of diabetes during surgery. Br J Anaesth 51:693, 1979.
2. Antimicrobial prophylaxis: Prevention of bacterial endocarditis. Med Lett Drugs Ther 19:40, 1977.
3. Arkins R, Smessaert AA, Hicks RG: Mortality and morbidity in surgical patients with coronary artery disease. JAMA 120:485, 1964.
4. Boundoulas H, Rittger SE, Lewis RP: Changes in diastolic time with various pharmacologic agents: Implication for myocardial perfusion. Circulation 60:164, 1979.
5. Buckberg GD, Fixler DE, Archie JP, Hoffman JIE: Experimental subendocardial ischemia in dogs with normal coronary arteries. Circ Res 30:67, 1972.
6. Coorlin R, Brachfeld N, MacLead C, et al: Effect of nitroglycerin on the coronary circulation in patients with coronary artery disease or increased left ventricular work. Circulation 19:205, 1959.
7. Crawford ES, DeBakey ME, Cooley DA, et al: Surgical consideration of aneurysms and atherosclerotic occlusive lesions of the aorta and major arteries. Postgrad Med 29:151, 1961.
8. Davidson MB: The case for control in diabetes mellitus. West J Med 129:193, 1978.
9. Davison JK: Anesthesia for peripheral vascular disease. Int Anesthesiol Clin 17:129, 1979.
10. DeBakey ME, Crawford ES, Cooley DA, et al: Aneurysm of abdominal aorta: Analysis of results of graft replacement therapy one to eleven years after operation. Ann Surg 160:622, 1964.
11. DeBakey ME, Crawford ES, Cooley DA, et al: Cerebral arterial insufficiency: One to 11 year results following arterial reconstructive operation. Ann Surg 161:921, 1965.
12. Egbert LD, Battit GE, Turndorf H, et al: The value of the preoperative visit by an anesthetist. JAMA 185:553, 1963.
13. Giesecke AH Jr, Spier CJ, Jenkins MT: Management

of diabetes mellitus during anesthesia and surgery. Tex J Med 60:840, 1964.

14. Goldman L: Supraventricular tachyarrhythmias in hospitalized adults after surgery: Clinical correlates in patients over 40 years of age after major noncardiac surgery. Chest 74:450, 1978.

15. Goldman L, Caldera DL: Risks of general anesthesia and elective surgery in the hypertensive patient. Anesthesiology 50:285, 1979.

16. Goldman L, Caldera DL, Nussbaum SR, et al: Multifactorial index of cardiac risk in noncardiac surgical procedures. N Engl J Med 297:845, 1977.

17. Goldman L, Caldera DL, Southwick FS, et al: Cardiac risk factors and complications in noncardiac surgery. Medicine (Baltimore) 57:357, 1978.

18. Goldman L, Marshall AW: The Heart and Circulation. In Vandam LD (ed): To Make the Patient Ready for Anesthesia: Medical Care of the Surgical Patient, 2nd Ed. Reading, Massachusetts, Addison-Wesley, 1983.

19. Gravenstein JS, Paulus DA: Monitoring Practice in Clinical Anesthesia. Philadelphia, JB Lippincott, 1982.

20. Guyton AC: Textbook of Medical Physiology, 7th Ed. Philadelphia, WB Saunders Co, 1986.

21. Hansson L, Hunyor SN: Blood pressure over-shoot due to acute clonidine (Capapres) withdrawal: Studies on arterial and urinary catecholamines and suggestions for management of the crisis. Clin Sci Mol Med 45:1815, 1973.

22. Harden WR, Barlow CH, Simson MB, Harken AH: Temporal relation between onset of cell anoxia and ischemic contractile failure. Am J Cardiol 44:741, 1979.

23. Hug CC: Pharmacology—anesthetic drugs. In Kaplan JA (ed): Cardiac Anesthesia. New York, Grune & Stratton, 1979.

24. Kaplan EL, Anthony BF, Bisno A, et al: Prevention of bacterial endocarditis. Circulation 56:139A, 1977.

25. Kaplan JA: Cardiovascular physiology. In Miller RD (ed): Anesthesia, 2nd Ed. New York, Churchill Livingstone, 1986, p 1165.

26. Katz RL, Bigger JT: Cardiac arrhythmias during anesthesia and operation. Anesthesiology 33:193, 1970.

27. Lager I, Blohmé G, Smith U: Effect of cardioselective and non-selective beta-blockade on the hypoglycaemic response in insulin-dependent diabetics. Lancet 1:458, 1979.

28. Laurent D, Bolene-Williams C, Williams FL, Katz LN: Effect of heart rate on coronary flow and cardiac oxygen consumption. Am J Physiol 185:355, 1956.

29. Maw DSJ: Emergency management of diabetes mellitus. Anaesthesia 30:520, 1975.

30. Meyer EJ, Lorenzi M, Bohannon NV, et al: Diabetic management by insulin infusion during major surgery. Am J Surg 137:323, 1979.

31. Miller J, Walts LF: Perioperative management of diabetes mellitus. Contemp Anesth Pract 3:91, 1980.

32. Nancarrow C, Mather LE: Pharmacokinetics in renal failure. Anaesth Intensive Care 11:350, 1983.

33. Page MM, Watkins PJ: Cardiorespiratory arrest and diabetic autonomic neuropathy. Lancet 1:14, 1978.

34. Foëx P, Prys-Roberts C: Anaesthesia and the hypertensive patient. Br J Anaesth 46:575, 1974.

35. Robinson BF: Relation of heart rate and systolic blood pressure to the onset of pain in angina pectoris. Circulation 35:1073, 1967.

36. Rubio R, Berne RM: Regulation of coronary blood flow. Prog Cardiovasc Dis 43:105, 1975.

37. Sarnoff SJ, Braunwald E, Welch GH Jr, et al: Hemodynamic determinants of oxygen consumption of the heart with special reference to the tension-time index. Am J Physiol 192:148, 1958.

38. Scribner BH, Burnell JM: Interpretation of the serum potassium concentration. Metabolism 5:468, 1956.

39. Skinner JF, Pearce ML: Surgical risk in the cardiac patient. J Chronic Dis 17:57, 1964.

40. Soncs FM Jr, Shirey EK: Cine coronary arteriography. Mod Concepts Cardiovasc Dis 31:735, 1962.

41. Sonnenblick EH, Ross J Jr, Covell JW, et al: Velocity of contraction as a determinant of myocardial oxygen consumption. Am J Physiol 209:919, 1965.

42. Clark NJ, Stanley TH: Anesthesia for vascular surgery. In Miller RD (ed): Anesthesia, 2nd Ed. New York, Churchill Livingstone, 1986.

43. Steinke J: Management of diabetes mellitus and surgery. N Engl J Med 282:1472, 1970.

44. Straver BE: Contractile responses to morphine, piritramide, meperidine, and fentanyl: A comparative study of effects on the isolated ventricular myocardium. Anesthesiology 37:304, 1972.

45. Taitelman U, Reece EA, Bessman AN: Insulin in the management of the surgical diabetic patient. JAMA 237:658, 1977.

46. Tarhan S, Moffitt EA, Taylor WF, et al: Myocardial infarction after general anesthesia. JAMA 220:1451, 1972.

47. Thomson IR, Dalton BC, Lappas DG, Lowenstein E: Right bundle-branch block and complete heart block caused by the Swan-Ganz catheter. Anesthesiology 51:359, 1979.

48. Vaisrub S: Low-dose intravenous infusions of insulin in diabetic coma. JAMA 230:11, 1974.

49. Walts LF, Miller J, Davidson MB, Brown J: Perioperative management of diabetes mellitus. Anesthesiology 55:104, 1981.

50. Wells PH, Kaplan JA: Optimal management of patients with ischemic heart disease for non-cardiac surgery by complementary anesthesiologist and cardiologist interaction. Am Heart J 102:1029, 1981.

51. Wheelock FC Jr, Marble A: Surgery and diabetes. In Marble A, White P, Bradley FR, Knall LP (eds): Jaslin's Diabetes Mellitus, 11th Ed. Philadelphia, Lea & Febiger, 1971, p 599.

52. Wong KC, Kawamura R, Hodges MR, et al: Acute intravenous administration of potassium chloride to furosemide pretreated dogs. Can Anaesth Soc J 24:203, 1977.

11

Amputations of the Foot and Ankle

F. William Wagner, Jr., M.D.

"...for the life of all flesh is in the blood thereof...."
LEVITICUS 17:14, KING JAMES VERSION

Gangrenous and pregangrenous lesions are the major reasons for amputation of the foot.[24, 31, 33, 50] These amputations are usually secondary to atherosclerotic lesions of the major vascular supply to the lower extremity. Improved vascular reconstructive procedures have increased limb salvage rates.[7, 14, 15, 22, 25, 49] The same atherosclerotic lesions are present in patients with diabetes mellitus as in nondiabetics and now appear to be responsible for 40 to 70% of major lower extremity amputations.[3, 8–10, 16, 17, 21, 24, 31, 33–35, 50, 51, 57]

Besides the macrovascular lesions, the diabetic patient suffers from thickening of the capillary basement membrane. This lesion is seen with aging in otherwise normal people but appears exaggerated in the diabetic.[1, 44] Its exact relationship to other pathological processes is still not clear, as the lesion does not appear to be obstructive. The author favors the theory that it somehow interferes with the natural anticoagulability of the endothelial lining of the capillary. This may account for the diabetic foot's failure to heal lesions and surgical procedures in the toes even though bounding pedal pulses are present.

Diabetic patients also appear to be more susceptible to infection. This is controversial, but when infection does occur, it appears to be more widespread, is associated with multiple aerobic and anaerobic organisms, does not drain readily, and usually requires surgical removal of affected tissues.[5, 17, 23, 26, 41, 43, 46]

In addition to vasculopathy and infection, neuropathy is a frequent complication of diabetes.[32, 48] It is found to some degree in virtually all patients who have had the disease over 20 years. It has many manifestations—central, autonomic, and peripheral. Diabetic neuropathy has been implicated in the formation of diabetic foot ulcers and gangrene; however, at Rancho Los Amigos Medical

Center, open lesions of an insensitive foot have not been seen except in the presence of bony deformity. These deformities are usually clawtoes, hammer toes, depressed metatarsal heads, and bunions.[21, 52, 53] In addition, mid- and hindfoot deformities can result from breakdown of the midfoot joints in Charcot's disease. Hyperkeratoses over or under such bony prominences lead to breakdown and ulceration unless protective shoes are used or prophylactic surgery is performed to remove the offending bone.[21, 52, 53] A plausible theory for the associaton of neuropathy and ulceration is that the patient is unaware of the pressure against the deformed bone; an open lesion results that would be severely painful in the non-neuropathic patient. Treatment is designed to relieve pressure at the bony deformity either with protective footwear or by reconstructive surgery.[53]

Although this section appears in a chapter on amputations, ideally, one should prevent amputation. Unfortunately no cure is known for diabetes mellitus, the major cause of lower extremity amputation. Except for changes in control of blood sugar levels by drugs or insulin therapy, no advances have been made in over 30 years.[27] Cloning of pancreatic beta cells with subsequent implantation will possibly be a means of blood sugar control; however, this still does not represent a cure. Since the diabetic foot is the site at which most problems begin, recent studies have shown a 50% reduction in major amputations with vigorous care in a clinical setting.[21, 34]

An additional difficulty is that the secondary problems of diabetes are progressive. The same general process is present in both legs, and bilateral amputations are a frequent result.[6, 10, 16, 51, 56, 57] Thus, the primary amputation should be at the lowest level possible, as ambulation is still efficient when at least both knees are spared.[51, 55, 57]

AMPUTATION LEVEL SELECTION IN THE DYSVASCULAR PATIENT

Despite the development of noninvasive vascular testing, clinical judgment and experience remain major parts of amputation level selection.[24, 38] In the diabetic, if amputation is emergent, the surgeon should have some concept of how blood sugar is controlled.[4, 40] Along with the decision to amputate should be a decision on the possibility of referral for revascularization procedures. The transcutaneous Doppler ultrasound flowmeter has been useful in mapping the vascular tree noninvasively and in evaluating the possible success of local healing (Figs. 11–1 to 11–5).[52, 54] Each operating surgeon should take a few minutes to examine the extremity with the Doppler ultrasound flowmeter. Listening to the sounds (Fig. 11–2) and taking two or three systolic pressure measurements give a clinical picture difficult to obtain any more readily (Figs. 11–3, 11–4). Figure 11–5 depicts 71 cases in which the Ischemic Index (systolic pressure at the level of amputation divided by the brachial artery pressure) was a factor in choosing the amputation site. The Ischemic Index has also been useful in determining the need for revascularization procedures. If the clinical appearance of the skin and tissues is good at the proposed amputation level but the vascular supply is inadequate on Doppler testing, revascularization may be feasible. After grafting to the infrapopliteal area, further grafting to the foot is possible.[7, 14, 22, 25, 49]

There are several articles citing the fallibility of the ankle/arm index in predicting toe and foot healing. Such a ratio is designed for use in predicting healing at the level of measurement only; therefore, ratios must contain

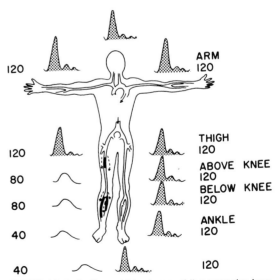

FIGURE 11–1. Outline of blockage of the vascular tree, obtained with a transcutaneous Doppler ultrasound flowmeter. The arrows indicate collateral flow.

FIGURE 11–2. Recording of Doppler ultrasound. The first tracing shows a normal pattern. The second tracing is higher in tone and, when heard, has a sharp "water hammer" effect that occurs just before a high-grade stenosis. The third tracing, just distal to the blockage, shows a low, broad wave, referred to as a wind tunnel effect when it is heard. The fourth tracing is an exaggeration of the wind tunnel effect, is louder, and represents greater collateral circulation. The fifth tracing is over a completely blocked vessel and shows little more than the noise of the instrument.

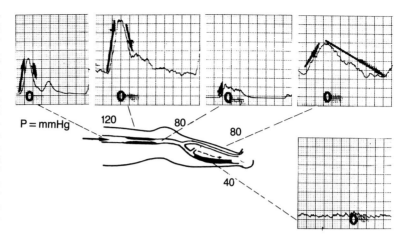

ARM B.P. = 120 mmHg

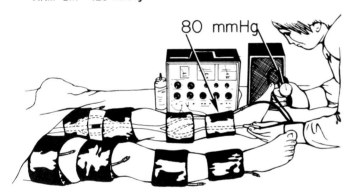

FIGURE 11–3. Using a Doppler ultrasound flowmeter as a sensitive stethoscope to obtain blood pressure at the ankle. The Ischemic Index is 80 divided by 120, equaling 0.67.

FIGURE 11–4. Use of a 9.4 MHz Doppler probe to examine the dorsalis pedis artery. Note the coupling gel at the tip of the probe.

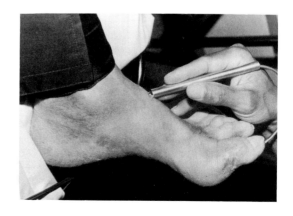

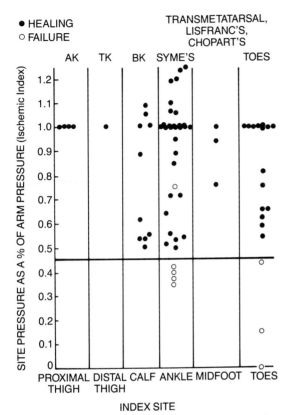

FIGURE 11–5. Scattergram showing the Ischemic Index as a factor in amputation level selection. Note that pressures are taken at the level of the amputation.

measurements from the toes and midfoot as well as from the ankle.[15, 29, 53, 54]

Nutritional status is also implicated in the healing of surgical wounds, especially in diabetic patients. If serum albumin is low and the total lymphocyte count is low, foot and ankle procedures will not heal, despite satisfactory circulation indicated by Doppler indices.[12] Proper preoperative alimentation increases healing rates.

There appears to be some reluctance among clinicians to close wounds in diabetic patients when infection is present. However, there is evidence of increased healing with wound closure if proper irrigation and drainage systems are implemented.[13, 23, 52–54] At Rancho Los Amigos Medical Center, the author obtained healing rates of approximately 60% in toe and ray resections when they were left open. If the granulating area was wide, skin grafting was performed. Otherwise, the wounds were left to heal by scarring. Since the author began closing these wounds over

Kritter's irrigation tubes,[23] he achieves over a 90% healing rate in the same type of wounds. Ecker and Jacobs report higher healing rates in closed wounds than in open ones.[13]

ADDITIONAL CAUSES OF FOOT AMPUTATION

Trauma is the second most common cause of foot amputation.[20, 30, 58] Powered road vehicles, industrial and farm machinery, powered lawn mowers, and similar objects that impart an unforgiving, unrelenting force produce amputations of the foot. In "police actions" around the world, low-velocity antipersonnel mines are producing a large number of partial foot amputations. These are occurring among nonmilitary, as well as military, personnel.

Primary and secondary neoplasms are relatively rare in the foot when compared with the rest of the body. The foot does not lend itself well to excision of compartments as neurovascular supplies may be lost. Occasionally, a longitudinal resection leaves a foot that can be used for walking.

Congenital and acquired deformities may result in a foot that is not amenable to reconstructive procedures. When a plantigrade foot does not result, a Syme's amputation or a long below-knee amputation produces a functional gait superior to that of the deformed foot.[52, 53]

SPECIFIC AMPUTATION LEVELS AND TECHNIQUES

Toe Amputation

The toes may be amputated at virtually any level as long as there is weight-bearing skin on the plantar surface and balanced muscle power. Toes may be disarticulated, amputated at any level in the phalanges, or removed along with metatarsals.

The great toe may be disarticulated for gangrene, infection, and injury. A fishmouth or racket incision may be used (Fig. 11–6). The incision is extended to the lateral side, staying away from the base of the second toe to protect its blood supply (Figs. 11–7, 11–

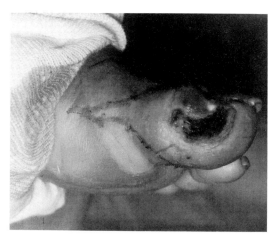

FIGURE 11–6. Fishmouth incision used to disarticulate the great toe.

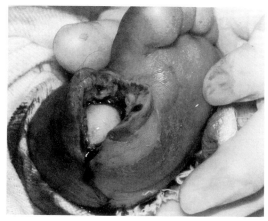

FIGURE 11–8. The lateral incision is well away from the base of the second toe. The tourniquet has just been released, and adequate blood flow is present.

8). An Esmarch bandage is used at the ankle for hemostasis; upon its release, blood flow is timed. If flow appears in 2 to 3 minutes, the wound will heal. Higher amputation is not considered unless no flow is present after 5 minutes. A Kritter drain is drawn into the wound through a separate stab incision (Fig. 11–9).[23] The wound is lavaged for 72 hours. The incision is closed through skin and subcutaneous tissue with nylon, polypropylene, or similar sutures (Fig. 11–10).

The lesser toes may be disarticulated at any of the joints, amputated through any of the phalanges, and removed along with metatarsals. The toe in Figure 11–11 became infected through a corn on the proximal interphalangeal joint of a clawtoe. On disarticulation of the toe, early osteomyelitis of the metatarsal head is noted (Fig. 11–12).

The metatarsal head is removed just proximal to the neck (Fig. 11–13). The wound is inspected for further signs of infection, and none are found. The tourniquet is released, and bleeding starts immediately (Fig. 11–14). All wound flaps are closed manually to ensure closure without tension (Fig. 11–15). A Kritter irrigation tube is inserted through a separate stab incision (Fig. 11–16). Closure of the wound is completed with simple through-and-through sutures. Irrigating fluid exits between the sutures, diluting the hematoma, debris, and bacteria (Fig. 11–17).

Removal of all of the lateral toes and portions of the rays provides a foot suitable for walking (Fig. 11–18). Patients who have the great toe and ray remaining and have had a transmetatarsal amputation on the opposite side report a strong preference for the resid-

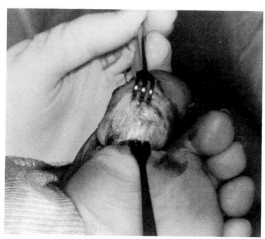

FIGURE 11–7. Plantar incision carried to the lateral side of the toe.

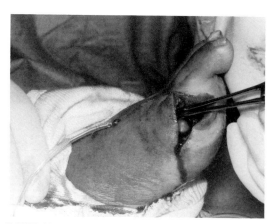

FIGURE 11–9. Placement of the Kritter irrigation tube. The fluid may be a physiological solution or may contain an antibiotic of the surgeon's choice.

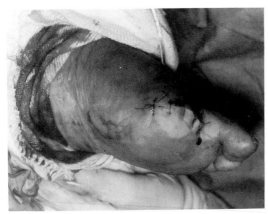

FIGURE 11–10. Closure in one layer with nonabsorbable sutures.

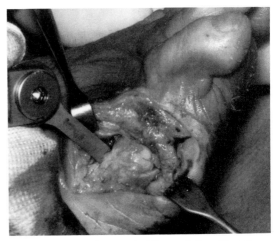

FIGURE 11–13. Removal of the metatarsal head.

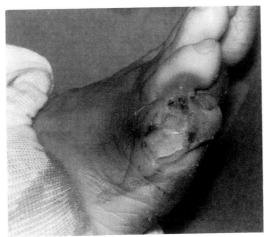

FIGURE 11–11. Clawtoe with infected corn and draining ulcer.

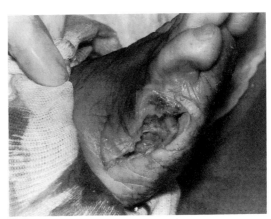

FIGURE 11–14. Release of the tourniquet. Note the capillary bleeding just starting at the lateral wound edge.

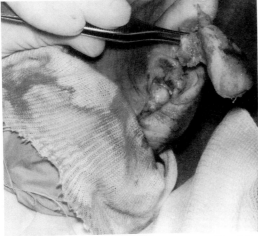

FIGURE 11–12. Disarticulated toe. Osteomyelitis of the metatarsal head is present.

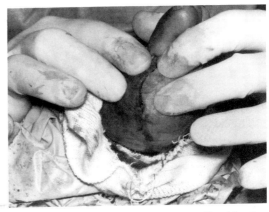

FIGURE 11–15. Test the flaps for closure without tension.

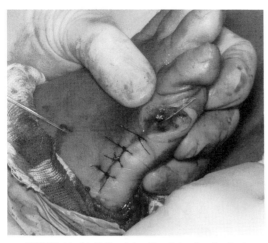

FIGURE 11-16. Kritter irrigation tube implanted.

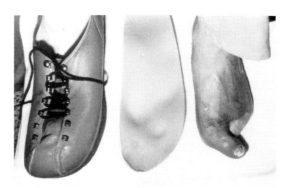

FIGURE 11-18. Foot with lateral toes and metatarsal heads removed. The patient requires no special inserts. The shoe is an extra-depth type with a polyethylene foam insert.

ual great toe type of amputation. Figure 11–19 depicts the feet of a 72-year-old patient with diabetes mellitus. Her right foot was amputated 18 months before, after several unhealed toe amputations performed at another hospital. She was quite pleased with her right foot amputation. One week before the surgery on her left side, she entered the hospital with infected second, third, and fourth toes. She demanded a single surgical procedure and did not want a series of "small cuts to see if they would heal." Amputation of the lateral toes and metatarsals provided her with another foot suitable for walking (Fig. 11–19).

Transmetatarsal Amputation

Although this amputation had been performed throughout the last century, it was popularized after Mc Kittrick and coworkers' article in 1949[28] and Pedersen and Day's article in 1954.[33] With improvements in vascular evaluation, the author's healing rate for this procedure is now over 95%. The amputation is long lasting, and few complications arise, most being from pressure areas at the ends of the metatarsals. A typical case is that of a 55-year-old diabetic with gangrene of the first and second toes with infection progressing toward the foot (Fig. 11–20). The metatarsals are divided at a 15° angle to approximate the motion at the metatarsophalangeal joints (Fig. 11–21). The distal foot is removed parallel to the plantar incision. In Figure 11–22, the tourniquet has been released, and bleeding is apparent at the most distal edges. The tendons and any devitalized fascial structures are removed. A Kritter ir-

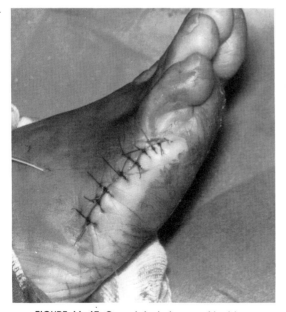

FIGURE 11-17. Completed closure of incision.

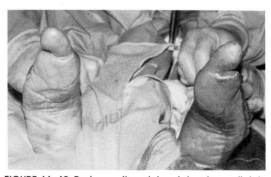

FIGURE 11-19. Postoperative picture taken immediately after removal of left lateral toes and metatarsal heads. Note the bloody drainage on the left from the Kritter irrigation tube.

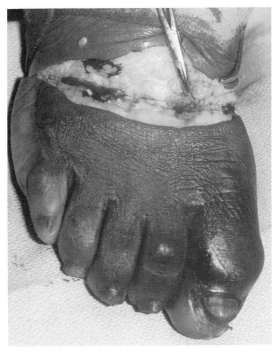

FIGURE 11–20. Early gangrenous changes of the first and second toes. The clamp is on the dorsalis pedis artery, which is sclerotic.

rigation tube is implanted. Note the plantar rounding of the metatarsals to relieve stress risers (Fig. 11–23). The wound is closed in one layer with nonabsorbable sutures (Fig. 11–24).

An excellent example of a transmetatarsal amputation in a 68-year-old diabetic man is

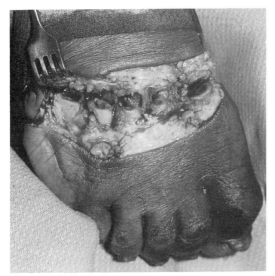

FIGURE 11–21. Division of the metatarsals on a 15° oblique line.

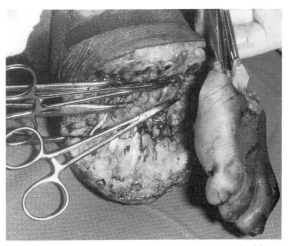

FIGURE 11–22. Removal of the distal foot by an incision parallel to the skin flaps.

depicted in Figure 11–25. When admitted to the hospital, the patient had no blood flow at the foot and had an Ischemic Index of 0.5 only at the hip. A sequential bypass graft from the aorta to the superficial femoral arteries to the posterior tibial arteries raised his Ischemic Index to 0.62 at the midfoot. This increase in circulation healed his amputation. In Figure 11–26, the residual effects of severe trauma are depicted. A compound fracture of the femur and laceration

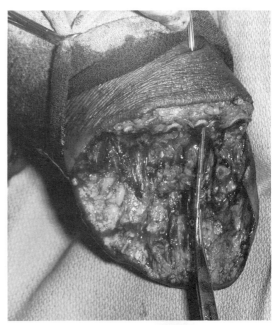

FIGURE 11–23. Placement of a Kritter irrigation tube after debridement of tendons and fascial structures. Note inferior rounding of the metatarsal osteotomies.

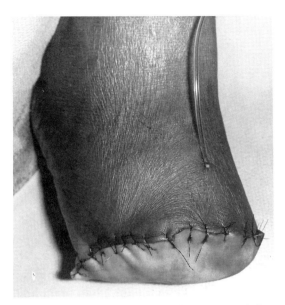

FIGURE 11–24. Completed transmetatarsal amputation.

of the femoral artery and sciatic nerve led to gangrenous toes necessitating a transmetatarsal amputation. The polypropylene ankle-foot orthosis protects the insensate foot while providing propulsive power.

Lisfranc's and Chopart's Disarticulations

These procedures were developed as disarticulations during wartime. They still have use when there is insufficient viable tissue for a short transmetatarsal amputation. When the amputations work well, they appear to be

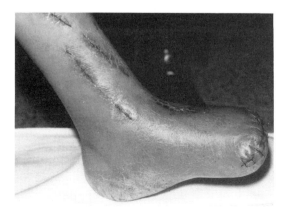

FIGURE 11–25. Transmetatarsal amputation after a successful vascular sequential bypass graft. Note the distal vascular incisions for evacuation of clots and harvesting of veins.

superior to those at a Syme's or below-knee level. Their major disadvantage is muscle imbalance, which leads to an equinovarus position of the residual foot; however, heel cord lengthening and transfer of tendons can be performed to correct the equinovarus when infection is not present.

The following case illustrates another technique for balancing the foot. Salvage of the base of the fifth metatarsal preserves the function of the peroneus brevis tendon. The patient is 55 years old with an ulcer at the first metatarsal head and an Ischemic Index of 0.65 at the midfoot (Figs. 11–27 to 11–29). Incisions are outlined for an attempt at a transmetatarsal amputation (Figs. 11–30, 11–31). Infected tissues are found medially (Fig. 11–32). The bases of the fourth and fifth metatarsals are then divided to allow

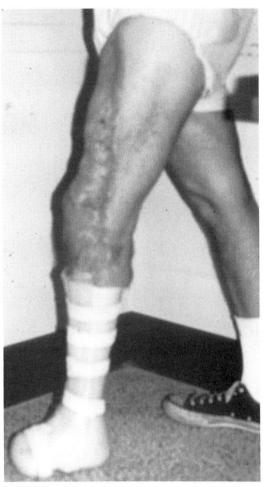

FIGURE 11–26. Ankle-foot orthosis to protect the insensate foot after fracture of the femor and laceration of the femoral artery and sciatic nerve.

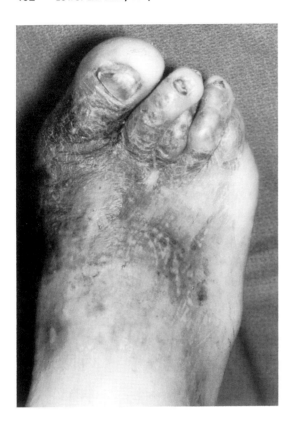

FIGURE 11-27. Dorsal view showing hallux valgus, bunion, and clawtoes.

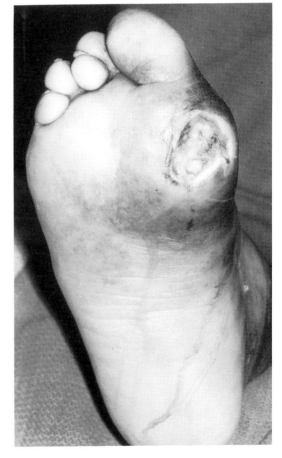

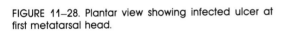

FIGURE 11-28. Plantar view showing infected ulcer at first metatarsal head.

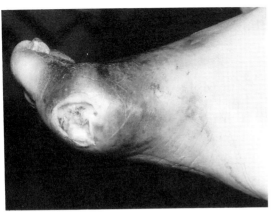

FIGURE 11–29. Medial view showing ulcer and surrounding thickened and discolored tissue.

retention of the peroneus brevis tendon (Fig. 11–33). The first, second, and third metatarsals are disarticulated (Fig. 11–34). A Kritter irrigation tube is implanted, the distal flap trimmed, and the incision closed in a single layer (Fig. 11–35). The patient walks in a polypropylene ankle-foot orthosis with a polyethylene foam toe block (Fig. 11–36).

Syme's Amputation

James Syme first described the ankle disarticulation amputation named for him in 1843.[47] Beause it retains the heel pad and the proprioceptive sense of the heel, the

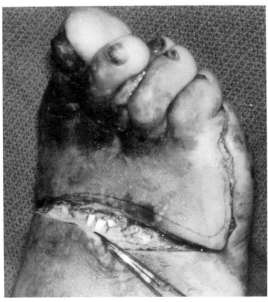

FIGURE 11–30. Incision outline for attempt at transmetatarsal amputation.

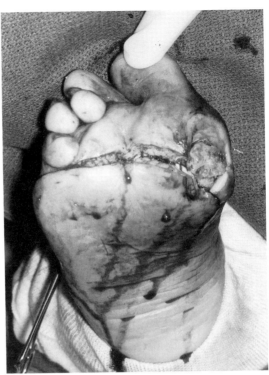

FIGURE 11–31. Plantar incision for attempt at transmetatarsal amputation.

author considers it a partial foot amputation. Its function also is superior to that of higher amputations in the leg.[55] Young healthy men, especially those in the military, adjust well to this amputation. It was rarely recommended for dysvascular and diabetic patients.[18–20, 36, 38, 39, 42] In 1954, Spittler and associates described the use of Hulnick's two-stage technique for infected war wounds. Whereas there was virtually 100% failure and infection

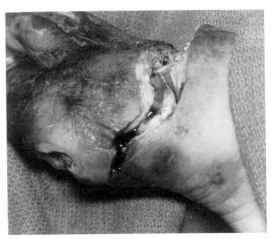

FIGURE 11–32. The medial tissues are infected and require debridement or excision.

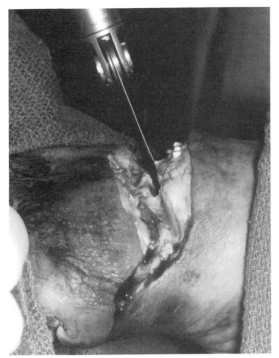

FIGURE 11–33. The fourth and fifth metatarsal bases are divided to retain action of the peroneus brevis tendon.

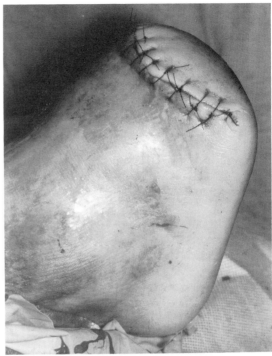

FIGURE 11–35. After the distal flap is trimmed, the wound is closed in one layer over a Kritter irrigation tube.

of the residual limb with a single-stage method, there was virtually 100% healing when the first stage was a disarticulation and the definitive second stage followed 6 to 8 weeks later.[45] This procedure was adopted on the Diabetic Service of the Los Angeles County Hospital in 1954. Additional patients were treated at Rancho Los Amigos Medical Center on the Ortho-Diabetes Service begin-

ning in 1969. With the author's private cases, over 800 patients have been treated. Series of 50 to 60 cases have been reviewed from time to time, and the success rate has varied from 85 to 86% to 93 to 94%. The first stage is considered a debriding procedure to remove an infected foot. If it heals, there is virtually 100% success in the second stage.

Single Stage

The single-stage method is used with un-infected feet. JC is 36 years of age and had incomplete cast treatment in Mexico for a clubfoot. He presented with a severe equi-

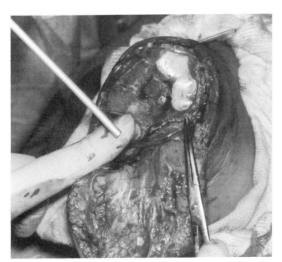

FIGURE 11–34. Disarticulation of the medial metatarsals: the fourth and fifth metatarsals are divided at the base.

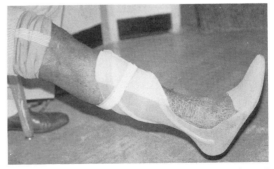

FIGURE 11–36. After final healing, the patient walks well in a polypropylene orthosis.

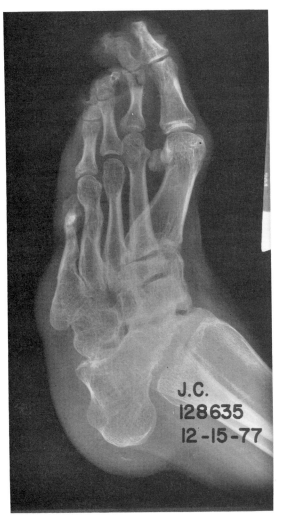

FIGURE 11–37. Severe clubfoot with residual painful equinovarus deformity.

novarus deformity of the foot with a stiff and painful ankle and midtarsal region (Figs. 11–37, 11–38). After many consultations, a Syme's amputation was performed in one stage. The flare of the distal tibia suspends the double-walled prosthesis (Figs. 11–39, 11–40).

Two Stage

The two-stage procedure is indicated in this 62-year-old diabetic woman who had a previous resection of her second toe (Fig. 11–41). Gangrene has recently spread from an infected fifth toe corn. Her Ischemic Index is 0.57 at the ankle and 0.37 at the midfoot. The incision starts 1.0 cm distal and 1.0 cm anterior to the tips of the malleoli. It crosses the dome of the talus and the sole of the foot

(Fig. 11–42). The collateral ligaments are cut alternately to allow dislocation of the talus (Fig. 11–43). A bone hook driven into the talus aids in control of the foot and in placing tension on the tissues to be cut (Fig. 11–44). Care must be taken not to damage the neurovascular structures just medial to the flexor hallucis longus tendon, which is used as a guide to the position of these structures (Fig. 11–45). Division of the Achilles tendon from the os calcis must be done carefully; there is always a small transverse ridge of bone that can deflect the knife blade, causing a buttonhole in the posterior skin (Fig. 11–46). The body of the calcaneus is freed by combined sharp and subperiosteal dissection (Fig. 11–47). Division of the plantar fascia completes

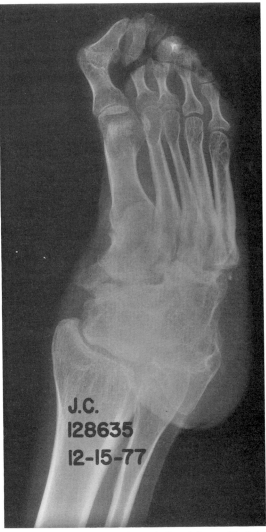

FIGURE 11–38. Note the irregularity of the ankle joint and marked deformity of the tarsus.

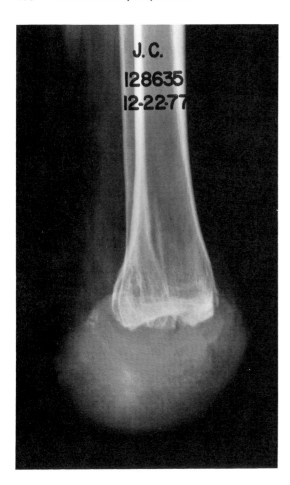

FIGURE 11–39. Syme's amputation: the plafond is left in place. Note the flare of the distal tibia, which aids in suspension of the prosthesis.

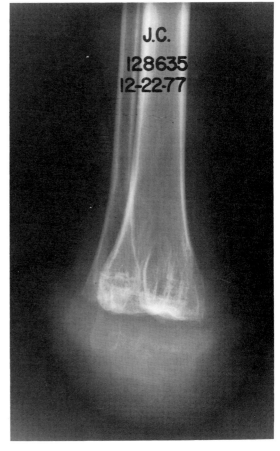

FIGURE 11–40. Syme's amputation: an anterior radiograph shows the broad surface needed for weight transmission.

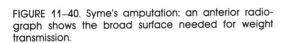

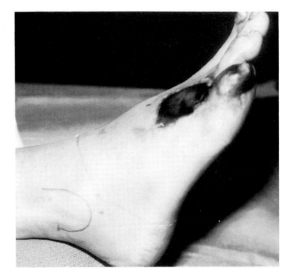

FIGURE 11–41. Two-stage Syme's amputation: infected, gangrenous forefoot in a diabetic patient. Note the outlines of the incisions.

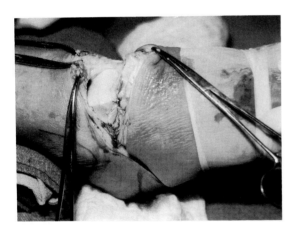

FIGURE 11–42. Two-stage Syme's amputation: an incision is made across the dome of the talus and sole of the foot.

FIGURE 11–43. Two-stage Syme's amputation: the collateral ligaments are divided.

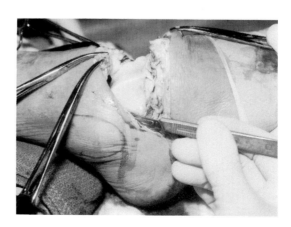

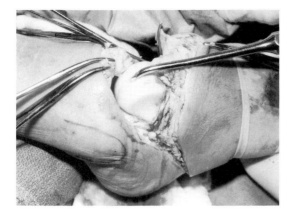

FIGURE 11–44. Two-stage Syme's amputation: a bone hook is placed in the talus.

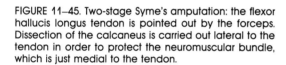

FIGURE 11–45. Two-stage Syme's amputation: the flexor hallucis longus tendon is pointed out by the forceps. Dissection of the calcaneus is carried out lateral to the tendon in order to protect the neuromuscular bundle, which is just medial to the tendon.

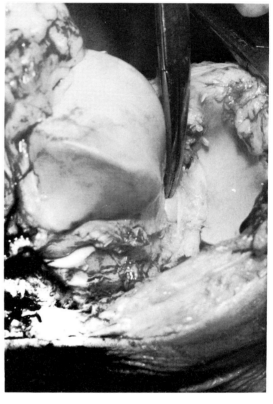

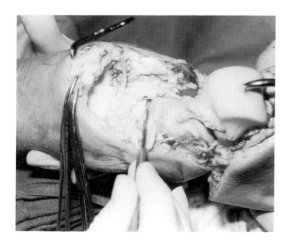

FIGURE 11–46. Two-stage Syme's amputation: a scalpel is used to divide the Achilles tendon.

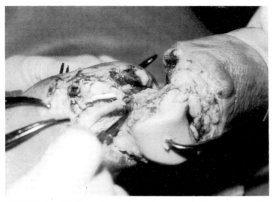

FIGURE 11–47. Two-stage Syme's amputation: sharp dissection begins the outlining of the os calcis.

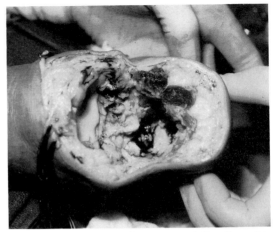

FIGURE 11–49. Two-stage Syme's amputation: the residual heel just at release of the tourniquet. Note the distal bleeding beginning on the lateral side of the sole.

the freeing of the amputated foot from the plantar pad (Fig. 11–48).

The tourniquet is released. It is rarely inflated for more than 20 minutes in most foot amputations. Bleeding is timed. With immediate bleeding, the healing rate is high (Fig. 11–49). To drain the resulting cavity, a Shirley two-lumen drain is modified by removing the filter and using the smaller tube for irrigation. No suction is used. The outflow tubing drains by gravity to a collecting bag. The irrigant can be a physiological or an antibiotic solution, depending on the surgeon's wishes (Fig. 11–50). Closure is in layers. An absorbable suture is used to anchor the deep fascia to the residual collateral ligaments (Fig. 11–51). The subcutaneous fat is sutured so as to level the skin edges (Fig. 11–52). Nylon or similar suture material is used to close the skin (Fig. 11–53).

Irrigation is continued for 48 to 72 hours, depending upon the degree of preoperative infection and the appearance of the tissues at surgery. The results of cultures taken at surgery dictate further antibiotic therapy.

The skin sutures are removed after 2 to 3 weeks. A walking cast is applied after 2 weeks. Healing is usually secure enough after 6 to 8 weeks to perform the second stage.

Second Stage. Instead of adhering to the original amputation procedure,[45] the second stage has been modified to remove the malleoli only through elliptical incisions and then smooth the residual bone edges.

The second stage Syme's amputation is demonstrated in the case of a 24-year-old girl who was severely burned on all extremities and her face. Multiple procedures remain to be performed on her face and hands. Syme's amputations have allowed her to walk with a virtually normal gait (Fig. 11–54). The resid-

Text continued on page 114

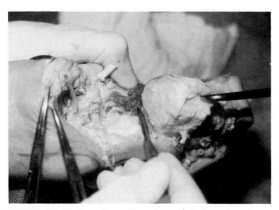

FIGURE 11–48. Two-stage Syme's amputation: the deep fascia is the only remaining structure holding the distal foot in place.

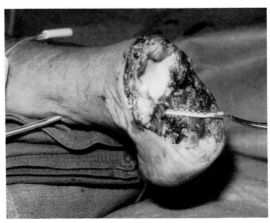

FIGURE 11–50. Two-stage Syme's amputation: placement of a modified Shirley drain.

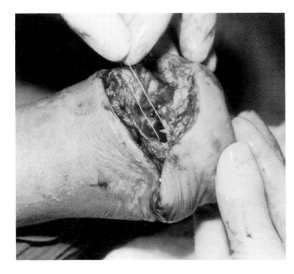

FIGURE 11–51. Two-stage Syme's amputation: the deep fascia is anchored to two collateral ligaments.

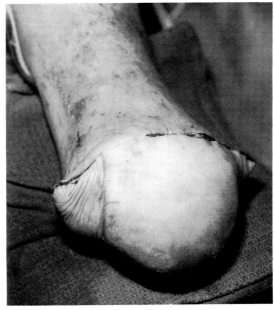

FIGURE 11–52. Two-stage Syme's amputation: the skin is leveled through closure of the subcutaneous tissue.

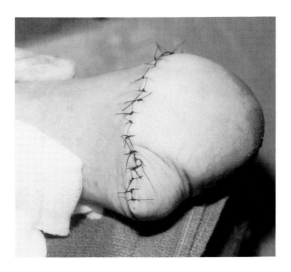

FIGURE 11–53. Two-stage Syme's amputation: the skin is closed with interrupted nylon sutures.

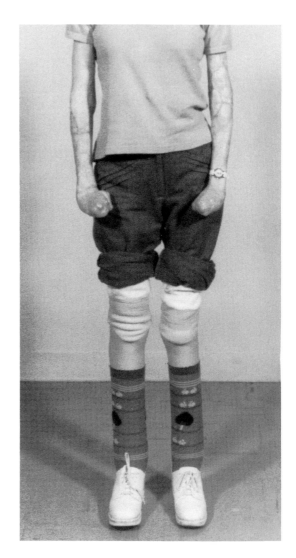

FIGURE 11–54. Severely burned girl in Syme's double-walled prostheses.

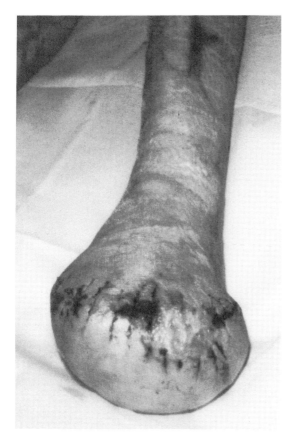

FIGURE 11–55. Two-stage Syme's amputation: healed residual limb from the first stage.

FIGURE 11–56. Two-stage Syme's amputation: a radiograph, taken after the first stage, shows a Shirley drain in place.

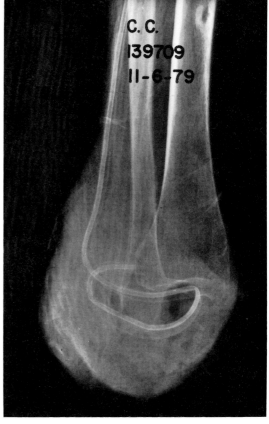

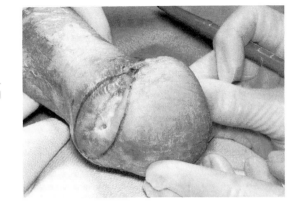

FIGURE 11–57. Two-stage Syme's amputation: the partially healed area is outlined and will be removed along with the dog-ear.

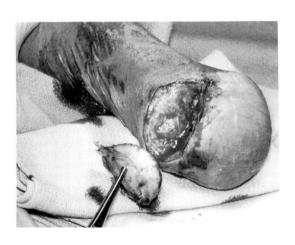

FIGURE 11–58. Two-stage Syme's amputation: the dog-ear is removed.

FIGURE 11–59. Two-stage Syme's amputation: the malleolus is removed level with the plafond.

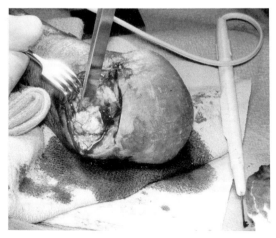

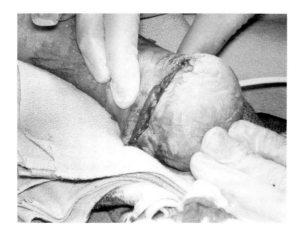

FIGURE 11–60. Two-stage Syme's amputation: the pad is centered.

ual limbs from the first stage are shown in Figures 11–55 and 11–56. The dog-ears are removed through elliptical incisions down to the malleoli (Figs. 11–57, 11–58).

The malleoli are outlined sharply and removed flush with the plafond (Fig. 11–59). The pad is then tested for tightness. If the pad centers satisfactorily, the deep fascia is sutured to the periosteum (Fig. 11–60). A similar procedure is performed on the opposite side, with removal of the dog-ear, malleolus, and flare of the bone (Fig. 11–61). The healed residual limb is shown several weeks later (Fig. 11–62).

Amputation of the Calcaneus

Large ulcers of the heel are not infrequent in elderly patients on bed rest for healing of fractures, treatment of pulmonary and abdominal diseases, and similar long-term procedures.[11] Removal of the ulcer and enough of the calcaneus to close the incision results in a foot suitable for walking. Split thickness skin grafts do not do well in this weight-bearing area. The expansions of the Achilles tendon bind it well to the residual calcaneus,

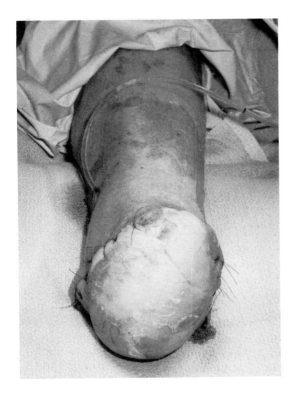

FIGURE 11–61. Completed two-stage Syme's amputation.

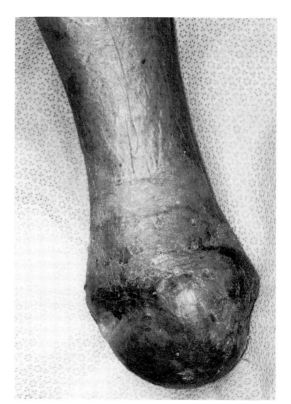

FIGURE 11–62. Completed two-stage Syme's amputation several weeks later.

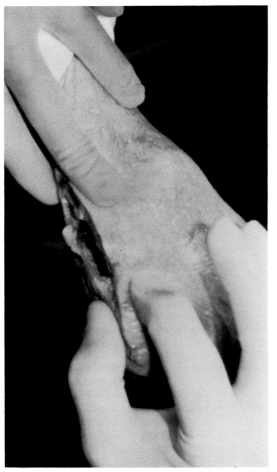

FIGURE 11–63. Excision of a heel ulcer along with a portion of the posterior os calcis.

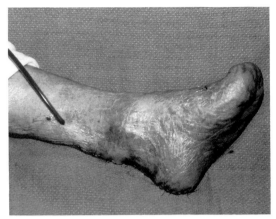

FIGURE 11–64. Shirley drain for evacuation of hematoma from raw bone surface.

and one year after surgery, a brace is no longer necessary. The patient pictured had a fractured distal femur and, during casting, developed a large ulcer on her left heel. The ulcer was removed along with the posterior half of the calaneus (Fig. 11–63). The wound was closed over a Shirley drain (Fig. 11–64). Nine months later, she is still using a polypropylene ankle-foot orthosis. Since she has a Syme's amputation of the right leg, she is extremely pleased not to have to undergo a below-knee amputation. The residual foot on the left gives her a stability she could not derive from a below-knee amputation.

REFERENCES

1. Banson BB, Lacey PE: Diabetic microangiopathy in human toes. Am J Pathol 45:41, 1964.
2. Barnes RW, Shanik GD, Slaymaker EE: An index of healing in below knee amputation: Leg blood pressure by Doppler ultrasound. Surgery 79:13, 1976.
3. Bell ET: Atherosclerotic gangrene of the lower extremities in diabetic and non-diabetic persons. Am J Clin Pathol 28:27, 1957.
4. Bessman AN: Management of the diabetic surgical patient. Compr Ther 5:57, 1979.
5. Bessman AN, Sapico FL, Tabatabai M, Montgomerie JZ: Persistence of polymicrobial abscesses in the poorly controlled diabetic host. Diabetes 35:448, 1986.
6. Brown OW: Rehabilitation of bilateral lower extremity amputees. J Bone Joint Surg 52A:687, 1970.
7. Buchbinder D, Pasch AR, Rolllins DS, et al: Results of arterial reconstruction of the foot. Arch Surg 121:673, 1986.
8. Carter Center of Emory University: Closing the gap—the problem of diabetes mellitus in the United States. Diabetes Care 8:391, 1984.
9. Carter SA: The relationship of distal systolic pressures to healing of skin lesions in limbs with arterial occlusive disease, with special reference to diabetes mellitus. Scand J Clin Lab Invest 31:Suppl 128:239, 1973.
10. Clark-Williams MJ: The elderly double amputee. Geront Clin 11:283, 1969.
11. Crandall RC, Wagner FW Jr: Partial and total calcanectomy: A review of thirty-one consecutive cases over a ten-year period. J Bone Joint Surg 63A:152, 1981.
12. Dickhaut SC, Dehee JC, Page CP: Nutritional status: Importance in predicting wound healing after amputation. J Bone Joint Surg 66A:71, 1984.
13. Ecker MD, Jacobs SS: Lower extremity amputations in diabetic patients. Diabetes 19:189, 1970.
14. Edwards WH, Mulheirn JL Jr: The role of graft material in femoral tibial bypass grafts. Am Surg 191:721, 1980.
15. Gibbons GW, Wheelock FC Jr, Hoar CS Jr, et al: Predicting success of forefoot amputations in diabetics by noninvasive testing. Arch Surg 114:1034, 1979.
16. Goldner MG: The fate of the second leg in the diabetic amputee. Diabetes 9:100, 1960.
17. Goodman J, Bessman AN, Teget BN, Wagner FW Jr: Risk factors in local procedures for diabetic gangrene. Surg Gynecol Obstet 143:587, 1976.
18. Harris RI: Syme's amputation—the technical details essential for success. J Bone Joint Surg 38B:614, 1956.
19. Harris RI: The history and the development of Syme's amputation. Artif Limbs 6:4, 1961.
20. Hunter GA: Results of minor foot amputations for ischemia of the lower extremity in diabetics and nondiabetics. Can J Surg 18:273, 1975.
21. Jacobs RL, Karmody AM, Wirth C, et al: The team approach in salvage of the diabetic foot. Surg Annu 9:231, 1977.
22. King TA, Yao JST, Flynn WR, et al: Extending operability by pre-bypass intraoperative arteriography. In Bergan JJ, Yao JST (eds): Evaluation and Treatment of Upper and Lower Extremity Circulatory Disorders. New York, Grune & Stratton, 1984.
23. Kritter AE: A technique for salvage of the infected diabetic gangrenous foot. Orthop Clin North Am 4:21, 1973.
24. Lempke RE, King RD, Kaiser GC, et al: Amputation for arteriosclerosis obliterans. Arch Surg 86:406, 1963.
25. Lo Gerfo FW, Corson JD, Mannick JA: Improved results with femoral popliteal vein grafts for limb salvage. Arch Surg 112:567, 1977.
26. Louie TJ, Bartlett JG, Tally FP, Sherwood LG: Aerobic and anaerobic bacteria in diabetic foot ulcers. Ann Intern Med 85:461, 1976.
27. Maurer AC: The therapy of diabetes. Am Sci 67:422, 1979.
28. Mc Kittrick LS, Mc Kittrick JB, Risley TS: Transmetatarsal amputation for infection or gangrene in patients with diabetes mellitus. Ann Surg 130:826, 1949.
29. Mehta K, Hobson RW 2d, Jamil Z, et al: Fallibility of Doppler ankle pressure in predicting healing of transmetatarsal amputation. J Surg Res 28:466, 1980.
30. Meyer LC: Lawnmower injuries in children. Orthop Trans 11:183, 1987.
31. Most RS, Sinnock P: The epidemiology of lower

extremity amputation in diabetic individuals. Diabetes Care 6:87, 1983.

32. Mulder DW, Lambert EH, Bastron JA, Sprague RG: The neuropathies associated with diabetes mellitus. A clinical and electromyographic study of one hundred and three unselected diabetic patients. Neurology 11:275, 1961.

33. Pedersen HE, Day AJ: The transmetatarsal amputation in peripheral vascular disease. J Bone Joint Surg 36A:1190, 1954.

34. A Plan for the Prevention of Lower Extremity Amputations of Persons with Diabetes. Division of Diabetes Control, Center For Prevention Services, Centers For Disease Control, November 1986.

35. Pratt TC: Gangrene and infection in the diabetic. Med Clin North Am 49:987, 1965.

36. Rentoul WW: Syme's amputation. J Bone Joint Surg 36B:672, 1954.

37. A Report of The National Diabetes Advisory Board. National Institute of Health Publication No. 81-2284, Bethesda, Maryland, November 1980, p 25.

38. Romano RL, Burgess EM: Level selection in lower extremity amputations. Clin Orthop 74:177, 1971.

39. Rosenman LD: Syme amputation for ischemic disease in the foot. Am J Surg 188:194, 1969.

40. Rossini AA, Hare JW: How to control the blood glucose level in the surgical diabetic patient. Arch Surg 111:945, 1976.

41. Sapico FL, Canawati HN, Wittie JL, et al: Quantitative aerobic and anaerobic bacteriology of infected diabetic feet. J Clin Microbiol 12:413, 1980.

42. Sarmiento A, Warren WD: A reevaluation of lower extremity amputations. Surg Gynecol Obstet 129:799, 1969.

43. Sharp CS, Bessman AN, Wagner FW Jr, Garland D: Microbiology of deep tissue in diabetic gangrene. Diabetes 25:385, 1976.

44. Siperstein MD, Unger RH, Madison LL: Studies of muscle capillary basement membranes in normal subjects, diabetic, and prediabetic patients. J Clin Invest 47:1973, 1968.

45. Spittler AW, Brenner JS, Payne JW: Syme amputation performed in two stages. J Bone Joint Surg 36A:37, 1954.

46. Spring M, Kahn S: Nonclostridial gas infections in the diabetic. Arch Intern Med 88:373, 1951.

47. Syme J: Amputation at the ankle joint. London and Edinburgh Monthly, Journal of Medical Science 2:93, 1843.

48. Thomas PK, Lascelles RG: The pathology of diabetic neuropathy. Q J Med 35:489, 1966.

49. Veith FJ, Moso CM, Daly V, et al: New approaches to limb salvage by extended anatomic bypass and prosthetic reconstruction to foot arteries. Surgery 84:6, 1978.

50. Vital and Health Statistics, Series 13, No. 32DHHS, Publication No. 85-1743, Public Health Service, Washington, DC, US Government Printing Office, March 1985.

51. Volpicelli KJ, Chambers RB, Wagner FW Jr: Ambulation levels of bilateral lower extremity amputees. An analysis of one hundred and three cases. J Bone Joint Surg 65A:599, 1983.

52. Wagner FW Jr: Amputations of the foot and ankle. Clin Orthop 122:62, 1977.

53. Wagner FW Jr: The dysvascular foot: A system for diagnosis and treatment. Foot Ankle 2:64, 1981.

54. Wagner FW Jr, Buggs H: Use of Doppler ultrasound in determining healing levels in diabetic dysvascular lower extremity problems. In Bergen JJ, Yao JST (eds): Gangrene and Severe Ischemia of the Lower Extremities. New York, Grune & Stratton, 1978, pp 131–138.

55. Waters RL, Perry J, Antonelli D, Hislop H: Energy costs of walking of amputees. The influence of level of amputation. J Bone Joint Surg 58A:42, 1976.

56. Watkins AL, Liao SJ: Rehabilitation of persons with bilateral amputation of lower extremities. JAMA 166:1584, 1958.

57. Whitehouse FW, Jurgensen C, Block MA: The later life of the diabetic amputee. Another look at the fate of the second leg. Diabetes 17:520, 1968.

58. Wood MB, Cooney WP, Irons GB: Lower extremity salvage and reconstruction by free tissue transfer. Clin Orthop 201:151, 1985.

12

Below-Knee Amputation

Wesley S. Moore, M.D.

The most common amputation level selected for the management of lower extremity pathology is below the knee. Its popularity is due to its superiority in prosthetic rehabilitation and healing for the most common indication, lower extremity ischemia.

Advances in prosthetic fabrication and rehabilitation, which have allowed bipedal ambulation, reflect the importance and increasing use of this amputation level.

INDICATIONS

Ischemic Gangrene

The most common indication for below-knee amputation is irreversible ischemia of the lower extremity, producing rest pain, limited infection, or gangrene. This accounts for 76% of amputations performed in Veterans Administration hospitals in 1964.[1] Although limited ischemia may be controlled with amputation of a toe, a ray, or part of the foot, the ischemic process is usually more extensive, and the next available amputation level will be below the knee. The reader is referred to the chapters on amputation level selection for a more extended discussion of the criteria for selecting a specific level.

In the past, below-knee amputation was rarely selected for ischemic gangrene; above-knee amputation was considered the level of choice because of the likelihood of healing. Previous surveys suggested that the ratio between above-knee and below-knee amputation for ischemic gangrene was as high as 2.4 to 1.[1] With the recognition of the importance of the knee joint and the likelihood of healing at the below-knee level, this ratio has markedly reversed, and now the below-knee to above-knee ratio is in the range of 2 or 3 to 1.[2] At present, it is easier to describe the contraindications to amputation at the below-knee level rather than specific indications. Contraindications to below-knee amputation include the presence of infection, ulceration, gangrene, or dependent rubor at the highest feasible below-knee amputation site. Other contraindications include knee joint pathology or a paretic extremity. A patient who has suffered a stroke and has hemiparesis on the side of the proposed amputation is probably not a good candidate for below-knee amputation because of the knee flexion deformity that will occur with the imbalance of muscle innervation. In the absence of one of the above contraindications and with one of the quantitative methods of determining the adequacy of skin blood flow, below the knee becomes the level of choice.

Other Indications

Other indications for below-knee amputation include congenital deformity, tumor, trauma, and infection. The indications for selecting the below-knee level for these conditions depend on the location and extent of the process, provided there is an adequate blood supply and good skin at the level of the below-knee amputation site.

ADVANTAGES

Healing Potential

Even in the absence of skin blood flow measurement, healing of a below-knee amputation is highly likely when performed for ischemic gangrene. Healing rates as high as 83% have been reported in cases in which test results did not contribute to amputation level selection. When the amputation level is selected on the basis of test results, healing rates approach 100%.[2, 4–6]

Prosthetic Fitting

Techniques for socket fitting and prosthetic fabrication rapidly advanced after the end of World War II. The techniques for prosthetic fitting of the below-knee amputation site have become highly advanced and will continue to progress with the use of computer modeling. The ability to achieve a comfortable and durable prosthetic fit is excellent.

Ambulation

It has been stated that if patients are able to walk before amputation, it is virtually guaranteed that they will walk with below-knee prostheses after successful healing; the likelihood of this approaches 100%, even in geriatric amputees.[2–6] Furthermore, there are series reporting successful bipedal ambulation in patients with bilateral below-knee amputations.[5]

Durability

Once a below-knee amputation heals and the patient is properly fit with a prosthesis, the frequency of late breakdown requiring higher revision is extremely low. A 96% durability rate throughout the life of the patient has been reported.[5]

PREOPERATIVE PREPARATION

On occasion, amputation must be done under emergency conditions. However, when time permits, proper preparation of the patient reduces morbidity and mortality and increases the likelihood of prosthetic rehabilitation. This is particularly true in the geriatric patient requiring amputation for lower extremity ischemia. There are several factors that can be addressed in order to improve overall outcome.

Nutrition

Patients with lower extremity ischemia, especially in the geriatric age group, may be severely malnourished owing to the consequences of ischemic pain and gangrene. Assessment of their nutritional status—judged by current compared with optimum weight, measurement of the serum albumin/globulin ratio, and skin testing for evidence of anergy related to a catabolic state—provides the clinician with ample information on the nutritional state of the patient. If there is evidence of severe nutritional depletion and time permits, this condition should be corrected before surgery. Pain and infection control may permit an improvement in oral alimentation and correction of a catabolic state. Parenteral hyperalimentation for 1 or 2 weeks before amputation may also be feasible and significantly contribute to the healing potential after amputation.

Physical Therapy

Even though the patient may not be ambulatory owing to the nature of the process requiring amputation, it is possible for the physical therapist to implement upper extremity conditioning exercises and work with the opposite lower extremity to maintain joint mobility, muscle tone, and strength. Time spent in physical therapy of the three unaffected extremities improves the rehabilitation potential and shortens subsequent hospitalization.

Infection Control

Patients who require amputation for primary infection, the infectious complications of diabetes mellitus, or infection complicating ischemic gangrene are at particular risk for amputation failure due to infectious complications at the below-knee amputation site. This risk can be significantly reduced by proper preoperative preparation and infectious disease control. This includes appropriate antibiotic management based on the identification of the organisms by culture and the selection of specific antibiotics by sensitivity testing. Space infection of the forefoot must be appropriately drained, debrided, or both. Finally, if there is extensive space infection of the forefoot that is not amenable to conservative debridement, an open guillotine amputation at the malleoli is a very effective means of controlling the source of sepsis from the foot. This preparatory guillotine amputation, in conjunction with systemic antibiotic therapy, permits primary below-knee amputation several days later.[7]

General Medical Management

The elderly patient requiring amputation for diabetic infection or ischemic gangrene is likely to have multisystem organ involvement. Time taken to optimize medical management of diabetes mellitus and to correct diabetic acidosis is of particular importance. Identification and correction of cardiac abnormalities, including congestive failure, arrhythmia, cardiac ischemia, and hypertension, significantly reduces morbidity and mortality. Assessment of pulmonary function and pulmonary physical therapy help to identify or prevent significant pulmonary complications after amputation. Finally, patients with lower extremity ischemia may have associated renal failure. Proper identification of this condition, followed by fluid and diuretic therapy, may be helpful in improving renal function before amputation.

SURGICAL TECHNIQUE

Several alternative approaches to residual limb length and skin flap configuration are available with below-knee amputation. Although variations are mentioned, details are given for only the approach most recommended.

Tourniquet

If below-knee amputation is being performed in a patient with a normal blood supply, the use of a tourniquet expedites the operation and reduces blood loss. The tourniquet is placed at the high thigh level before preparation of the extremity; a pressure setting of 250 mmHg at the time of inflation provides a dry field. The tourniquet should not be inflated until the surgeon is ready to make the incision.

Preparation of the Extremity

After satisfactory anesthesia has been induced, the extremity can be positioned on an elevated foot rest or stirrup. If the indication for operation is ischemic gangrene or infection, the foot of the extremity can be placed in a sterile plastic bag and the drawstring tied (Fig. 12–1). In patients with a normal blood supply, the hair of the extremity can be removed by either careful shaving or the use of a depilatory. In cases of ischemia, the amount of hair present on the extremity is minimal, and it is probably safer not to remove it.

The antiseptic preparation of the skin can be left to the usual choice of the surgeon. Povidone-iodine (Betadine) soap followed by povidone-iodine skin preparation is commonly employed. The author's preference is to use 2% tincture of iodine; there is no preparatory scrub, and the iodine is simply painted on once without scrubbing. The extremity is then placed in a tubular stockinette, and two split sheets—one placed proximally with the split ends down and the other placed distally with the split ends up—are an excellent way to provide maximum exposure of the extremity with coverage of the field (Fig. 12–2).

Skin Flaps

Before marking the incision, the surgeon should decide the appropriate length of the

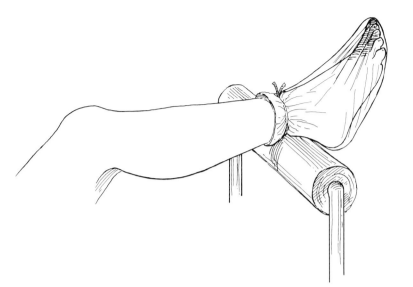

FIGURE 12–1. The patient's leg is elevated on a transverse bar, and the gangrenous portion of the extremity is enclosed in a sterile plastic bag with the drawstring tied.

residual limb. Often the indication for amputation, such as tumor or trauma, dictates the residual limb's length. However, if the surgeon has a choice, while attempting to encompass the involved tissue and maximize the available blood supply, a relatively long residual limb is desirable for prosthetic fitting and stability in ambulation. A length of 7 to 8 inches below the knee joint is ideal.

There are three primary configurations for skin flaps, which can be further modified depending on the available tissues. A circular skin incision is closed transversely, using no flaps (Fig. 12–3). A fishmouth incision creates equal anterior and posterior flaps (Fig. 12–4). However, a long or total posterior flap (Fig. 12–5) has been shown to be the most effective configuration in patients with lower extremity ischemia, the most common indication for amputation.

Once the residual limb's length has been determined, a mark is made on the anterior line of the skin incision, approximately 1.5 cm distal to the point of anticipated division of the tibia. This line is continued around the circumference of the calf medially and laterally to points representing approximately one half of the circumference. The anteroposterior diameter of the calf at that level is measured, and this diameter plus approximately 1.5 cm represents the length needed for the posterior flap. This point is marked on the posterior aspect of the calf, and the marking is continued medially and laterally, encompassing approximately one half of the available circumference at that point. The distal portion of the proximal circumferential skin marking is now connected with a longitudinal line to the proximal part of the distal circumferential mark,

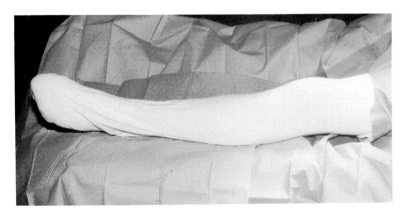

FIGURE 12–2. After the extremity has been appropriately prepared, a stockinette is drawn over the entire length of the leg, and it is draped with a double split sheet.

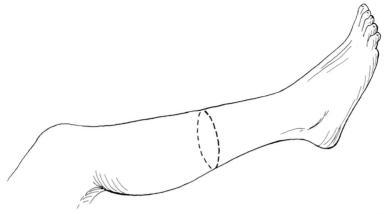

FIGURE 12–3. Artist's rendition of a circular skin incision that will be closed in a transverse fashion. No flaps are used.

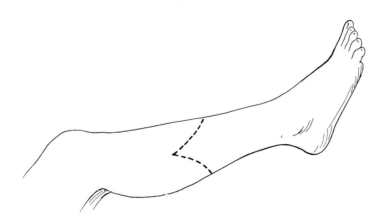

FIGURE 12–4. Typical appearance of a fishmouth incision.

FIGURE 12–5. Outline of the skin incision used for a total long posterior flap. The anterior skin incision is approximately one-half the transverse diameter. The horizontal portion of the posterior skin incision is measured as the total diameter of the calf at the level of the anterior skin incision plus 1.5 cm.

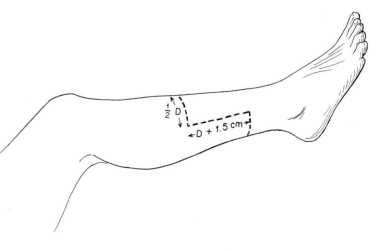

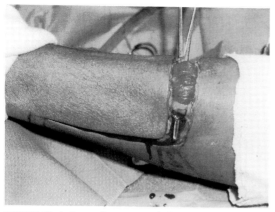

FIGURE 12–6. Operating room photograph demonstrating encirclement of the muscles of the anterior compartment with the clamp before division.

medially and laterally. This constitutes the proposed line of skin incision for a long posterior flap (Fig. 12–5). The skin incision is then made along the outline through the skin, subcutaneous tissue, and fascia. This skin incision effectively divides the long and short saphenous veins, which should be clamped and ligated.

Muscle and Bone Division

An early division of the tibia and fibula permits easier exposure of the tibial neurovascular structures. The muscles of the anterior compartment, including the tibialis anterior, extensor hallucis longus, extensor digitorum longus, and peroneus tertius, are bluntly mobilized and divided at the same level as the anterior skin incision (Figs. 12–

6, 12–7). The anterior tibial neurovascular bundle is found coursing along the interosseous membrane. This neurovascular bundle can be encircled, clamped, divided, and ligated (Fig. 12–8). With the muscles of the anterior compartment divided, the tibia can be mobilized in a subperiosteal plane. The tibia is initially divided 2 cm proximal to the skin incision (Fig. 12–9). The fibula is then mobilized in a subperiosteal plane and is divided in a convenient location (Fig. 12–10). It will later be resected back approximately 1 cm proximal to the tibial division. Once both bones are divided, the distal end of the extremity can be displaced posteriorly, and the muscles adhering to the posterior aspect of the tibia and fibula—the flexor digitorum longus, the tibialis posterior, and the flexor hallucis longus—are sharply separated from the tibia and fibula, down to the level of the proposed muscle division at the distal end of the posterior flap (Fig. 12–11). At this point, the remaining portion of the flexor digitorum longus and tibialis posterior are debrided off the posterior myocutaneous flap and resected flush with the distal cut edge of the tibia. The posterior tibial artery, nerve, and vein are identified at the distal end of the myocutaneous flap. The posterior tibial nerve is separated from the neurovascular bundle. The vascular bundle is then clamped, divided, and ligated. Similarly, the peroneal vascular bundle is identified, mobilized, clamped, divided, and ligated (Fig. 12–12). The muscles of the posterior compartment are then divided flush with the distal cut edge of the skin flap; this includes the flexor hallucis longus and the gastrocnemius-soleus

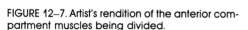
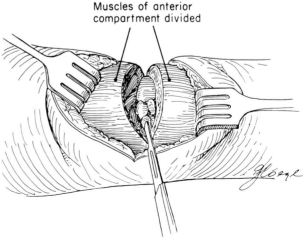

Muscles of anterior compartment divided

FIGURE 12–7. Artist's rendition of the anterior compartment muscles being divided.

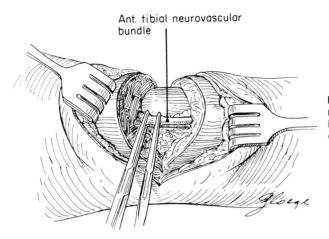

Ant. tibial neurovascular bundle

FIGURE 12–8. After the anterior compartment muscles are divided, the neurovascular bundle is identified, mobilized, and divided between clamps before ligation.

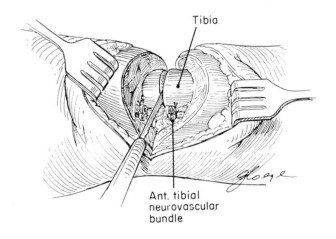

Tibia

FIGURE 12–9. The tibia is mobilized in a sub-periosteal plane and divided approximately 2 cm proximal to the line of skin incision.

Ant. tibial neurovascular bundle

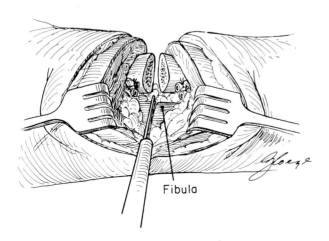

FIGURE 12–10. The fibula is divided at a convenient location at this time. It will later be shortened in the final preparation for bone division.

Fibula

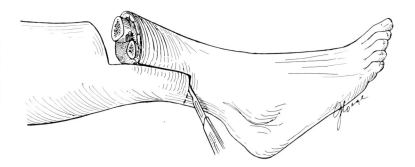

FIGURE 12–11. After the tibia and fibula are divided, the distal, or specimen, end of the extremity can be dislocated posteriorly as the posterior muscles are stripped off the bones and the division of the posterior skin flap is completed.

muscle group. The amputated limb is then passed off. The posterior tibial nerve is mobilized proximal to a point beneath the tibia, where it is clamped, divided, and ligated. This places the subsequent neuroma well proximal to the end of the bone and keeps it from being traumatized. The sural nerve is also mobilized from the posterior skin flap and divided well proximal to the bone. This keeps the neuroma out of weight-bearing contact.

Attention now returns to finishing bone division. The periosteum on the anterior lateral and medial aspect of the tibia is mobi-

lized to permit the anterior border of the bone to have a 60° bevel. The plane of the bevel is parallel with the patella. After the tibia is beveled, the cut edges are filed smooth and rounded (Fig. 12–13). The periosteum of the fibula as then mobilized allows transverse smooth division of the fibula approximately 1 cm proximal to the tibia. The objective is to obtain a residual limb that has a cylindrical, as opposed to a conical, configuration (Fig. 12–14). The wound is then copiously irrigated with an antibiotic-saline mixture, and meticulous hemostasis is achieved. If the operation is done in a patient

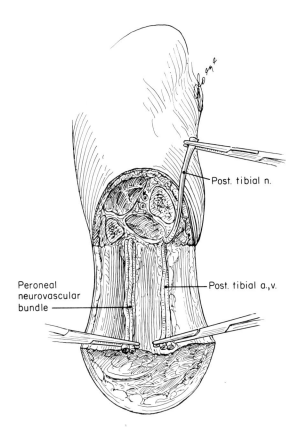

Post. tibial n.

Peroneal neurovascular bundle

Post. tibial a.,v.

FIGURE 12–12. Control of the vascular bundles of the peroneal and posterior tibial compartment (artist's conception). The posterior tibial nerve is separated, freed to the point where it emerges underneath the tibia, and then divided high to avoid positioning the neuroma at a point of prosthetic contact.

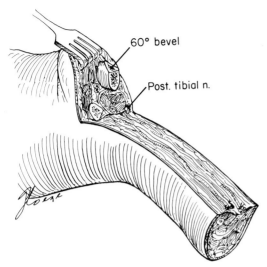

FIGURE 12–13. The tibia is beveled at a 60° angle, and the edges are rounded.

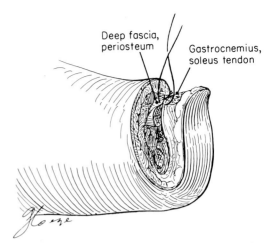

FIGURE 12–15. The initial sutures between the tendons of the gastrocnemius and soleus muscles and the anterior periosteum of the tibia, with overlying fascia, effect a myoplasty.

with a normal blood supply, a suction catheter drain is placed and brought out through a separate stab wound before closure. If the operation is done for ischemia and the wound is relatively dry, no drain is required.

Closure

With the muscles remaining attached to the posterior skin flap, the closure is performed to effect a myoplasty. Absorbable sutures are used to attach the fascia and tendinous portion of the gastrocnemius-soleus group to the periosteum and fascia at the anterior tibial line (Fig. 12–15). This is performed with interrupted sutures, then the remaining portion of the fascial edges are approximated with interrupted sutures (Fig. 12–16).

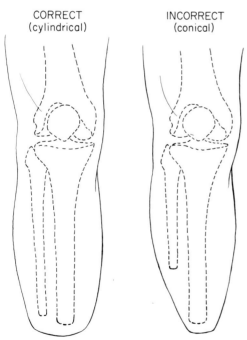

FIGURE 12–14. The fibula is then divided at its definitive location, just slightly shorter than the tibia, in order to maintain a cylindrical configuration of the residual limb. This provides optimal characteristics for prosthetic fitting. A conical shape of the residual limb, occurring with a high division of the fibula, is to be avoided.

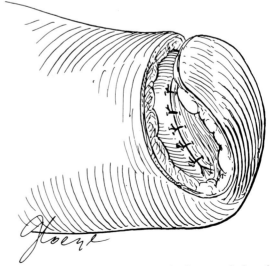

FIGURE 12–16. Following myoplasty, the remainder of the deep fascia is closed with interrupted sutures.

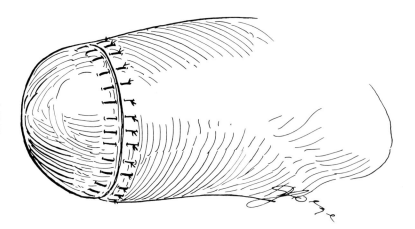

FIGURE 12–17. Perfect edge-to-edge skin coaptation is achieved with carefully placed vertical mattress sutures.

Closure of the skin is particularly critical in patients undergoing amputation for ischemia. A careful edge-to-edge coaptation is mandatory. The author discourages the use of any toothed grasping forcep to avoid traumatizing the skin edges. Interrupted vertical mattress sutures effect a perfect edge-to-edge coaptation (Fig. 12–17). If significant dog-ears remain on the medial and lateral aspects of the residual limb, they can be trimmed to create a well-molded residual limb.

Dressing

The author prefers to use some form of a rigid dressing, either alone or as part of an immediate postoperative prosthesis.[4–6, 8] The rigid dressing has the advantage of immobilizing the wound to improve healing, control edema, avoid knee flexion contracture, and protect the incision from extrinsic trauma.

A nonadhering fine mesh silk is applied over the incision site (Fig. 12–18). One ounce of fluffed-out lamb's wool is placed over the end of the residual limb for a soft interface material (Fig. 12–19). This is held in place by a Lycra-Spandex stocking that is drawn over the end of the residual limb and up the thigh (Fig. 12–20).

At this point, the prosthetist can apply a rigid dressing or an immediate postoperative prosthesis, as described in Chapter 16.

POSTOPERATIVE MANAGEMENT

The objectives of postoperative care include quick recovery, minimization of complications, and rapid achievement of bipedal ambulation on a prosthesis.

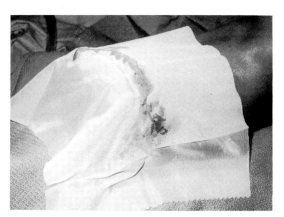

FIGURE 12–18. The initial phase of the dressing begins with the placement of a nonadherent, fine mesh silk over the suture line.

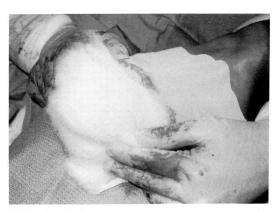

FIGURE 12–19. Fluffed-out lamb's wool placed over the end of the residual limb will serve as a soft, compressible interface material.

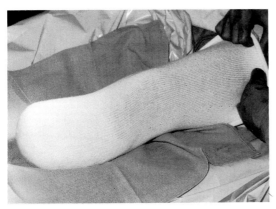

FIGURE 12–20. A Lycra-Spandex stocking is drawn over the lamb's wool and up the leg before placement of the immediate-fit prosthetic cast.

Nutritional Support

As soon as the patient has recovered from anesthesia, a progressively calorie-intensive diet should be implemented in anticipation of increasing physical activity and the need for caloric support.

The excessive use of narcotics for pain management interferes with activity and alimentary function. Use of a rigid dressing and early ambulation appear to minimize postoperative pain and requirements for narcotic medication.

Antibiotic Therapy

If the indication for amputation was infection or gangrene, organism-specific antibiotics should be continued for a full therapeutic course of 7 to 10 days.

Pulmonary Function

One of the major causes of postoperative morbidity and mortality in the geriatric amputee is pulmonary dysfunction in the form of either atelectasis or pneumonia. As soon as the patient wakes from anesthesia, deep-breathing exercises and coughing should be actively encouraged to clear secretions and open atelectatic air spaces. Use of the incentive spirometer and, if necessary, intermittent positive pressure breathing is recommended; once the patient begins ambulation, this will be the most potent stimulus for increasing respiratory activity.

Venous Thromboembolism

In the past, one of the common complications of lower extremity amputation was pulmonary embolism. The incidence of this complication varies from center to center but seems, in general, to be on the decline. Patients who are at high risk for deep venous thrombosis and pulmonary embolism should be treated with subcutaneous low-dose heparin; other treatments include the use of an elastic support stocking on the opposite extremity and early ambulation.

Physical Activity and Ambulation

Physical therapy should resume the morning after amputation. The extent of physical activity is determined, in part, by the patient's general condition and by the technique of rigid dressing application, specifically, whether an immediate postoperative prosthesis with a pylon and foot has been used. Exercise involving the upper extremities, the opposite leg, and hip flexion with quadriceps-tensing on the opposite side should be initiated.

As soon as patients are strong enough, and certainly no later than the second or third postoperative day, they should be encouraged to get out of bed with assistance and stand on the opposite (sound) lower extremity. This can be facilitated with a portable walker and ultimately advanced to the use of parallel bars in the physical therapy department. If an immediate postoperative prosthesis has been applied, the program of progressive, limited weight-bearing ambulation is initiated.

Dressing Changes

Whether or not an immediate postoperative prosthesis is employed, the dressing should be a rigid cast immobilizing the knee joint. Unless there is some compelling reason to remove the cast early, such as an unusual amount of pain or unexplained fever, the first cast change is performed 7 to 10 days after operation. At this time, the residual limb is inspected for healing. If healing is satisfactory, a second cast is applied. This remains in place for an additional 10 days, then a third cast is applied. At the end of the 27th to 30th postoperative day, if healing is satisfactory, there should be sufficient residual limb maturation to proceed with the fitting of an intermediate prosthesis—a below-knee, patellar tendon-bearing socket that allows full knee joint function.

POSTOPERATIVE COMPLICATIONS

Death

In younger, otherwise healthy patients requiring lower extremity amputation for tumor or trauma, the procedure's mortality rate is very low. Most mortality associated with lower extremity amputation occurs in geriatric patients requiring amputation for ischemia or complications of diabetes mellitus. Most of these deaths are due to cardiovascular complications, including myocardial infarction, congestive heart failure, stroke, and visceral ischemic complications. Approximately one half of the deaths due to cardiovascular disease are related to myocardial infarction.

Pulmonary Complications

Pulmonary complications include varying degrees of atelectasis, pneumonia, or pulmonary embolism.

The incidence of septic pulmonary complications has been approximated as 8%.[5] It should be emphasized that this complication rate is maximized in patients who are kept on bed rest, have limited activity, and are maintained in a debilitated state.

The incidence of pulmonary embolism has been estimated to range from 4 to 38%.[5, 9] Deep venous thrombosis and pulmonary embolism may be particularly prevalent in patients after amputation. Division of major veins leads to stagnation of blood flow and thrombosis. If the patient is kept on bed rest, these conditions are further aggravated, and the risk of deep venous thrombosis is markedly augmented.

Wound Hematoma

The presence of a hematoma in a below-knee amputation site is a major complication. Every effort should be directed at avoiding this complication, and for the most part, it is preventable.

The patient undergoing amputation for lower extremity ischemia usually has a hemostatic wound before closure. If the wound is moderately "wet," a drain or suction catheter should be placed in the depth of the wound to prevent hematoma formation. If a hematoma is discovered because of complaints of pain leading to early cast removal, it is probably best to return the patient to the operating room for drainage under sterile conditions and repeat primary closure.

Skin Necrosis

At the time of the first cast change, if there are minimal edges of skin necrosis that are dry, they can be treated expectantly with continued application of a rigid dressing but minimal vertical loading of the residual limb on a prosthesis. However, if areas of major flap necrosis are seen, it is probably best to return the patient to the operating room for an early revision and new primary closure. This avoids the problem of necrotic breakdown and secondary infection.

Wound Infection

Since one of the major indications for lower extremity amputation is infection and gangrene, the potential for wound infection is high. The incidence ranges from 1.8 to 28%, depending on the preoperative indication.[5, 10]

If the infection is manifested by cellulitis and skin erythema, systemic antibiotic therapy should be initiated. However, if there is evidence of a deep wound infection with abscess formation, the only option is to open the process and drain it widely. In the case of the patient with a compromised blood supply, this procedure may well jeopardize the potential of ultimate healing at the below-knee level. However, a trial of conservative therapy should be initiated before making a decision to reamputate at a higher level.

Flexion Contracture of the Knee Joint

This complication is usually seen in patients who are treated with a soft dressing after amputation. In this instance, when the patient awakes from anesthesia and senses the pain, the first response is to flex the knee and the hip joint. Once this happens, it is virtually impossible to get the patient to relax sufficiently to re-extend the knee joint. If this condition is allowed to persist, a knee flexion contracture ultimately develops and may not be reversible with active physical therapy. This complication is best prevented by the use of a rigid, knee-immobilizing dressing.

RESULTS

A good result of below-knee amputation can be defined as a live patient who proceeds to rapid primary healing, is fit with a comfortable prosthesis, returns to bipedal ambulation, and is able to continue the same type of activity that was feasible before amputation. In general, these objectives are easily achieved in patients in the younger age group who undergo amputation unrelated to vascular disease. The challenge is to achieve these objectives in the geriatric amputee in whom the amputation was performed for the complications of advanced vascular disease or diabetic infection.

Mortality

The trend away from above-knee amputation for vascular disease to below-knee amputation has had its most major impact in the reduction of in-hospital mortality. Previous reports of above-knee amputation indicate a mortality rate of up to 35% following that operation.[1-3, 6, 9, 10] However, with the increasing use of below-knee amputation, the mortality rate has dropped to an average of 7% with a range of 4 to 17%.[1, 10-12] Furthermore, with the use of immediate postoperative prostheses, the author has reported on three separate occasions his experience with below-knee amputation with no deaths. The initial report documented 20 consecutive below-knee amputations.[4] The second report details 113 below-knee amputations with immediate postoperative prosthesis placement, which were also performed without a death.[5] Finally, a combined study at two Veterans Administration hospitals reports 142 below-knee amputations, also performed without a death.[6]

Wound Healing

A considerable range of healing rates are reported in the literature before the use of immediate postoperative prosthesis. The primary healing rate ranged from 62 to 75%.[1, 3, 13-17] Some of these patients went on to secondary healing with an ultimate eventual healing rate averaging 82%. With the use of immediate postoperative prosthesis and amputation level selection by xenon clearance, healing approached 100%.[2, 4-6, 8]

Prosthetic Rehabilitation

Before the use of immediate postoperative prosthesis, the average rate of prosthetic rehabilitation in the geriatric amputee was 64%, with a range of 29 to 83%.[1, 3, 10-12] With the advent of immediate postoperative prosthesis, a 100% prosthetic rehabilitation rate was achieved in unilateral amputees who had been ambulatory before amputation.[2, 4-8]

Time Interval Between Amputation and Fitting of Prosthesis

Before the use of immediate postoperative prosthesis, the average time interval between amputation and prosthetic rehabilitation was 133 days. With the advent of immediate postoperative prosthesis, the average time interval between amputation and ambulation with an intermediate prosthesis was 32 days.[2]

SUMMARY

Below-knee amputation is the most commonly employed, most durable, and most functional amputation level. With the use of quantitative preoperative amputation level selection, meticulous surgical technique, and application of a rigid prosthesis with immediate postoperative ambulation; mortality rates of 0%, healing rates of 97%, and prosthetic rehabilitation rates of 100% have been achieved in patients requiring amputation for ischemic gangrene or complications of diabetes mellitus.

REFERENCES

1. Warren R, Kihn RB: A survey of lower extremity amputations for ischemia. Surgery 63:107, 1968.
2. Malone JM, Moore WS, Leal JM, Childers SJ: Rehabilitation for lower extremity amputation. Arch Surg 116:93, 1981.
3. Lim RC Sr, Blaisdell FW, Hall AD, et al: Below knee amputation for ischemic gangrene. Surg Gynecol Obstet 125:493, 1967.
4. Moore WS, Hall AD, Wylie EJ: Below knee amputation for vascular insufficiency: Experience with immediate postoperative fitting of prosthesis. Arch Surg 97:886, 1968.
5. Roon AJ, Moore WS, Goldstone J: Below-knee amputation: A modern approach. Am J Surg 134:153, 1977.
6. Malone JM, Moore WS, Goldstone J, Malone SJ: Therapeutic and economic impact of a modern amputation program. Ann Surg 189:798, 1979.
7. McIntyre KE Jr, Bailey SA, Malone JM, Goldstone J: Guillotine amputation in the management of nonsalvageable lower extremity infection. Arch Surg 119:450, 1984.
8. Moore WS, Hall AD, Lim RC: Below the knee amputation for ischemic gangrene. Comparative results of conventional operation and immediate postoperative fitting technic. Am J Surg 124:127, 1972.
9. Huston CC, Bivins BA, Ernst CB, Griffen WO Jr: Morbid implications of above-knee amputations. Report of a series and review of the literature. Arch Surg 115:165, 1980.
10. Berardi RS, Keonin Y: Amputation in peripheral vascular occlusive disease. Am J Surg 135:231, 1978.
11. Baur GM, Porter JM, Axthelm S, et al: Lower extremity amputation for ischemia. Am Surg 44:472, 1978.
12. Wray CH, Still JM Jr, Moretz WH: Present management of amputations for peripheral vascular disease. Am Surg 38:87, 1972.
13. Harris PO, Schwartz SI, DeWeese JA: Midcalf amputation for peripheral vascular disease. Arch Surg 82:381, 1961.
14. Lempke RE, King RD, Kaiser GC, et al: Amputation for arteriosclerosis obliterans. Arch Surg 86:406, 1963.
15. Dale WA, Jacobs JK: Lower extremity amputation: Results in Nashville, 1956–1960. Ann Surg 155:1011, 1962.
16. Tolstedt GE, Bell JW: Failure of below-knee amputation in peripheral arterial disease. Arch Surg 83:934, 1961.
17. Vankka E: Study on arteriosclerotics undergoing amputations. Acta Orthop Scand Suppl 104:1, 1967.

13

Knee Disarticulation and Above-Knee Amputation

Ernest M. Burgess, M.D.

Lower limb function is critically dependent on the contribution of the knee joint. Static and dynamic studies of all phases of bipedal gait emphasize this fact. Loss of the knee joint by knee disarticulation and above-knee amputation radically changes the environment in which the residual limb and the prosthetic substitute act. After amputation at the above-knee level, weight bearing can no longer be largely or completely transferred from the residual limb to the prosthesis. Varying and often major weight increments must be taken by the soft tissues and underlying bony structures of the pelvis proximal to the hip joint. Although knee disarticulation does permit considerable, though never complete, weight bearing by the end of the residual limb—as the amputation level progressively leaves a shorter remaining thigh segment—weight bearing and prosthetic control increasingly depend on the pelvis and trunk for stability and voluntary movement. Consequently, it is primary that amputation provide, whenever feasible, a strong and dynamic muscle-controlled residual limb with all available muscle function preserved to assure stable, comfortable, and energy-efficient prosthetic control.

The nearly 100 artificial knees designed for knee disarticulation and above-knee amputation prostheses attest to the engineering challenge presented by mechanically duplicating normal knee function. Even the most advanced swing and stance phase hydraulic and pneumatic artificial knee controls coupled with state-of-the-art sockets and suspension systems cannot compensate for a poor quality amputation, one with inadequate muscle stabilization, which permits excessive lateral and anterior drift of the femur.

Amputation surgery at the through-knee and above-knee levels is not difficult. It is, however, exacting and is not considered a casual endeavor to be undertaken by a relatively inexperienced staff. It is just as important that the operating surgeons, when performing amputation, understand in detail the anatomy and functional physiology of the limb as they understand the function of the pancreas or adrenal gland when performing surgery on these organs. At no level in the upper or lower limb is a reconstructive approach to amputation more important than at the thigh and knee joint levels. No matter how excellent the prosthetic rehabilitation, the quality of the surgery will largely determine the physical quality of life; this is particularly true with the young, active amputee.

It is rewarding to see a young unilateral above-knee amputee run, play baseball, participate in racket sports, ice skate, and roller skate. This level of function is attainable only when the surgery is performed as a reconstructive and physiological procedure based on a working knowledge of prosthetic rehabilitation and not simply on limb ablation.

KNEE DISARTICULATION

The knee has had varying degrees of surgical acceptance as an elective site for amputation. Surgeons have generally appreciated knee disarticulation's advantages over amputation through the femur. Until recently, prosthetists have discouraged its use, finding it difficult to fit with a satisfactory, functional and cosmetic substitute. In the last two decades, there have been significant improvements in knee disarticulation prosthetics. This level is now a favored elective site for amputation, especially when circumstances permit appropriate techniques leading to a muscle-stabilized, well-healed, and properly contoured residual limb. It is also a useful amputation level for treating limb ischemia, both in the older marginally ambulating person and in the nonambulating patient.

The advantages of knee disarticulation have been outlined on many occasions in the surgical literature. The orthopedic surgeon Perry Rogers, himself a through-knee amputee, emphasized these positive and favorable features:

1. Maximal femoral lever arm length for active, strong prosthetic control.

2. Residual limb/socket stability, a result of the large interface surface and irregular contour of the distal residual limb end.

3. Significant end-bearing capacity, transferring considerable weight longitudinally through the femur to the pelvis and trunk, i.e., physiological weight-bearing.

4. Improved contour prosthetic suspension as compared with the above-knee level. Muscle activity within the residual limb and residual limb contour suspension characteristics decrease the need for ancillary suspension.

5. The surgery itself is in general low risk, with blood loss easily controlled; bone transection is not required. Division of muscle mass is also minimized, since the soft tissue surgery is carried out largely through tendons, fascia, and aponeuroses contiguous to the joint.

The disadvantages attributed to this amputation are largely related to prosthetic fit. The standard conventional prosthesis requires external knee hinge joints rather than intrinsic knee mechanisms, including the more modern and physiological hydraulic and pneumatic types. Many prosthetists feel that the artificial limb is difficult in cosmesis and unsightly due to the width and bulk at the distal end of the femur. The length of the residual limb can create difficulty in placing the prosthetic knee symmetrically with the opposite normal knee, adding to the unsightliness on the prosthetic side, especially when the amputee is sitting.

Modern prosthetic designs have largely negated many of these objections. Current knee disarticulation prostheses can incorporate intrinsic knee joints with specific hydraulic and pneumatic damping as well as refined polycentric and multiaxial mechanical types. The leather thigh-lacer socket with simple unicentric external hinges and thigh bars has largely been replaced with composite flexible or rigid sockets. Nonrigid sleeve socket inserts can be used when indicated. The entire limb can be covered with attractive cosmetic skin, permitting the wearing of shorts and skirts. Endoskeletal or exoskeletal below-knee structures are available with a variety of ankle/foot mechanisms.

Prosthetic improvements are continuing. The high level of function that most younger individuals with knee disarticulation can accomplish rewards the surgeon and prosthetist for their effort and ingenuity.

Indications

Knee disarticulation is indicated when the knee is the most distal level at which a satisfactory, durable, and functional residual limb can be obtained. It has been stated that retention of knee function is the single most important aspect of major lower limb amputation. This is true for patients of all ages. It is particularly true in the elderly in whom retention of a functional knee—even though the below-knee amputation may be short— will often allow prosthetic fit and comfortable weight bearing, whereas a higher amputation, including knee disarticulation, decreases the chance of successful prosthetic use. This decision depends, of course, on the retention of a functional knee joint. Fixed knee contractures, extensive adherent scarring about the knee, or loss of voluntary muscle control may justify a knee disarticulation even though a below-knee amputation might successfully heal. Frequently under these circumstances, the healed below-knee limb may be complicated by pain, fixed knee contractures, and awkward positioning in beds and wheelchairs, with the threat of terminal residual limb injury with skin breakdown. Patients who will not ambulate may benefit by knee disarticulation rather than an attempt at a lower level.

Because amputation through the knee is functionally superior to that through the femur, the surgeon must carefully weigh the advantages this level offers and make the decision with a full understanding of the prosthetic and rehabilitative implications. Although each circumstance must be individualized, there are certain well-defined factors that assist in making the appropriate decision.

Special Considerations

Infancy and Childhood

Knee disarticulation in children must leave the adjacent distal femoral epiphysis undisturbed whenever possible. Amputation at this level is used when severe congenital deformity of the distal leg is present and reconstruction for useful plantigrade bipedal gait is not attainable. The classic example is congenital absence of the tibia (paraxial tibial hemimelia) (Fig. 13–1). Occasionally, a functional limb distal to the knee can be salvaged by tibiofibular synostosis in the presence of a residual short tibial segment and by other surgical techniques. In general, individuals born with a major or complete loss of the tibia perform much better with knee disarticulation than with attempted fibular centralization or other related reconstructions. Excellent skin coverage is routinely accomplished.

Muscle stabilization is mandatory when there are active muscle groups with which to work. The femoral condyles are not disturbed surgically, since the distal femoral epiphysis should be left to obtain maximal femoral length with growth.

When other congenital limb deficits that will leave great inequality of leg length or a functionally inadequate limb distal to the knee joint are present, knee disarticulation should be considered.

In the presence of neoplasms, infection of the proximal tibia extending into the knee joint, or trauma with extensive destruction of the proximal tibial area to a degree that a functional knee cannot be restored, the knee is generally the level of choice for amputation in children and adults. Children adapt rapidly to this amputation level, particularly when the opposite limb is normal.

Growth irregularities that alter the bony contours of the distal femur may require revision of the amputation at the completion of growth. In general, no attempt should be made before epiphyseal closure to correct deformity by localized epiphysiodesis or other surgical intervention. If necessary, reconstruction based on prosthetic needs, including the recontouring of a bulbous terminal femur, should await skeletal maturity.

The Active Adult

When trauma, infection, or neoplasm justifies its use, knee disarticulation is highly effective as an amputation level during the active adult years. The most common situation seen involves a crushing injury to the limb distal to and extending into the knee, eliminating the below-knee level as an option. In such a case good knee disarticulation is generally more satisfactory than a short below-knee amputation with scarring, deformity, recurrent infection, severe loss of knee function, and pain. This preference is substantiated by the excellent function, endurance, and comfort that are the hallmarks of a well-performed knee disarticulation that is followed by proper prosthetic fitting and physical therapy.

Occasionally, bilateral limb loss results in a knee disarticulation on one side and a higher through-knee amputation on the opposite side. The response of individuals who have experienced this situation invariably indicates the superiority of the through-knee level. This clinical information from amputees outweighs data received from gait and energy studies based on objective tests.

The Elderly

It has been stated earlier that salvage of a functional knee is the single most important

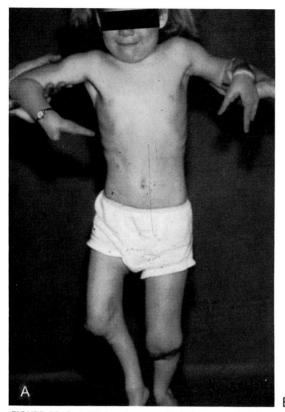
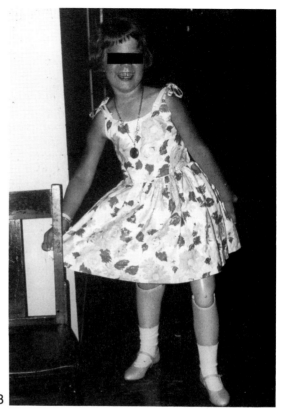

FIGURE 13–1. *A*, Bilateral congenital absence of tibia (paraxial tibial hemimelia). A series of reconstructive surgical procedures have not restored the ability to stand or walk unsupported. *B*, Bilateral knee disarticulation. The child walks well without supports and attends regular school.

factor in lower limb amputation level selection. This is especially true in the elderly patient in whom diminished balance, strength, and visual acuity, together with an often compromised opposite leg, make walking difficult. With current below-knee amputation techniques for long posterior, vertical, or skewed flaps, it is possible to salvage a functional knee joint and obtain healing at short below-knee levels 6 to 10 cm in length. If complete or near complete knee extension is present and an active quadriceps mechanism is intact, these short amputations can be well fitted and will function with more stability than those at the through-knee level. Therefore, the decision to perform knee disarticulation is particularly critical in this age group. Careful evaluation of skin healing potential indicates whether one should attempt a short amputation distal to the knee or proceed to knee disarticulation. Preference for the short below-knee level has greatly reduced the number of knee disarticulations used in older persons with vascular

disease. When functional evaluation definitely indicates that the individual has no standing or walking potential and will be bed- or wheelchair-confined, knee disarticulation or above-knee amputation foregoes difficulties in transferring the patient from bed to wheelchair and prevents complications such as knee joint contractures and residual limb breakdown due to pressure from weight bearing.

Surgical Procedure

The patient is placed supine on the operating table. A pneumatic tourniquet is used unless ischemia of the tissues is present. Skin flaps are developed as dictated by local skin conditions about the knee and the proximal part of the leg. The classic long anterior skin flap is neither necessary nor especially desirable unless good, very viable skin can be incorporated into the flap with this traditional technique. When kneeling, one normally rests on the skin over the anterior aspect of the proximal tibia in the region of the patellar tendon. These tissues tolerate well the pressure of weight bearing when they are healthy.

There is no contraindication to the use of equal anterior and posterior flaps, irregularly placed incisions, or mediolateral skin flaps (i.e., sagittal closure), any of which can make an excellent and acceptable scar. The important aspect of skin management is the necessity of a well-vascularized, nontender, nonadherent scar, rather than a specific, fixed position of scar placement. A common error in skin management is tight closure. With anterior-posterior flaps, the posterior skin flap, especially, should be left sufficiently long to permit comfortable closure without tension, since it has a tendency to retract (Fig. 13–2).

Dissection is carried down directly to the proximal anterior tibia and the insertion of the patellar tendon. The tendon is severed at its most distal insertion site and retracted proximally as the surgery continues. Deep dissection on the inner side includes division of the tendons of the inner hamstrings as they are exposed. They are also sectioned low, at the level of their insertion. The deep fascia is reflected with the skin and tendon flap. No attempt is made to dissect each level. On the lateral side of the knee, the tendon

of the biceps femoris muscle and the iliotibial band are also sectioned low. The knee joint is entered anteriorly, the knee flexed, and division of the cruciate ligaments carried out at their tibial insertions (Fig. 13–3). The posterior structures are divided, and the popliteal artery is sectioned and divided distal to the superior geniculate branches. The tibial and peroneal nerves are identified, retracted under moderate tension, ligated, and sectioned with a sharp knife. The remaining posterior soft tissues are divided, and the leg is removed.

After removal of the leg, the thigh muscles are stabilized under normal tension by suture of the patellar tendon to the remaining cruciate ligaments in the femoral intracondylar notch (Fig. 13–4). It is not necessary to remove the patella unless the patellofemoral joint is pathologically involved. In that instance, the patella is carefully removed, and a reconstruction of the quadriceps/patellar mechanism is carried out in the usual manner. The patellar tendon is now pulled down under *mild* tension well into the intracondylar notch and is sewn to the stump of the cruciate ligaments. The semitendinosus and biceps tendons are likewise pulled into the notch, tailored appropriately, and sewn to the stump of the patellar tendon and to the cruciate ligaments. In this way, thigh muscle stability is achieved (Fig. 13–5).

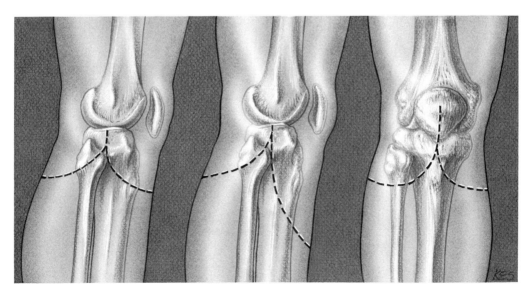

Equal   Long anterior   Sagittal

FIGURE 13–2. Standard skin incisions for knee disarticulation: equal, long anterior, and sagittal. The equal anteroposterior or sagittal flaps are preferred.

FIGURE 13–3. Anterior dissection.

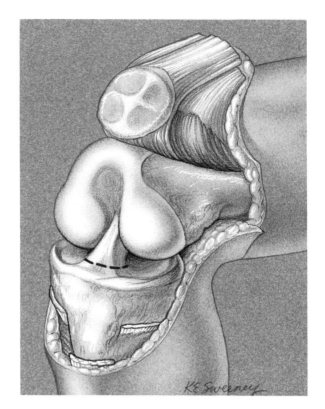

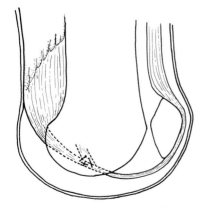

FIGURE 13–4. Intercondylar muscle stabilization. P = posterior; A = anterior.

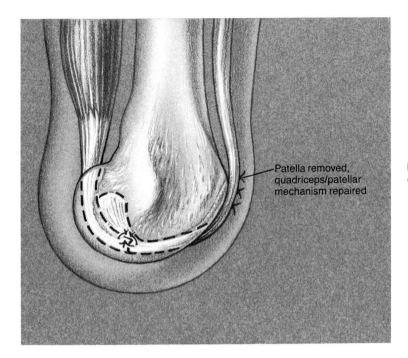

Patella removed, quadriceps/patellar mechanism repaired

FIGURE 13–5. Muscle stabilization combined with patellectomy.

Reduction osteoplasty, as advocated by Mazet and Burgess, reduces somewhat the bulk of the distal femoral condyles to form a less bulbous terminal configuration. It is important that when the condyles and particularly the medial and lateral condylar surfaces are trimmed, the bone contour is tailored very carefully and the distal broad weight-bearing surface is left essentially intact. In this way, the advantage of end bearing is preserved. When the operation is performed on individuals who will not ambulate, it is not necessary to modify the distal femur; the primary goal in such cases is prompt wound healing.

Closure

Routine closure in layers over through-and-through or suction drainage, or both, is accomplished by a rigid or semirigid dressing (Fig. 13–6). Postoperative rehabilitation begins immediately, the day after surgery if possible. The drains are removed at the appropriate time, usually in 24 to 48 hours.

Postoperative Management

Immediate postsurgical rigid dressings provide the appropriate early wound-healing environment. A number of systems are available, including elastic plaster of Paris or one of a number of quick-setting cast materials, i.e., polyurethane-coated bandages. The operative site is routinely drained by suction, through-and-through drainage, or both. Hematomas with collection of synovial fluid arising from remaining synovial tissue occur often if adequate drainage and postsurgical compression dressings are not used. The classic plaster-of-Paris dressing—elastic plastic reinforced by surface application of regular plaster wrapped over an Orlon stocking and a polyurethane end pad—continues to be an excellent and efficient system. The suction drain can be removed without disturbing the cast. If the operative site is also drained by through-and-through wick-type drainage, a small window is cut in the cast, the drain removed, and the window replaced. Suspension of the cast, which is essential to maintain good terminal pressure over the amputation site, is accomplished by means of cast contouring around the condylar region and by application of chemical adhesive between the upper two thirds of the Orlon stocking and the skin. Additional suspension can be obtained by a light flexible pelvic belt attached to or near the brim of the cast.

In most instances, the patient can be out of bed the day after surgery. Weight bearing

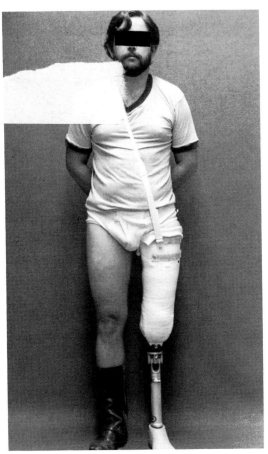

FIGURE 13–6. Immediate postoperative rigid dressing for knee disarticulation and above-knee amputation levels (with pylon attached).

not occur. Poorly applied dressings can produce a tourniquet effect, causing wound breakdown. It may be necessary to rewrap the elastic or compressive part of the soft dressing several times a day to prevent proximal constriction. The rigid dressing is far more secure, comfortable, and efficient as a terminal, gentle pressure support system.

When healing is uneventful, a preliminary prosthetic limb can usually be fitted by the fifth to sixth week. This is particularly true of younger, active amputees. Hip range of motion and muscle strengthening exercises are started early in the convalescent period to maintain comfortable, free hip joint function. Isometric conditioning of the stabilized thigh muscles is also an important part of effective physical rehabilitation. Voluntary thigh muscle exercise is slowly graduated to maintain and improve strength but not sufficiently to stress the myoplasty fixation at the intercondylar notch. Three to four weeks after surgery, progressively resistive exercises for the thigh and hip should be vigorously pursued. Active unilateral amputees are encouraged to engage early in vocational and recreational activities, including those involving considerable bipedal skills. Social activities such as dancing are encouraged. The healthy, older unilateral through-knee amputee often may be able to play golf and bowl. Custom prostheses allow diverse recreation as well as workplace performance.

on a temporary prosthesis is "touch down" only or is *withheld* until the first cast change, which is usually at the eighth to fourteenth postoperative day. If wound healing is progressing uneventfully at that time, a new cast can be applied, and a distal pylon and foot can be fitted to the end of the rigid dressing and properly aligned.

The temporary prosthesis may be removable. Early supported minimal weight bearing *under supervision* improves the patient's physical and psychological progress.

When soft dressings are used, a compressible material, such as sterile polyurethane or carefully fluffed gauze, should be placed over the distal end of the amputation site, then a supportive compression dressing is applied. The shape of the thigh creates difficulty in maintaining the soft dressings and distal compression without proximal "choking" and limb constriction. Proximal constriction must

ABOVE-KNEE AMPUTATION

Indications

The indications for above knee-amputation are in most circumstances well defined. It is reserved for conditions in which surgery at a lower level would not provide satisfactory healing and a stable, functional, comfortable, relatively pain-free residual limb. Selection of this level in the presence of trauma, tumors, congenital anomalies, and infections is, in most cases, self-evident. In the presence of peripheral vascular disease, level determination can require careful screening on the basis of the physical findings and the general condition and potential mobility of the patient, including the condition of the other leg and specific assay of the limb viability as it relates to primary healing.

The importance of knee retention has already been stressed. The patient coming to amputation with peripheral vascular disease with or without diabetes is particularly in need of knee retention when possible. Many thousands of older individuals have sustained a primary above-knee amputation when careful consideration of limb viability, healing potential, and appropriate surgical and postsurgical management would have salvaged a functional knee.

Elsewhere in this text are described the evaluation procedures that assist in establishing amputation level. The surgeon should understand and consider level determination on the basis of this information. Statistics from many surgical centers throughout the world indicate a knee salvage rate of 50 to 85% in all patients coming to major above-knee amputation for peripheral vascular disease. This salvage percentage can be achieved without multiple surgeries attributable to faulty level selection.

Because well over half of all patients coming to major limb amputation for vascular problems will heal a below-knee amputation, the number of above-knee amputations being performed is relatively decreasing as appropriate limb viability information, experience, and state-of-the-art techniques achieve widespread usage. Above-knee amputations for ischemia after vascular reconstruction require incorporation of pre-existing thigh surgical scars into the amputation incision. The principles of plastic surgery prevail. A small number of patients, generally elderly, require above-knee amputation after failed, septic, total knee joint replacement. Surgical considerations will be defined later.

Special Considerations

Infancy and Childhood

With rare exception, above-knee amputations in children with immature skeletons result from trauma, tumors, congenital anomalies, and infection. The principles of surgical technique are essentially the same as in the active adult. The level of thigh amputation depends on the extent of the disease or trauma and the availability of suitable tissues for healing. All length is saved consistent with good surgical technique and with the healing capacity of the tissues. The longer

the lever arm provided by the thigh down to the knee disarticulation level, the more effective is the fit and the use of the prosthesis.

In keeping with this principle, bone length is sacrificed only occasionally, as in the very short thigh amputation just below the level of the intertrochanteric line at the hip. In this circumstance, it may be advisable to remove the small proximal bone segment to prevent a hip flexion and abduction deformity that will complicate prosthetic fit.

Of all the major levels of amputation in the upper and lower limbs, muscle stabilization is most critical at the above-knee level. Left unstabilized, the muscles retract, allowing the femur to drift laterally and anteriorly in the surrounding muscle and soft tissues. Failure to control and stabilize the femur by the activity and strength of the remaining hip and thigh muscles results in weakness no matter how carefully and correctly the prosthesis is fabricated, aligned, and fitted. A strong, muscle-stabilized residual limb allows transfer of forces from the body through the prosthesis, to better control the prosthetic knee. Prosthetic function is thus greatly enhanced. The favorable kinesiology associated with well-stabilized above-knee amputations is particularly appreciated by the young amputee. In such patients, blood supply is not usually a problem. Healing can be accomplished with skin and muscle management, which are optional and elective. A lack of understanding of the kinematics and kinetics involved in above-knee amputation is unfortunately seen not infrequently in the operating theater. The orthopedic surgeon takes meticulous care in properly performing a prosthetic hip replacement. The detail with which limb length, orientation, and muscle management are determined all evidence the surgeon's concern for end-result function. This same surgeon too often performs an above-knee amputation with little or no attention to similar surgical management of the muscles and other supportive tissues when, in fact, the functional response may depend even more critically on correct surgical technique than it does in thigh or hip joint replacement.

The Active Adult

Trauma is the cause of thigh amputation in most adults. As with young people, in adults, muscle stabilization is a necessity when surgically obtainable. The same general amputation principles apply and are of maximal importance when the amputee is still actively engaged in work, particularly when that work requires significant standing and walking. Above-knee amputees have a high rehabilitation potential. They can perform many of the vocational and recreational activities enjoyed by the general population. Appropriate rehabilitation to a level of maximal achievable function begins with proper presurgical evaluation and state-of-the-art surgical technique.

The Elderly

By far, most above-knee amputations performed in the western world result from ischemia and gangrene. Associated physical and mental deficits common to patients with these conditions limit the potential of more than one half of unilateral above-knee amputees to wear a prosthetic device successfully. Bilateral above-knee limb loss in the elderly essentially eliminates ambulation.

The primary surgical objective is a healed, stable amputation site. The desirable features incorporating *muscle stabilization* and maximal *residual femoral length* are of secondary importance unless the wound heals. Most through-thigh amputations for limb ischemia, gangrene, diabetes, neuropathic disorders, and related pathological conditions are, therefore, directed toward ablation through viable tissues, usually the middle two thirds of the thigh.

Rehabilitation should be aggressive. Life expectancy is generally short. The remaining limb, if present, is often at risk. Recumbency and prolonged bed rest soon render the individual physically incompetent for even limited walking. Aware of these facts, the amputee rehabilitation team encourages mobility, with a wheelchair or otherwise, as soon as possible. If the individual is a potential walker, a temporary device to permit upright bipedal stance—usually with assistance—should be used as promptly as wound healing allows.

Evaluation of rehabilitation potential is particularly significant with these patients. This assessment should be constructive and positive but not unrealistic. Patients with strokes; Alzheimer's disease; and severe impairment of pulmonary, cardiac, and renal function should not be expected to expend the energy required to ambulate simply for the satisfaction of walking a few steps with assistance. On the other hand, every reasonable attempt should be made to improve the quality of life as it relates to mobility and particularly bipedal gait. Compassion and sensitivity combined with realistic expectations allow the most effective approach.

Surgical Procedure

The operation is performed with the patient supine and with the hip in a neutral position. When tissue ischemia is *not* present, a tourniquet can be placed proximal to the site of surgery.

When the level of bone amputation has been determined, slightly fish-mouthed equal skin flaps are made; the anterior flap can also be designed slightly longer than the posterior flap (Fig. 13–7). The skin incision should be almost guillotinelike and placed at the lowest available skin level. Long, tongue-like flaps, which tend to compromise central skin blood supply, should be avoided. Scars from previous surgery or trauma are incorporated into the incision following plastic surgical principles.

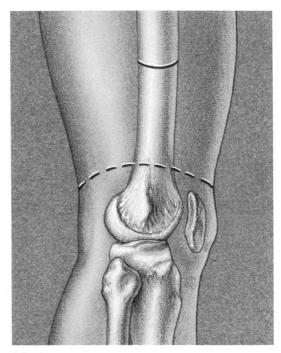

FIGURE 13–7. Skin and bone section for classic above-knee amputation.

Incisions through the skin can be made in any appropriate manner consistent with available skin and soft tissues. Equal flaps, oblique flaps, and sagittal flaps, when healed, present no hazard to the fit of a prosthetic socket, provided the scar is nonadherent, nontender, and under no tension (Fig. 13–8).

After the skin flaps are completed, dissection is carried directly down anteriorly through the quadriceps muscles to the bone. If any portion of anterior knee synovial tissue remains, it should be selectively excised. The periosteum is divided circularly around the femur and is stripped proximally to expose the bare femoral shaft.

The level of bone section as compared with the division of muscles depends on the thickness of the soft tissues. As a general rule, the bone should be divided proximal to the skin and muscle incision by one and one half times the diameter of the thigh at the level of amputation. The edges of the femur are made smooth and slightly rounded. Closure of the soft tissues under excess tension is a common mistake in thigh amputations. This error is particularly common if muscle stabilization has been carried out. The added distal bulk resulting from tying down muscles and from preserving adequate length of the sectioned muscles relative to the bone requires additional skin for coverage.

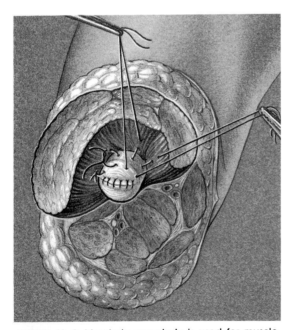

FIGURE 13–8. Myodesis; myoplasty is used for muscle stabilization when indicated.

After division of the bone from the anterior aspect, a bone hook is placed in the medullary cavity of the distal femur. It is lifted forward, and the soft tissues are divided posteriorly with isolation and ligation of the various vessels and nerves. At thigh level, it is important to retract the sciatic and femoral nerves into the field with moderate tension, then to section them with a knife distal to the site of ligation before allowing them to retract. If the sciatic nerve has divided into the popliteal and peroneal branches at the level of section, each branch is treated similarly. Thus, the neuromas are kept well away from pressure exerted by the prosthesis.

Muscle stabilization is a key part of thigh amputations (Fig. 13–9). Unless the major muscle groups are stabilized at or near the site of amputation, they will retract. The resulting residual limb is weak and often painful. Weight transfer through the residual limb socket interface permits the femur to drift laterally and forward to lie against the wall of the prosthetic socket. Unapposed, unbalanced muscle pull causes femur drift even in the nonambulating amputee.

Fascial closure alone is used when ischemia necessitates the surgery or when extensive scarring is present. Both factors can compromise wound healing when coupled with the additional surgery necessary to provide muscle stabilization.

When muscles are stabilized, one of two techniques or a combination is used. One, *myoplasty,* calls for suturing the major muscle groups to each other and to the periosteum over the distal end of the femur with interrupted appropriate sutures. A slinglike effect must be avoided by tying down the muscle groups. After periosteal closure of the end of the bone, the major muscle groups—quadriceps, hamstring, and adductors—are pulled down and are sewed to each other across the end of the bone; the sutures are extended into the periosteum to prevent their sliding over the end of the bone, a source of pain and bursae formation. If muscle coverage distally is unstable, myoplasty will be ineffective.

Myodesis involves stabilizing the thigh muscles directly to the femur just proximal to the bone amputation level. Small drill holes are placed through the femur to allow a through-and-through suture of the quadriceps muscles, the knots being tied in the medullary

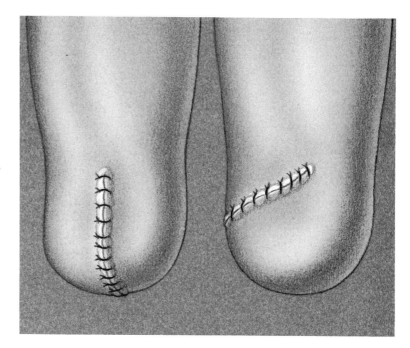

FIGURE 13–9. Equal and long anterior flap closures.

cavity. The thigh muscles are carefully balanced. It is critical to avoid sewing the quadriceps muscles under tension or with the hip flexed; otherwise, permanent hip flexion contracture will ensue, and this is very difficult to correct when the muscles have been sewn under undue tension.

The hamstrings, both medial and lateral, and especially the adductors are likewise folded into the myodesis site and are carefully stabilized with through-bone sutures to opposing muscle groups. The adductor muscle mass can be stabilized under moderate tension, since the hip abductors are a strong opposing force and adduction contracture is rarely seen in above-knee amputations.

The hamstring muscles or tendons and the tensor fascia should also be sewn under moderate tension, since a balance of these muscles allows active residual limb control with prevention of fixed deformity of the hip. Careful distal muscle stabilization and reconstruction provide what has come to be known as physiological amputation (Fig. 13–10). The surgical technique under these optimal conditions is critical for maximal functional restoration. It is indeed gratifying to observe the almost normal gait and the endurance and comfort the amputee experiences when fitted with a modern, narrow M/L flexible brim socket, a stance/swing phase knee, and an energy-storing shank and foot. There are

few limb reconstructions that are more gratifying to the health care team as well as, of course, to the patient.

Myodesis and myoplasty are not performed in the presence of ischemia or gan-

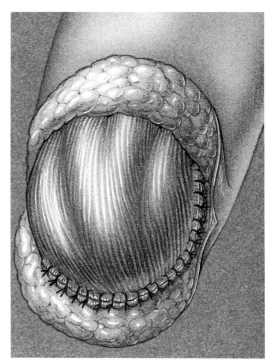

FIGURE 13–10. Completed muscle stabilization.

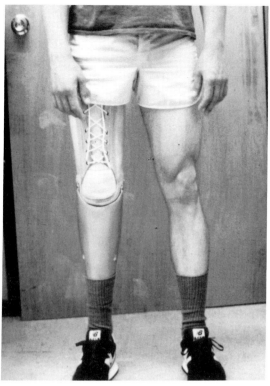

FIGURE 13–11. Conventional knee disarticulation prosthesis with single-axis knee hinge joints and thigh lacer. (*Courtesy of* Wayne Koniuk, CP, San Francisco Prosthetic Orthotic Service, Inc, San Francisco, California.)

grene. When an amputee has compromised circulation and low healing potential, the primary goal of uneventful wound healing is best accomplished by a simple fascial closure. The periosteum should be closed with purse string sutures around the end of the bone after the sharp bone edges are beveled. A myofascial closure is then carried out in one or two layers, with the femur centered in the muscle mass as well as possible but without any attempt to formally stabilize the muscles. The additional surgery required for muscle stabilization may add sufficient surgical trauma to cause tissue death and wound breakdown.

Complications of knee joint reconstructive surgery, specifically total knee replacement, occasionally dictate above-knee amputation. Individuals with such complications are generally in the older age bracket. Associated disabilities, including polyarticular arthritis and limited mobility due to muscle weakness, compromise functional restoration. When these factors are combined with a prolonged surgical course with sepsis, removal of the implant components, and multiple surgeries, those few individuals who come to amputation present a severe rehabilitation challenge.

The amputation is done at the appropriate site, usually just above the level of the tip of

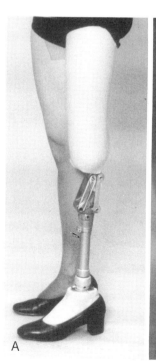
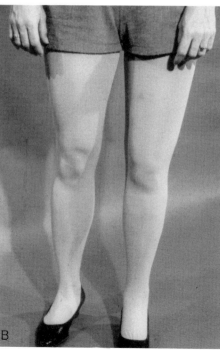

FIGURE 13–12. *A,* Modern knee disarticulation prosthesis with a multiaxial knee and plastic laminate suction socket. *B,* Same with cosmetic cover. (*Courtesy of* Al Pike, CP, Otto Bock Industries, Inc, Minneapolis, Minnesota.)

A   B

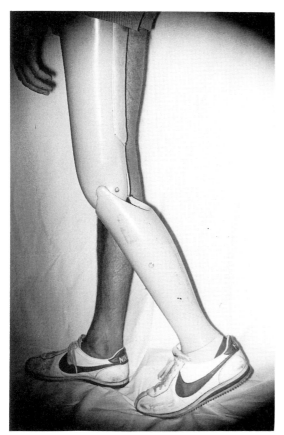

FIGURE 13–13. Conventional above-knee prosthesis with suction socket and hydraulic knee.

for above-knee amputation (see Fig. 13–6). This method requires some additional equipment but is justified on the basis of the improved healing environment, reduced pain, easy mobility of the patient, and early rehabilitation. A rigid dressing is strongly recommended whether or not one allows the patient to walk in the early postoperative period.

In debilitated and cachectic patients, simple soft dressings with a compression bandage, rather than a rigid dressing, are advisable. In such cases, the compression dressing is carried up over the pelvis in a spica configuration to prevent its slipping off or displacing and constricting blood flow and fluid exchange. It is inspected and adjusted as necessary.

Drains are removed within 48 hours. Flexion contractures of the hips are prevented by a carefully supervised and vigorous postoperative therapy regimen.

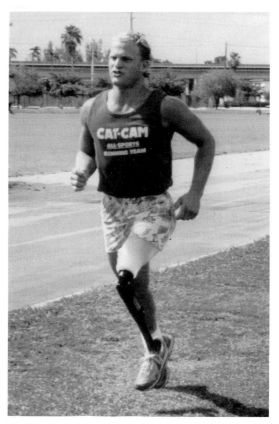

FIGURE 13–14. State-of-the-art above-knee (Endolite) prosthesis, narrow M/L socket, hydraulic (Mauch) stance/ swing phase knee control, graphite shank, and energy storage foot (cosmetic cover not shown). (*Courtesy of George DePontis, CAT-CAM Team, Miami, Florida.*)

the femoral component. If component stabilization with methyl methacrylate has been carried out, any residual methyl methacrylate should be removed from the medullary cavity at the time of amputation. The amputation may require staging with secondary closure owing to the proximity of the infection. The same principles apply although muscle stabilization is generally not feasible and simple fascial closure is preferred. This author has performed amputation under these circumstances in eight patients. Six of these patients subsequently became successful prosthesis users.

Postoperative Management

Postoperative dressings consist of a layer of Owen's silk over the operative site, with fluff gauze and additional compressive materials distally. The author recommends a rigid dressing for knee disarticulation and

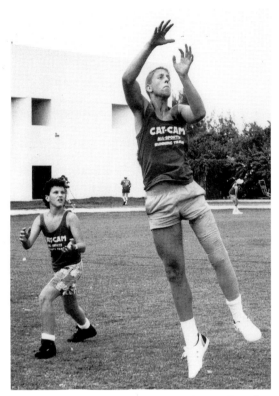

FIGURE 13–15. Endoskeletal, narrow M/L socket, suction above-knee prosthesis (CAT-CAM). (*Courtesy of* George DePontis, CAT-CAM Team, Miami, Florida.)

Selected types of available prostheses for knee disarticulation and above-knee amputation levels are illustrated in Figures 13–11 through 13–15.

SUGGESTED REFERENCES

American Academy of Orthopaedic Surgeons: Atlas of Limb Prosthetics: Surgical and Prosthetic Principles. St Louis, CV Mosby Co, 1981.

Banerjee SN (ed): Rehabilitation Management of Amputees. Baltimore, Williams & Wilkins, 1982.

Batch JW, Spittler AW, McFaddin JG: Advantages of knee disarticulation over amputations through the thigh. J Bone Joint Surg 36A:921, 1954.

Burgess EM: Immediate postsurgical prosthetic fitting: A system of amputee management. J Am Phys Ther Assoc 51:139, 1971.

Burgess EM: Major amputations. *In* Nora PF (ed): Operative Surgery—Principles and Techniques. Philadelphia, Lea & Febiger, 1972.

Burgess EM: Disarticulation of the knee: A modified technique. Arch Surg 112:1250, 1977.

Burgess EM, Romano RL, Zettl JH: The Management of Lower Extremity Amputations. Bulletin TR 10–6. Washington, DC, US Government Printing Office, 1969.

Fulford GE: The surgery of the AK-amputation. *In* Murdock G (ed): Prosthetic and Orthotic Practice. London, Edward Arnold Publishers, 1970.

Hierton T (ed): Amputations Kirurgi och Proteser. Uppsala, Tiden/Folksam, 1980.

Howard RS, Chamberlain J, McPherson AFS: Through knee amputation in peripheral vascular disease. Lancet 2:240, 1969.

Kjøble J: The surgery of the through-knee amputation. *In* Murdock G (ed): Prosthetic and Orthotic Practice. London, Edward Arnold Publishers, 1970.

Kostuik JP (ed): Amputation Surgery and Rehabilitation. The Toronto Experience. New York, Churchill Livingstone, 1981.

Mazet R Jr, Hennessy CA: Knee disarticulation: A new technique and a new knee joint mechanism. J Bone Joint Surg 48A:126, 1966.

Mensch G, Ellis PM: Physical Therapy Management of Lower Extremity Amputations. Rockville, Aspen Publishers, 1986.

Murdock G: Levels of amputation and limiting factors. Ann R Coll Surg Engl 40:204, 1967.

Nickel VL (ed): Orthopedic Rehabilitation. New York, Churchill Livingstone, 1982.

Rogers SP: Amputation at the knee joint. J Bone Joint Surg 22:973, 1940.

Slocum DB (ed): An Atlas of Amputations. St Louis, CV Mosby Co, 1949.

Zettl JH: The team—preoperative planning. *In* Gerhardt JJ, King PS (eds): Amputations: Immediate and Early Prosthetic Management. Vienna, Hans Huber, 1982, pp 26–39.

14

Hip Disarticulation

Paul H. Sugarbaker, M.D.

Evolution of the commonly used technique of hip joint disarticulation may be traced to the report of Kirk, who in 1943 described his experience with amputations through the hip joint.[3] All muscles except those normally belonging in the buttock were removed from the residual limb, except one muscle flap, which was conserved to fill the acetabulum. In general, nearly all the muscles were transected at their origins. Improvements in the technique were presented by Boyd, who in 1947 described an "anatomic disarticulation of the hip" designed to reduce blood loss by dividing all muscles at either their origin on the pelvis or at their insertion on the femur.[2] Muscles (other than those of the buttock) that remained attached to the pelvis were the iliopsoas and obturator externus. Slocum, in his *Atlas of Amputations* published in 1949, described a technique in which a long posterior skin flap was used to resurface the operative site.[4] If a prosthesis were to be used, weight bearing would be on the posterior myocutaneous flap rather than on a suture line. Slocum also emphasized high ligation of the femoral, obturator, and sciatic nerves so that they would retract out of the weight-bearing areas. An elastic bandage was used to provide compression and thereby minimize postoperative hematoma. Bickel and Koch described a technique for hip disartic-

ulation but did not amplify further previously described techniques.[1]

The description of hip disarticulation in this chapter incorporates the concepts that have developed over the last 4 decades. A surgical plan is presented whereby

1. The incision does not lie over bony prominences or weight-bearing areas so that local pain with use of a prosthesis is minimized.

2. All muscles are transected at either their origin or insertion to minimize blood loss and postoperative wound complications.

3. Viable musculature is preserved for use as a myodesis to cover the protruding acetabulum.

INDICATIONS

Hip joint disarticulation is indicated for malignant bony tumors (usually osteosarcomas) of the femur below the lesser trochanter and for malignant soft tissue tumors (usually sarcomas) of the middle and lower thigh.[5] Often, small osteosarcomas of the lower femoral epiphysis without skip osseous metastases can be managed by high above-knee amputation. Tumors at or above the lesser trochanter in either bone or soft tissue must be treated by hemipelvectomy (Chapter 15).

PROCEDURE

Patient Position. Before preparation of the operative site, a Foley catheter is placed in the bladder, and the opposite lower extremity is covered by an elastic wrap to prevent venous pooling. The patient is placed in the lateral position and secured with pads anterior and posterior to the torso; there should be a slight posterior tilt. The skin is prepared from midchest to midcalf and the leg draped free.

Incision. Bony landmarks to be identified include the pubic tubercle, anterosuperior iliac spine, anteroinferior iliac spine, ischial tuberosity, and greater trochanter (Fig. 14–1). The anterior portion of the incision commences one fingerbreadth medial to the anterosuperior iliac spine. It descends to the pubic tubercle then over the pubic bone to two fingerbreadths distal to the ischial tuberosity and gluteal crease. If the buttock flap is extremely thick, the anterior portion of the incision should be moved laterally. The posterior portion of the incision extends two fingerbreadths anterior to the greater trochanter then around the back of the leg, distal to the gluteal crease. The distance the incision is made beyond the gluteal crease is directly proportional to the anteroposterior diameter of the patient's pelvis.

Exposure of the Femoral Triangle. The skin is incised, and the dissection is extended through the subcutaneous fat and Scarpa's fascia until the external oblique aponeurosis is seen. Multiple venous bleeding points from branches of the saphenous vein are clamped, divided, and ligated. A moderate-sized artery, the superficial epigastric, and multiple branches of the external pudendal vessels must be secured. The superficial inguinal lymph nodes should be moved laterally with the specimen, and the round ligament in the female or the spermatic cord in the male should be exposed but not included in the specimen (Fig. 14–2).

An Adair clamp is placed securely on the apex of the skin specimen for traction. By incising just below the inguinal ligament into the fossa ovalis, the femoral vein, artery, and nerve are widely exposed below the inguinal ligament.

Division of the Femoral Vessels and Nerve. Individual silk ties are placed around the femoral vessels; first the artery, then the vein, is tied in continuity. Right-angled clamps are placed between the ties, and the vessels are severed. The proximal ends of the vessels are further secured by a silk suture ligature

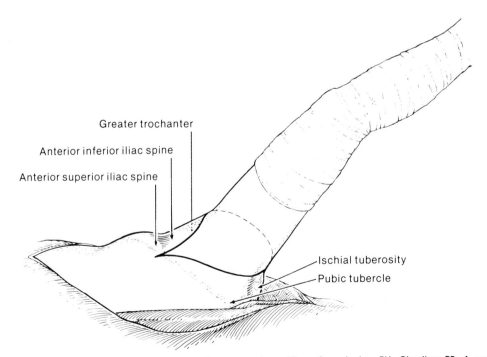

FIGURE 14–1. Skin incision for the hip disarticulation procedure. (*From* Sugarbaker PH, Chretien PB: A surgical technique for hip disarticulation. Surgery 90:546, 1981.)

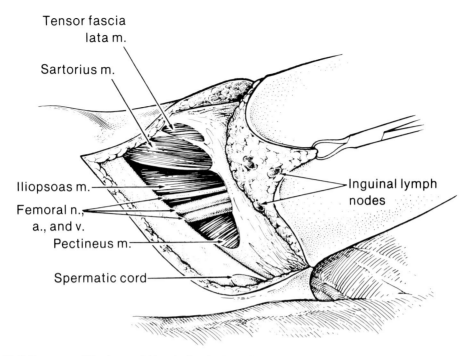

FIGURE 14–2. Exposure of the femoral triangle for division of the femoral vein, artery, and nerve. (*From* Sugarbaker PH, Chretien PB: A surgical technique for hip disarticulation. Surgery 90:546, 1981.)

placed proximal to the right-angle clamps. The femoral nerve is placed on gentle traction and is ligated at its point of exit from beneath the inguinal ligament. When the femoral nerve is severed, it retracts beneath the external oblique aponeurosis; thus, if a neuroma forms, it will not be in a weight-bearing portion of the residual limb.

Division of the Sartorius Muscle at Its Origin and the Femoral Sheath beneath the Femoral Vessels. The sartorius muscle is located as it arises from the anterosuperior iliac spine. It is dissected free from the surrounding fascia then transected from its orgin on the spine with electrocautery. Also using electrocautery, the femoral sheath and fibroareolar tissue posterior to the femoral vessels are incised. This dissection exposes the hip joint capsule.

Division of the Iliopsoas Muscle at Its Insertion. The hip is flexed slightly to relax the iliopsoas muscle. It is then possible to pass a finger around the muscle in a medial to lateral blunt dissection. If an attempt is made to pass the finger beneath the muscle from lateral to medial, the very intimate attachments between the iliopsoas muscle and the rectus femoris muscle prevent this from being done with ease. The entire iliopsoas muscle is dissected in a sharp and blunt manner until its insertion on the lesser trochanter is clearly defined. Several vessels of prominent size pass from the anterior surface of this muscle, and care should be taken to secure these vessels before their division. The iliopsoas muscle is severed at the level of its insertion on the lesser trochanter.

Transection of the Pectineus Muscle at Its Origin. Now attention is turned to the adductor muscles and their release from the pelvis (Fig. 14–3). It is important to note that this dissection proceeds from lateral to medial around the extremity. To preserve the obturator externus muscle on the pelvis, locate its prominent tendon arising from the lesser trochanter. The location of this tendon identifies the plane between the pectineus and obturator externus muscles; a difference in the direction of the fibers of these two muscles is also apparent. A finger is passed beneath the pectineus muscle, which is released at the level of its origin from the pubis with electrocautery. Beneath the pectineus muscle, numerous branches of the obturator artery, vein, and nerve can now be visualized; these are clamped, divided, and ligated.

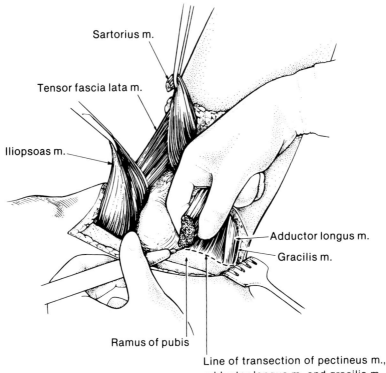

Sartorius m.

Tensor fascia lata m.

Iliopsoas m.

Adductor longus m.

Gracilis m.

Ramus of pubis

Line of transection of pectineus m.,
adductor longus m. and gracilis m.

FIGURE 14–3. Transection of the anteriorly placed muscles from lateral to medial at their origin or insertion. (*From* Sugarbaker PH, Chretien PB: A surgical technique for hip disarticulation. Surgery 90:546, 1981.)

Transection of the Gracilis and Adductor Longus, Brevis, and Magnus Muscles from Their Origin; Division of the Obturator Vessels and Nerve. The remainder of the adductor muscles are transected at their origin on the symphysis pubis; these include the gracilis, adductor longus, adductor brevis, and adductor magnus muscles. Note that the obturator vessels and nerves usually bifurcate around the adductor brevis muscle. It is important that branches of the obturator artery be identified and secured during the dissection to prevent accidental rupture and retraction of the proximal ends up into the pelvis. Progressive abduction of the extremity facilitates exposure of the adductor magnus muscle.

Division of the Obturator Externus Muscle at Its Insertion. A finger is passed around the obturator externus muscle, which is isolated as it arises from the obturator foramen. Its tendon is severed at its insertion into the lesser trochanter with electrocautery (Fig. 14–4).

Release of the Flexor Muscles from the Ischial Tuberosity. The extremity is hyperabducted to help localize the ischial tuberosity and also to retract the cut ends of the adductor muscles. The flexor muscles, sciatic nerve, and quadratus femoris muscle are now identified (Fig. 14–5). The large circumflex femoral vessels are nearby and should be avoided. The semimembranosus and semitendinosus muscles and the long head of the biceps femoris muscle are transected from their origin on the ischial tuberosity, while the quadratus femoris muscle and sciatic nerve are preserved.

Incision of the Anterior Portion of the Hip Joint Capsule. At this point, all the anterior and posterior muscle groups have been divided. The joint capsule overlying the head of the femur is incised, and the ligamentum teres is transected with electrocautery.

Completion of the Skin Incision. The surgeon now moves from a position anterior to one posterior to the patient. The patient's torso is tilted from posterolateral to antero-

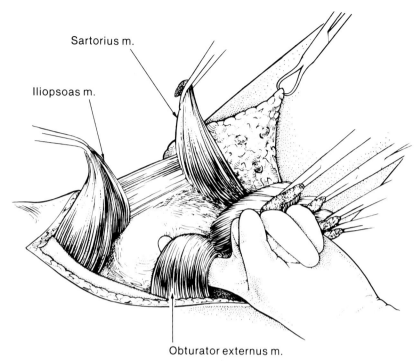

Sartorius m.

Iliopsoas m.

Obturator externus m.

FIGURE 14–4. Division of the obturator externus muscle at its origin. (*From* Sugarbaker PH, Chretien PB: A surgical technique for hip disarticulation. Surgery 90:546, 1981.)

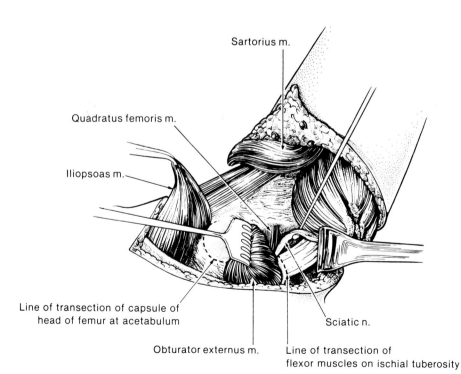

Sartorius m.

Quadratus femoris m.

Iliopsoas m.

Line of transection of capsule of head of femur at acetabulum

Obturator externus m.

Sciatic n.

Line of transection of flexor muscles on ischial tuberosity

FIGURE 14–5. Division of the flexor muscles. (*From* Sugarbaker PH, Chretien PB: A surgical technique for hip disarticulation. Surgery 90:546, 1981.)

lateral, and the skin incision is completed down through the gluteal fascia.

Division of the Tensor Fascia Lata, Gluteus Maximus, and Rectus Femoris Muscles. The tensor fascia lata and gluteus maximus muscles are divided in the depths of the skin incision (Fig. 14–6). These are the only muscles not divided at either their origin or insertion in the procedure. Directly beneath these muscles is the rectus femoris muscle, which is transected at its origin on the anterior inferior iliac spine with electrocautery.

Transection of the Muscles Inserting into the Greater Trochanter. After division of the gluteus maximus muscle, the common tendon that contains the multiple muscles inserting into the greater trochanter is exposed (Fig. 14–7). This tendon receives contributions from the gluteus medius, gluteus minimus, piriformis, superior gemellus, obturator internus, inferior gemellus, and quadratus femoris muscles. These muscles are divided close to their insertions on the greater trochanter with electrocautery.

Release of the Specimen. Transection of the hip joint capsule is completed by incising its posterior portion. The sciatic nerve is disssected free of surrounding muscle, transected, and allowed to retract beneath the piriformis muscle.

Approximation of the Quadratus Femoris and Iliopsoas Muscles over the Joint Capsule. After the specimen is removed from the operative field, the area is copiously irrigated with saline, and all bleeding points are secured. The basic principle in closure is coverage of the protruding acetabulum with the muscles that have been preserved. The quadratus femoris muscle is secured to the iliopsoas muscle over the joint capsule with interrupted sutures. Often the lower portion of the iliopsoas can be used to fill the empty joint capsule.

Approximation of the Obturator Externus and Gluteus Medius Muscles over the Joint Capsule. To help provide soft tissue coverage of bony prominences, these muscles are sutured together over the acetabulum (Fig. 14–8).

Approximation of the Gluteal Fascia to the Inguinal Ligament and Pubic Ramus. The gluteal fascia is elevated and secured to the inguinal ligament and pubic ramus (Fig. 14–9). When this is done, it becomes apparent that the posterior myocutaneous flap is much longer than the anterior fascia. Therefore,

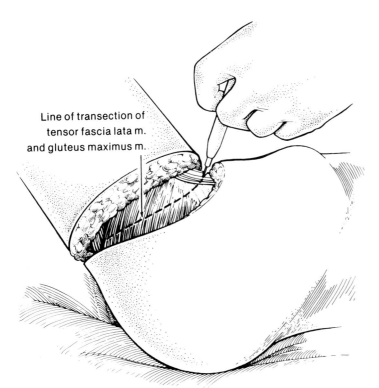

Line of transection of
tensor fascia lata m.
and gluteus maximus m.

FIGURE 14–6. Posterior skin incision and division of the tensor fascia lata, gluteus maximus, and rectus femoris muscles in the depths of the skin incision. (*From* Sugarbaker PH, Chretien PB: A surgical technique for hip disarticulation. Surgery 90:546, 1981.)

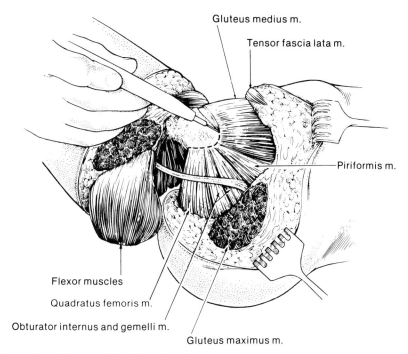

FIGURE 14–7. Transection of the conjoined tendon. (*From* Sugarbaker PH, Chretien PB: A surgical technique for hip disarticulation. Surgery 90:546, 1981.)

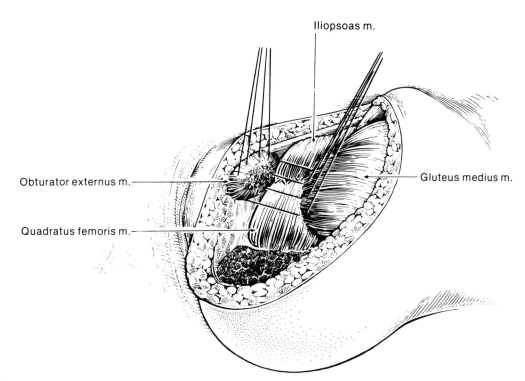

FIGURE 14–8. Muscular coverage of the hip joint capsule. (*From* Sugarbaker PH, Chretien PB: A surgical technique for hip disarticulation. Surgery 90:546, 1981.)

Inguinal ligament

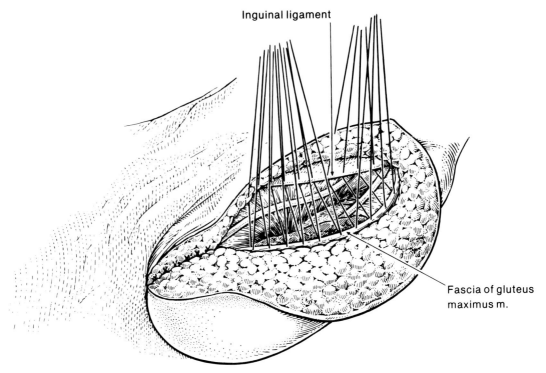

Fascia of gluteus
maximus m.

FIGURE 14–9. Fascial closure. (*From* Sugarbaker PH, Chretien PB: A surgical technique for hip disarticulation. Surgery 90:546, 1981.)

Drainage catheter

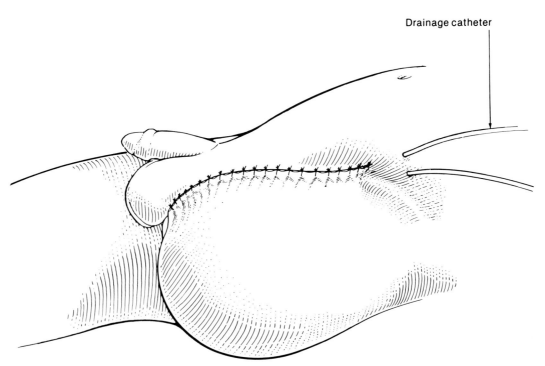

FIGURE 14–10. Skin closure with generous suction drainage. (*From* Sugarbaker PH, Chretien PB: A surgical technique for hip disarticulation. Surgery 90:546, 1981.)

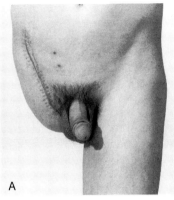
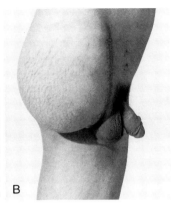
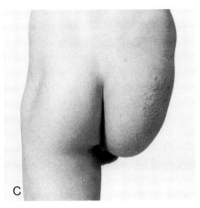

FIGURE 14–11. Anterior *(A)*, lateral *(B)*, and posterior *(C)* views of the stump constructed in a hip disarticulation procedure. Note the prominent stump; bone protuberances are covered with muscle so that prolonged weight bearing is well tolerated. (*From* Sugarbaker PH, Chretien PB: Hip disarticulation. *In* Sugarbaker PH, Nicholson T: Atlas of Extremity Sarcoma Surgery. Philadelphia, JB Lippincott Co, 1984, p 124.)

multiple stitches are made that bisect the fascial edge and uniformly gather the gluteus fascia as it is secured to the inguinal ligament. Sutures are individually placed and then tied. Before closure, a suction catheter is placed beneath the gluteal fascia.

Skin Closure. The skin is closed with interrupted sutures; again, one must make sure that there is equal distribution of the excess tissue on the posterior flap (Fig. 14–10). Not infrequently, additional suction catheters must be used to obliterate space within the subcutaneous tissue when the buttock flap is thick. Patency of the suction catheter must be maintained until drainage is diminished. Ambulation may proceed on the first postoperative day if the patient's hemodynamic status permits.

DISCUSSION

The hip disarticulation procedure as performed here is technically demanding. Considerable knowledge of the musculature around the hip and accurate dissection are required to preserve iliopsoas, obturator externus, and quadratus femoris muscles. These muscles, used to cover the protruding acetabulum, provide a generous cushion capable of bearing weight over extended time periods (Fig. 14–11).

Hip disarticulation is a well-tolerated procedure. Virtually none of the many problems seen after hemipelvectomy occur after this procedure. Wound infection may occur but

is much less frequently seen. Phantom limb pain is often noted but is of less severity than that after hemipelvectomy.

One problem more frequently encountered in female patients concerns the discrepancy of the thick buttock subcutaneous tissue as compared with that of the abdominal wall. When this tissue is closed, considerable tension on the abdominal wall skin may result. Preservation of a small flap of skin extending over the inguinal ligament provides a simple solution to this problem.

SUMMARY

Hip disarticulation is usually elected for malignant bony and soft tissue tumors below the lesser trochanter of the femur and for soft tissue sarcomas of the medial thigh. After incision of the skin and division of the femoral vessels and nerve, muscles of the anterior thigh are transected off the pelvic bone from lateral to medial, starting with the sartorius and finishing with the adductor magnus. Muscles are divided at their origin, except for the iliopsoas and obturator externus, which are divided at their insertion on the lesser trochanter of the femur. The quadratus femoris muscle is identified and preserved, then the flexor muscles are transected at their site of origin from the ischial tuberosity. The gluteal fascia, tensor fascia lata, and gluteus maximus muscle are divided and dissected free of their posterior attachments to expose the muscles inserting by way of a common tendon onto the greater trochanter. These muscles are then transected at their insertion on the bone. The posterior aspect of the joint capsule is now exposed and transected. Finally, the sciatic nerve is divided and allowed to retract beneath the piriformis muscle. To close the wound, the preserved muscles are approximated over the joint capsule, and the gluteal fascia is secured to the inguinal ligament over suction drains. The skin is closed with interrupted sutures.

REFERENCES

1. Bickel WH, Koch M: Amputations about the Shoulder and about the Hip. Boston, Little, Brown & Co, 1971.
2. Boyd HB: Anatomic disarticulation of the hip. Surg Gynecol Obstet 84:346, 1947.
3. Kirk NT: Amputations. Hagerstown, Maryland, WF Pryor Co, 1943.
4. Slocum DB: An Atlas of Amputation. St Louis, CV Mosby Co, 1949.
5. Sugarbaker PH, Nicholson T: Atlas of Extremity Sarcoma Surgery. Philadelphia, JB Lippincott Co, 1984.

15

Hemipelvectomy and Translumbar Amputation

Lawrence D. Wagman, M.D.
José J. Terz, M.D.

Hemipelvectomy

Radical amputations, including hemipelvectomy, are an important part of the diverse armamentarium of the surgical oncologist.[5] The trauma surgeon and the vascular surgeon also find themselves faced with difficult problems of tissue destruction and are forced to resort to similar aggressive amputations as emergent, lifesaving procedures. The hemipelvectomy (hindquarter amputation or sacroiliac disarticulation), first described by Girard in 1895, is an operative resection of the lower extremity, including the ipsilateral pelvic bones up to the sacroiliac joint and pubic symphysis. Variable amounts of soft tissue are resected and convenient flaps are constructed to close the defect. In the last decade, the expanding use of limb-sparing procedures and rational use of radiation therapy and chemotherapy as adjuvants have reduced the number of ablative amputations performed. The justification for such extensive operative procedures is a potential curative effect or an improvement in disease-free survival. Often, amputation is used palliatively to control lifestyle-limiting pain when other modalities of treatment have been exhausted. As hemipelvectomy becomes a less common procedure, variations to improve the operative management, reduce the postoperative complications, provide for improved survival, and maximize the postoperative rehabilitation potential of the patient become critical. With greater long-term experience, surgeons better understand the technical aspects of the procedure, reduce intraoperative blood loss, and decrease operative time.

INDICATIONS AND PRINCIPLES

Hemipelvectomy is primarily an elective procedure, although at times it must be performed in emergency situations. Whether the operation is done when the patient is near death or is performed in a more routine fashion, general guidelines for ultimate success can be identified. When there is a malignancy that is technically resectable, a complete preoperative evaluation for the presence of metastatic disease should be performed. For the soft tissue and bony sarcomas, this work-up usually includes whole lung tomograms or a computed axial tomographic (CAT) scan of the chest, evaluation of the liver, and often a CAT scan of the bony and soft tissue components of the primary tumor. With some tumors (e.g., melanoma) in which the potential for spread includes nodal disease that may not be detected on preoperative and diagnostic evaluation, a diagnostic celiotomy may be incorporated into the hemipelvectomy operation. In the more extreme setting, in which the operation is performed for control of life-threatening hemorrhage or sepsis,[6] preoperative evaluation is limited by the underlying clinical problem. It is important in these situations for the surgeon to evaluate the extent of the malignant disease intraoperatively to ensure that the surgical procedure adequately and rapidly controls both the acute life-threatening problem and the underlying malignant condition. In general, when hemipelvectomy is considered, five specific indications can be defined:

1. Bony tumors involving the proximal femur and hip joint; unilateral pelvic bones, including the symphysis pubis, pubic bones, and ischium; and iliac bones up to and including the sacroiliac joint.

2. Soft tissue sarcomas of the proximal thigh and buttocks and those arising in the true pelvis.

3. Extensive soft tissue sarcomas (melanoma, squamous cell carcinoma) of the lower extremity.

4. Vascular disease with tissue loss and progressive gangrene.

5. A dysfunctional lower extremity with nonreconstructible decubitus ulcers, massive trauma, or life-threatening sepsis.

The difficult question of whether to perform radical amputation solely for palliation is best decided on an individual patient basis. Besides the acute life-threatening situations in which palliative surgery may allow treatment of distant disease (e.g., pulmonary metastases), despite its failure to cure the patient, other situations arise in which palliation is important. Patients with severe pain and intractable wound complications (tumor necrosis, large fungating tumor masses) are also candidates for palliative surgery. The magnitude of the surgical procedure, the extent of possible rehabilitation, and the inevitable outcome of the disease must be carefully weighed when patients are considered for palliation by hemipelvectomy.

PROCEDURE

The technical aspects of performing hemipelvectomies are related to the location of the primary tumor; therefore, multiple variations of the procedure have emerged to comply with these restrictions. Variations are possible in the level of division of the vascular and neural structures, maintenance of a portion of the bony pelvis, and construction of an appropriate soft tissue flap to provide coverage of the operative defect. Such additional procedures as exploratory laparotomy and resection of associated pelvic structures, including the bladder, colon, and female reproductive organs, are related to the goal of completely resecting the primary disease. Regardless of the handling of the soft tissue and bony resection, several principles of preparation are universal for the procedure. The patients must be adequately hydrated, be treated with prophylactic antibiotics for skin and soft tissue pathogens, have adequate blood available (6 units of packed red blood cells) at the beginning of surgery, and be in a nutritional condition consistent with good wound healing and a psychological condition that will allow postoperative rehabilitation. The operation is performed with the patient in a partial lateral decubitus position. The bladder is drained with a Foley catheter. The anus is sewn closed. The entire lower extremity on the affected side is prepared and draped to allow intraoperative manipulation for adequate exposure and to set appropriate tension for muscular and bony division. If a large fungating tumor or an area of tissue necrosis secondary to compression (decubitus ulcer) exists, it should be excluded with an occlusive transparent adhesive dressing after preparation of the skin. This reduces contamination by bacteria or malignant cells during the operation.

Posterior Flap Technique

The posterior flap composed of skin and subcutaneous tissue overlying the buttock muscles (primarily the gluteus maximus) is the most widely used flap design for hemipelvectomy (Fig. 15–1). It is the simplest to

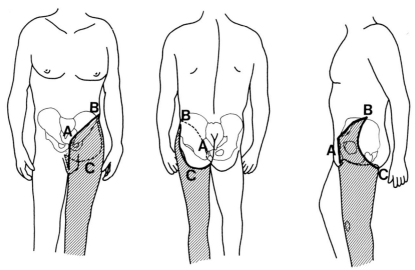

FIGURE 15–1. The posterior hemipelvectomy flap is illustrated in the anterior, posterior, and lateral positions. The shaded area represents that portion to be excised. The solid line defines the incision in the view shown, and the dotted line, the incision from the opposite side. Representative bony and soft tissue landmarks are the symphysis pubis (A), posterior superior iliac spine (B), and buttocks crease (C).

construct and is useful in covering the defect after hemipelvectomy for tumors of the more distal portion of the extremity and of the anterior structures of the soft tissue and bony hemipelvis.[1] Placement of the patient in a lateral position improves access to the incision and development of the posterior flap. This is best effected by placing sandbags or elevation devices under the patient's ipsilateral side at the time of initial positioning. A contralateral axillary roll may be necessary for patients whose surgery is performed in the true lateral position. The ability to move the leg across to the contralateral side promotes the ease in elevation of the flap.

The posterior portion of the skin and subcutaneous tissue flap begins at the level of the posterior superior iliac crest and extends laterally, roughly along the level of the gluteus maximus' insertion into the iliacus, to the greater trochanter. At the level of the greater trochanter, the incision courses medially along the gluteal crease to a point 1 to 2 cm lateral to the anus. This incision is, in turn, joined by the anterior incision along the perineum.

An extrafascial plane, based medially on the sacrum, is then developed. Use of tenacula or towel clamps to generate tension in raising the flap has been suggested. Inclusion of the gluteus maximus muscle in the flap when it is raised provides for a thicker flap; however, the blood supply to the gluteus

maximus is divided with transection of the common iliac artery at the level of the pelvic rim. Obviously, in some situations, the gluteus maximus provides the soft tissue margin for disease in the pelvis; therefore, unless the disease is clearly anterior in nature, it is prudent to include this muscular boundary on the specimen. The anterior portion of the skin incision begins at the posterior superior iliac spine, extends anteriorly to the anterior superior iliac spine, and continues to the pubic tubercle about 1 to 2 cm above the inguinal ligament.

Anterior Flap Technique

The anterior flap was developed to compensate for lesions that require resection of the soft tissue of the buttock along with the standard hemipelvectomy (Fig. 15–2). It is either a myocutaneous flap or one similar to the previously described posterior flap made up of skin and subcutaneous tissues. The primary difference is that a distinct blood supply (i.e., the superficial femoral artery) and draining vein are preserved. This definitive vascular supply is said to be of value in reducing perioperative flap complications.[4]

When the anterior flap is raised, an initial incision is made either at the pubic tubercle or at the anterior superior iliac spine and extends down into the anterior portion of

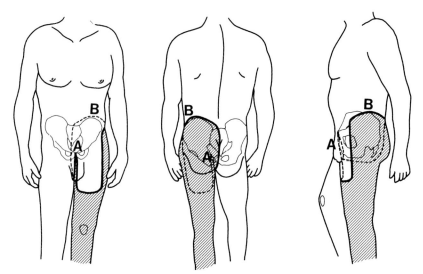

FIGURE 15–2. The anterior flap is illustrated in the anterior, posterior, and lateral positions. The shaded area represents that portion to be excised. The solid line defines the incision in the view shown, and the dotted line, the incision on the opposite surface. The symphysis pubis (A) and the posterior superior iliac spine (B) are the important bony landmarks. Longer myocutaneous flaps can be constructed that extend to the level of the suprapatellar bursa.

the thigh to a level just above the patella. Variation in the lateral or medial displacement of the initial incision is dictated by the location of the primary tumor. After completion of the skin and subcutaneous tissue incision, a plane may be developed beneath the tensor fascia lata and carried down to the level of the femoral vessels as they enter the adductor canal. Location of this deep margin further develops a plane for the subsequent cephalad dissection of the flap from the underlying muscles. Again, the medial portion of the skin incision is made as dictated by the location of the primary tumor and is extended up to the level of the inguinal ligament.

The vascular supply to the flap must be raised to the level of the bifurcation of the common iliac artery and may be divided at this time from the hypogastric artery. Care must be taken at the ligation point to ensure that no vascular compromise occurs owing to narrowing of the external iliac vessels. Further mobilization of the common iliac artery and vein to the aortic and caval bifurcation is required to ensure complete mobility at the time of bony transection. Branches from the external iliac and common femoral vessels to the flap should be carefully preserved throughout this dissection. However, the major branches of the superficial femoral artery, which provide the blood supply to the muscles of the thigh, require individual ligation during flap elevation.

In planning a myocutaneous flap based on the quadriceps muscle group (Fig. 15–3), a more extensive dissection is required. After the skin on the anterolateral aspect of the thigh is incised, the soft tissues and muscles are divided at a level above the patella. After this division, the superficial femoral artery

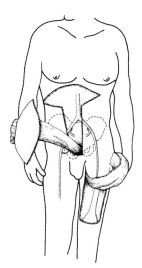

FIGURE 15–3. The elevation of the rectus abdominis myocutaneous flap is determined on the basis of the location of the contralateral inferior epigastric vessels. A skin flap of the correct size to cover the hemipelvectomy defect can be designed. The quadriceps femoris myocutaneous flap is an extension of the anterior skin and subcutaneous flap. The vascular supply is from the femoral artery and vein. The value of this flap is its reliability, bulkiness, and length.

and vein in the adductor canal are controlled, and the muscle insertion sites are sharply dissected off the femoral shaft with a knife or electrocautery. The lateral circumflex iliac artery and the proximal portion of the profunda femoris artery are preserved in the cephalad portion of the dissection, and the external iliac artery is traced to its origin. Careful control and ligation of the internal iliac artery are performed, and completion of the mobilization of the common iliac artery prepares the patient for the balance of the soft tissue and bony resection.

The use of customized flaps is sometimes necessary.[10] The authors have, on occasion, constructed rectus abdominis flaps based on the inferior epigastric artery's distribution (see Fig. 15–3) to cover resectional defects.

Whether anterior or posterior flaps are used, it is imperative that the flap be covered with warm, moist laparotomy pads after elevation and carefully protected against crushing, bony, or manipulative injury during the completion of the operative procedure.

Vascular Dissection

Division of the blood supply to the hindquarter involves a transection of either the common or the internal iliac artery. In either instance, the critical features are adequate mobility of structures and vascular control with suture ligature technique. No particular survival advantage or increased risk has been associated with early or late ligation of the vascular structures. At times, large lesions with the pelvis or involvement of contiguous structures (bladder, rectum, uterus) requires division of the major vascular structures after division of the bony pelvis to allow for "opening" of the pelvis.

The ureter is best identified and carefully protected early in the procedure at the time of identification of the aorta at its bifurcation to the common iliac arteries. If the ureter is swept medially, it can be protected during the division of the blood supply existing from the internal iliac artery to the pelvic structures.

The middle hemorrhoidal, superior vesical, and inferior vesical arteries are sequentially divided to provide mobility of the structures they supply and to prevent excessive backbleeding at the time of removal. In addition, the division of the vascular structures allows access to musculature of the hemipel-

vis (primarily the pelvic floor) in preparation for its ultimate division. Simultaneous with mobilization of the rectum and bladder, protection of the ureter, and division of the arterial or venous structures, the sacral nerve roots existing from the first through fifth sacral vertebrae (S1 through S5) can be divided just medial to the sacroiliac joint. This allows the operator to clean the soft tissues overlying the sacrum down to the planned bony resection margin.

Bony Resection

The bony resection is guided by the extent of the primary disease process, but significant variation is possible.[8] Maintenance of the pubic bone anteriorly (Fig. 15–4), the ischial tubercle, and the iliac crest posteriorly (Fig. 15–5) has become important to improve the overall rehabilitative potential of the patient. Resection extending beyond the midline anteriorly to involve the contralateral pubic bone may be performed for soft tissue and bony tumors in this area. If the tumor is juxtaposed or involves the sacroiliac joint, a bony resection including a portion of the ipsilateral sacrum can provide tumor-free bony margins. In general, for bony tumors, a 5 cm margin is favorable because it is most likely to include all tumor tissue and provide for a negative margin. Preservation of the posterior portion of the iliac crest allows for a more natural contouring of the body after resection. The amputee will sit more comfortably if the ischial tuberosity is salvaged.

In the standard hemipelvectomy, the pubic symphysis is divided with a Gigli saw or a knife through the cartilaginous articulation. The key point of this portion of the resection is to protect the urethra as it runs just under the bone. This is done by careful dissection, performed just posterior to the pubic symphysis with either a right-angle clamp or another blunt instrument, to find the appropriate plane. A malleable retractor may be placed behind the pubic bone to protect the urethra before division. Division of the sacroiliac joint is performed with a Gigli saw, a knife, or a chisel. Complete preparation of the bone anteriorly and posteriorly with division of the sacral vessels and the sacral venous plexus allows for rapid, controlled division of this structure at the appropriate time. If the technique using the Gigli saw is chosen, the saw is passed through the greater

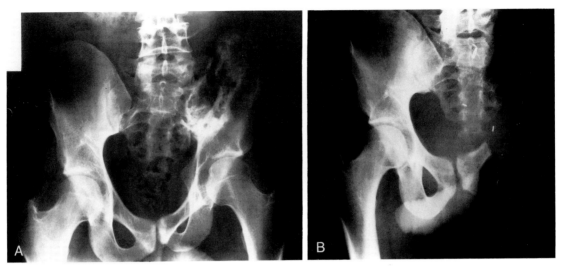

FIGURE 15–4. PB, a 20-year-old with osteogenic sarcoma of the left iliac bone, extending to the sacroiliac joint *(A)*. A modified hemipelvectomy, sparing the ischial tuberosity on the left and resecting a portion of the sacrum *(B)*, was performed.

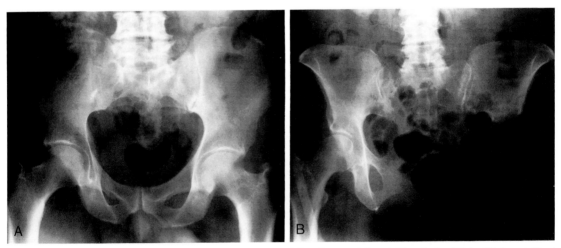

FIGURE 15–5. JB, a 60-year-old with a malignant fibrous histiocytoma of the right anterior thigh *(A)*. A modified hemipelvectomy, sparing the superior portion of the iliac bone and division of the symphysis pubis, *(B)* was performed.

sciatic notch, and a cephalad division of the sacroiliac joint is performed. Techniques using sharp division with a knife or chisel provide for a more accurate, complete disarticulation of the sacroiliac joint. However, in older patients, this area may be calcified and may not be amenable to a simple knife or chisel dissection. Here again, the Gigli saw technique aids in disarticulation. When modified procedures are performed, a Gigli saw or a power saw may be used to customize the resection.

Soft Tissue Resection

The soft tissue resection is performed in a stepwise fashion. Anteriorly, after the initial skin incision (for the posterior flap), the muscles of the anterior abdominal wall are released without transection from the pubic tubercle and anterior superior iliac spine. Muscles are not divided in this area but are left intact, unless the position of the tumor requires extension of the incision up onto the anterior abdominal wall. This is particularly the case for tumors overlying the femoral vessels and the inguinal crease. Release of the anterior musculature allows the surgeon to reach the retroperitoneal area for dissection of the vascular, neural, and bony structures when the anterior flap hemipelvectomy is performed.

After the posterior flap is raised, the rotator muscles of the hip and the muscles of the true pelvis may be divided off the sacrum; these include the gluteus maximus and medius, piriformis, obturator internus, and gemelli. This division exposes the sciatic nerve, which is controlled and divided as it exits beneath the sacrum. The sacrotuberous ligament at the inferior aspect of the sacrum is also divided during this portion of the dissection. Division of the psoas muscle completes the posterior release of the soft tissues. Of note is the iliolumbar ligament, which is divided as it courses from the transverse process of the fifth lumbar vertebra (L5) to the posterior superior iliac spine. Division of the soft tissues of the pelvic diaphragm completes the soft tissue resection in the anterior inferior location. Great care must be taken during division of these muscles to protect the critical pelvic structures, including the ureter, rectum, and bladder. These muscles are best divided from within the pelvis after complete division of the skin and subcutaneous tissues.

Use of the anterior or anterolateral myocutaneous flap for reconstruction is different only in that the anterior incision extends not across the area of the inguinal ligament but down onto the thigh. The muscles of the anterior abdominal wall and the flexors of the hip are similarly released from the pubic tubercle and anterior superior iliac spine to provide the anterior flap's vascular pedicle, which is supplied by the external iliac and, subsequently, the femoral arteries.

Internal Hemipelvectomy

The internal hemipelvectomy[2, 3] is a variant of the more standard hindquarter amputation but more accurately represents the name of the procedure. In the internal hemipelvectomy, a portion of the pelvic bone and adjacent musculature is resected without sacrifice of the ipsilateral lower extremity. This procedure is made possible by careful mobilization of the neurovascular structures to the ipsilateral lower extremity with division of the femoral neck and iliac bone at points appropriate to resect the tumor. Proponents of this technique point out its ability to maintain the leg's form with good cosmetic results despite an obligate ipsilateral leg shortening. After a prolonged period of hospitalization and skeletal traction and an aggressive physical therapy program, patients may be able to walk with a cane only; however, many still require the use of crutches. In either case, the use of the cumbersome energy-inefficient prosthesis is avoided. Despite its attractiveness, this procedure is rarely adequate for resection of a primary tumor.

Other Considerations

Because of the close association of the pelvic structures with adjacent pelvic tumors, more extensive resection of intrapelvic organs may be required. The surgical goal is creation of a negative microscopic margin and complete control of local disease. The pushing nature of the border of a sarcoma with indiscrete boundaries dictates that a clear margin be defined beyond the limits of the tumor. Hemipelvectomy, therefore, has been combined with cystectomy, hysterectomy, and intestinal resection to ensure that these primary surgical principles are preserved. It is often valuable to assess the status of the intra-abdominal organs, especially the liver, for metastatic disease at the time of hemipelvectomy. The peritoneum may be opened and explored after the anterior portion of the incision has been made. Although this is often an inadequate approach for biopsy or extensive resection, it provides the necessary "diagnostic window" early in the operative procedure before any irreversible surgical maneuvers are performed.

COMPLICATIONS

The complications of hemipelvectomy can be divided into those related to intraoperative, postoperative, and long-term morbidity. With care and appropriate intraoperative protection of the structures in the pelvis, such untoward complications as injuries to the ureter, bladder, and rectum can be easily avoided. The intraoperative blood loss usually ranges between 2000 and 5000 ml. Because of this, preoperative provisions must be made for adequate amounts of blood for transfusion during the operation to avoid episodes of hypotension; these may be anticipated at the times of division of large vascular structures, disarticulation of the sacroiliac joint with the sacral branches of the hypogastric vein, division of the infrapubic vessels, and division of the musculature of the pelvic floor, which is filled with multiple small venous and arterial plexuses. In the immediate postoperative period, complications of the flap and those related to the wound are of primary concern. Although much discussion has ensued as to the ideal flap for hemipelvectomy reconstruction, none appears to significantly improve survival or reduce complications. The principles of flap and wound closure must be adhered to, i.e., reduction of devascularized soft tissue, reduction of bacterial concentration, minimization of tension along the wound, and careful approximation of healthy, viable tissues. The use of drains prevents the collection of seromas and hematomas under the flap. The surgeon must be aware of distal ischemia in the flaps and be prepared to debride and revise these problematic areas.

Because of the extensive dissection in the pelvis with mobilization of the rectum and bladder from the pelvic sidewall and interruption of the pelvic splanchnic nerves, problems with defecation, urination, and sexual function may appear. Patients who lose their ability to sense fullness in the rectum or who have abnormalities in sphincter control should be placed on regular bowel protocols that provide for stools daily. An increase in dietary bulk, use of stool softeners, interval use of enemas, and bowel training re-educate the sluggish rectum. Denervation of the bladder may lead to long-term problems with voiding. Initial drainage with a Foley catheter is, of course, required, both for fluid management and because of patient immobility. Long-term bladder dysfunction is rare, but occasionally it may need to be managed with a long-term indwelling Foley catheter or with the use of intermittent catheterization. Finally, sexual functional difficulties based on vascular abnormalities have little potential for cure or rehabilitation. Protection of the nervi erigentes is the best method of reducing neural sexual dysfunction postoperatively. In either case, patients with sexual dysfunction can be treated with indwelling prosthetic devices as dictated by the patient's desire and the severity of the underlying disease process.

Because of the obvious change in weight bearing after hemipelvectomy, patients are likely to experience scoliotic changes in the spine. This may become especially problematic in those patients who have extended survival after a curative procedure.

Also, the problems of phantom limb pain and sensation plague the hemipelvectomy patients in whom they appear. Multiple medications, including chlordiazepoxide, carbamazepine, and standard pain medications (aspirin, nonsteroidal anti-inflammatory drugs, or codeine), have been prescribed for these untoward sensations. Unfortunately, the response is highly variable, and the physician is left with experimentation to provide the best method of symptom control in individual patients. Implantable and transcutaneous devices that provide stimulation to the nerve roots and operate on the "gate theory" have also been tried. The results are disappointingly similar to medicinal manipulations. Fortunately, much of the initial symptomatology resolves over time, and assuring the patient of this and supporting the complaints and fears during the recovery phase aid in the ultimate resolution of the problem. No precise surgical technique has been identified that prevents phantom sensation. Suggestions have been made that the nerve be cut sharply, clamps not be placed across tissue left in situ, and a variety of suture materials be used for control of the neural vascular plexus. Again, successes with these individual treatments are highly anecdotal and not reproducible.

REHABILITATION

The responsibility of the surgeon does not end with closure of the operative wound or even with the discharge of the patient from the hospital. One must be concerned not only with the reduction of morbidity but also with the return of the patient to a functional lifestyle. To this end, extensive preoperative counseling and postoperative planning for a prosthesis that will allow the patient both cosmetic and functional recovery are imperative. The early sense of loss for the amputated body part can be ameliorated with a well-fashioned prosthesis that returns form to the lower extremity and allows the patient, even in a static state, to "look normal." This, however, is merely the beginning, and return to a functional state is critical. Research has shown that a high percentage of patients with amputations for bony and soft tissue sarcomas return to the normal workplace and a lifestyle similar to the preoperative one.[9, 11] Aiding patients in these endeavors becomes the primary postoperative imperative for the surgeon.

Because a large number of the patients are of young or middle age, the ability to function with the somewhat bulky three-part hemipelvectomy prosthesis is still possible (Fig. 15–6). The increased energy expenditure for a hemipelvectomy patient using a prosthesis and walking at a normal place has been established.[7] These patients have two times the normal energy expenditure compared with normal subjects walking at their fastest possible rate. Of interest is that when patients using crutches after hemipelvectomy are compared with those patients who have not undergone amputation, walking at a normal pace, the hemipelvectomy patients can travel as fast, if not faster, and with a similar oxygen consumption. Therefore, it must be understood that patients not only must invest a significant amount of time learning to use the prosthetic device but also must invest significant extra energy to function with the prosthesis. This may preclude use of the prosthetic devices by older patients who have myocardial or pulmonary dysfunction limiting their exercise tolerance. In light of such information, patients need a complete evaluation of their exercise tolerance postoperatively, with such stress parameters as arm ergometry to rule out myocardial ischemia. This evaluation is particularly important in the older age group and in those patients who have taken some myocardial toxic chemotherapeutic agent before amputation (e.g., doxorubicin [Adriamycin]).

The sexual dysfunction attending hemipelvectomy with destruction of the nervi erigentes in the male can be treated with various indwelling penile protheses. It is of interest that in studies comparing those patients who have undergone amputation with those whose limbs were salvaged, the sexual function appears to be better preserved in the amputees. The reason for this is uncertain and may be related to the other treatment modalities offered to the patient with limb-sparing procedures.

RESULTS

Hemipelvectomy continues to be an uncommon surgical procedure. In the last 10 years, approximately 20 such procedures have been performed at the City of Hope National Medical Center. Eighteen of the 20 patients are available for evaluation. In this group of patients, the mean age was 43 years, with a range of 12 to 76 years. Thirteen patients received the standard hemipelvectomy described in the procedural portion of this chapter, and an additional five received modifed hemipelvectomies. Most patients had soft tissue sarcomas (9/18); many had bony tumors of the pelvis (7/18). One patient had a chronic infection in a high above-knee amputation, and another had a metastatic thyroid tumor known to be present only in the iliac wing. One patient died in the early postoperative period of sepsis and pulmonary failure, yielding a surgical mortality rate of 6%.

Complications involving the bladder were present in five patients, four of whom had postoperative neurogenic bladders and one of whom had fistula tract formation secondary to breakdown of a bladder wall closure after an en bloc resection that included a

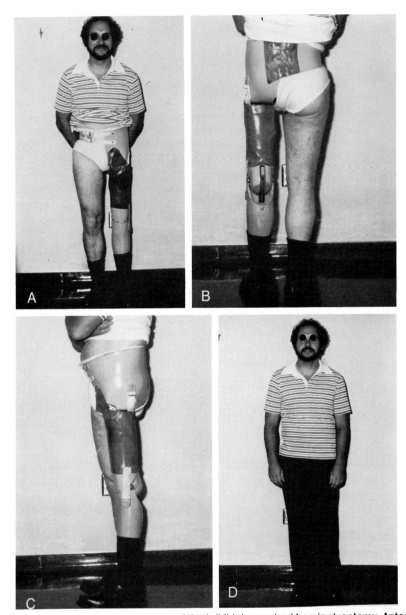

FIGURE 15–6. CS, a 32-year-old with a liposarcoma of the left thigh, required hemipelvectomy. Anterior *(A)*, posterior *(B)*, and lateral *(C)* views of the standing patient illustrate the prosthesis. When the patient is standing, the cosmetic effect is excellent and comfortable *(D)*.

portion of the bladder. Wound problems occurred in eight patients: two with abscesses, three with separation of the wound, and three with areas of frank flap necrosis. Drainage and secondary closure was required for the abscesses. Wound separation was treated then allowed to heal by secondary intention. Flap necrosis was treated with debridement and either delayed primary or secondary closure. Problems with phantom pain and phantom sensation are described by all hemipelvectomy patients, and this group was not different in that respect. The patients spent approximately 3 to 4 weeks in the hospital from day of admission until day of discharge. Most patients were fitted with prostheses, although few used them on a long-term basis.

SUMMARY

Hemipelvectomy is used in patients whose disease is in the proximal thigh, inguinal crease, or buttocks areas. Tumors are the most common indication for hemipelvectomy, but massive traumatic injury and extensive vascular disease occasionally warrant hemipelvectomy for management. The surgical goals are extirpation of disease, closure of the wound with healthy tissue, and rapid rehabilitation of the patient. Complications are few and primarily relate to the operative procedure. Excellent long-term results can be anticipated if the underlying disease is controlled locally and systemically.

Translumbar Amputation

Translumbar amputation (TLA), also known as hemicorporectomy, is a radical surgical procedure that is indicated only as a measure of last resort for patients with a life-threatening diagnosis but with an otherwise normal life expectancy if the current disease process can be corrected. This surgical procedure entails the transection of the lumbar spine at or below the third lumbar vertebra, with subsequent loss of the bony pelvis, rectum, bladder, genitalia, and both lower extremities. The significant physical and functional disability resulting from this procedure demands a careful patient selection.

INDICATIONS

The basic premises that determine which patients will benefit from this procedure are

1. An expected normal life span after extirpation of the life-threatening disease.

2. The emotional and psychological maturity to understand and cope with the extensive physical, functional, and emotional disability resulting from the loss of the lower one half of the body.

3. The mental determination and physical strength to undergo the intensive rehabilitation programs that are required of such physically disabled patients to attain at least 95% of functional independence in the activities of daily living.

Of patients with neoplastic diseases, those with locally advanced sacral chordomas are potential candidates. These tumors are slow growing and have a very low incidence of distant metastases. These metastases usually develop after many years and repeated attempts at local control. Most of these patients eventually die as a result of complications associated with locally advanced pelvic tumors (sepsis, bleeding, and urinary and intestinal obstruction) and not of metastatic disease.[12, 13] On the other hand, patients with advanced neoplasms (carcinomas or sarcomas) arising from pelvic structures should not be considered as operative candidates; invariably, these patients die of metastatic disease.[18]

Paraplegic patients with intractable decubitus ulcers, with or without osteomyelitis of the pelvic bones, also should be considered capable of benefiting significantly from TLA.[20] This procedure removes nonfunctional parts of the body that cause repeated hospital admissions (sepsis, bleeding, complex wound care) and bed confinement, which deprive these patients of the benefits from the established rehabilitation programs for well-compensated paraplegics. Also included in this group are patients who develop epidermoid cancer in chronic decubitus ulcers.

Decision Process

The process that the patient and family undergo in accepting this procedure is the gradual realization that the progressive physical and emotional deterioration of the patient is due to an illness confined to organs that have already ceased to function. For the paraplegic patient who has developed multiple and intractable complications, the presence of epidermoid cancer in the decubitus ulcer introduces a new life-threatening factor and enhances the urgency of the decision.

In patients with sacral chordomas, continuous and severe pain dominates the clinical picture, which is followed years later with loss of function of the pelvic organs and lower extremities. The patient comes to understand the progressive nature of the tumor, the severity of the disability, and the reality of death in the immediate future. At this point, the patient must seriously consider a radical surgical procedure as the only solution to arrest the progressive physical debility, control the emotional deterioration, and provide an attempt at disease cure.

A multidisciplinary, integrated team—led by a surgical oncologist and supported by a neurosurgeon, social worker, psychologist, occupational therapist, physical therapist, stomal nurse, and clinical nurse specialist—provides the physical and emotional structure needed to carry the patients and their families through these procedures. Many extensive and detailed discussions of all aspects of the surgical procedure and all possible complications and outcomes facilitate understanding and minimize all the expected apprehensions. The patient and family must meet at various times with different members of the team. Careful description of the parts of the anatomy to be removed and the physical rehabilitation to take place, and an interview with a patient who has had a similar procedure facilitate comprehension of the procedure.

PROCEDURE

Anesthesia Considerations

A central venous catheter and radial artery line are inserted for accurate hemodynamic monitoring, to guide fluid replacement, and to prevent fluid overload with the readjustment of body mass.[19]

Incision

The skin incision is carefully outlined, with consideration that maximal skin coverage is needed to accomplish wound closure (Fig. 15–7). The integrity of the abdominal contents is totally dependent on the careful closure of the subcutaneous tissue and skin. Anteriorly, the skin incision comes across the pubis and follows the inguinal ligaments bilaterally. The incision may be brought distal to the inguinal ligaments if necessary. Laterally, it should go below the iliac crest and, posteriorly, should include skin over the buttocks. The incision is tailored depending on the amount of viable skin and degree of soft tissue involvement. At this point, the skin is dissected from the bony pelvis and retracted superiorly.

Once the skin incision is completed, the abdominal rectus muscles are detached from the pubis, and the oblique muscles are detached from the femoral canal, iliac crest, and posterior iliac spine. The abdominal cavity is entered, and the aorta and vena cava are divided above the bifurcation and closed with 4-0 monofilament vascular sutures. The ureters are divided below the pelvic rim. The psoas muscle and lumbar plexus are divided bilaterally. The sigmoid colon is mobilized and divided, leaving the lumbar spine as the only place of continuity.

Division of the Spinal Canal (Transabdominal Approach)

Once all intra-abdominal structures are divided, the appropriate intervertebral space is exposed, and the disc is divided with a knife; then, with an osteotome, the spine is completely severed, separating the specimen. The procedure tends to avulse the dura mater and elements of the cauda equina, resulting in bleeding, which is controlled with packing. At this point, the spinal canal is exposed. All bleeding vessels are cauterized. The dura mater is repaired and closed. The canal is packed with pieces of fat and muscle. It is recommended that the spinous process and lamina of the last remaining lumbar vertebra be removed to avoid pressure points on the prothesis when the patient assumes a sitting position.

Laminectomy

When there is an unknown element of extension of the tumor along the spinal canal, the abdominal procedure is preceded by a laminectomy to gain access to the spinal canal. The patient is placed in a prone position, and the lumbar spine is exposed two intervertebral disc spaces above the expected level of amputation. The dural sac is opened, and frozen sections of the dural edges and tissues from the canal are obtained to determine the presence of tumor extension. The cauda equina is divided, and the proximal

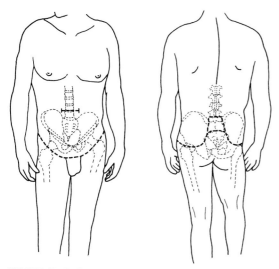

FIGURE 15–7. Outline of the anterior and posterior skin incision for translumbar amputation. The posterior skin flap is designed according to the extent of skin involvement over the sacrum and buttocks.

and distal segments of the dural sac are closed. The laminectomy wound is then closed, and the patient is placed in the supine position; the abdominal procedure is performed as previously described.

Ostomies

When feasible, the urinary conduit is constructed with a segment of distal sigmoid colon; otherwise, a segment of ileum is used. Because the lower third of the abdominal wall is used to support the intra-abdominal contents, both ostomies must be brought out through the upper half of the abdominal wall, close to the costal margin, but leaving the necessary space to fit the appliances.

The abdomen is closed by approximating the oblique muscles laterally and the subcutaneous tissue and skin of the posterior flap to the fascia, skin, and subcutaneous tissue of the anterior abdominal wall.

REHABILITATION

The rehabilitation process is initiated before surgery.[14, 16, 17] The core treatment team is composed of the surgeon, clinical nurse specialist, floor nurse, occupational therapist, physical therapist, enterostomal therapist, prosthetist, psychologist, pharmacist, dietician, social worker, and discharge planner. The patient and family members attend a presurgical conference with all team members present. Patient questions are answered, misconceptions addressed, and facts presented concerning the proposed surgery and its functional ramifications. This is done in an unhurried and comfortable setting outside the clinic area. The patient's anxieties are lessened by meeting with the staff before surgery. A comprehensive rehabilitation team approach reduces feelings of hopelessness and isolation and acknowledges the family's role in the restorative process. The staff is able to assess the patient's level of motivation and the support available to the patient. After the information sharing meeting, the patient is scheduled for evaluations with physical and occupational therapy. Performance abilities are assessed for range of motion, muscle strength, endurance, and activities of daily living.

Deep-breathing exercises are taught to reduce the potential of postoperative pulmonary complications. Beginning strengthening and bed mobility exercises early in the postoperative course appears to benefit the patient physically and psychologically. Use of a multicompartment air mattress to minimize pressure over bony prominences and to help maintain body temperature equilibrium is suggested. An overhead trapeze system allows the patient to participate in repositioning, transfers, and bed mobility activities. Amputation site desensitization exercises are provided to alleviate postoperative and phantom pain. Occasionally, a transcutaneous electric nerve stimulation unit is used to assist in pain reduction. Each patient is shown a video tape chronicling the phases of rehabilitation after translumbar amputation. The tape serves as a motivational tool. The film depicts donning and doffing prostheses, transferring to chairs, cars, and bathtubs, and ambulating in wheelchairs.

Rehabilitation treatment goals are outlined in Table 15–1. During the first postoperative month, these goals include establishing the patient's ability to lift the full body weight with the use of the overhead trapeze; independence in rolling, scooting, supine and prone lying, dressing, and managing ostomy

Table 15–1. OUTLINE OF POSTOPERATIVE PHYSICAL REHABILITATION PROGRAM FOR TRANSLUMBAR AMPUTEES

Activities	Assessment	Goal
Bathing	Unable	Independent with device
Feeding	Independent	Independent
Dressing	Unable	Independent
Grooming	Assisted	Independent
Bed mobility	Moderate assistance	Independent with device
Transfers	Moderate assistance	Independent
Wheelchair mobility	Moderate assistance	Independent
Ambulation	Unable	Not a goal
Driving	Unable	Independent with device

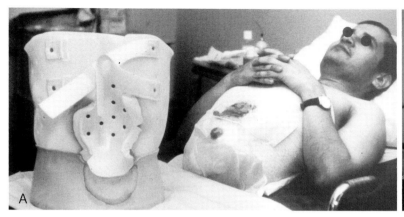
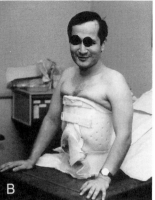

FIGURE 15–8. A, A patient 6 months after translumbar amputation, with a prosthetic bucket. B, The patient seated in the prosthetic bucket.

appliances; transferring from bed to a semi-reclining wheelchair or an adapted bath bench; and wheelchair propulsion of 1000 feet on level surfaces. The wheelchair is weighted to prevent tipping and is initially a reclining type, as the patient must reacclimate to the upright position. Careful monitoring of blood pressure, heart rate, and respiratory rate during the initial phases of rehabilitation is necessary. The patient can approximate a fully upright position but cannot maintain one without the use of a prosthetic bucket.

Depending on the status of the wound healing, a cast of the stump can be taken as early as the fourth postoperative week. Prosthetic considerations include an allowance for the pronounced protuberance of the spinal column, the amount of soft tissue at the distal stump, and the placement of the ostomy appliances.[15] The ideal goal is a total contact prosthesis that does not exert pressure on the spine or ostomies. A major prosthetic difficulty is managing the large amount of soft tissue at the distal end of the stump. This is demonstrated by comparing casting results from the supine and suspended positions. The supine cast is found to be more effective, but fitting problems still exist. Shrinkage of the stump postoperatively is also a consideration in regard to the timing of the prosthetic fitting.

The design and construction of the prosthesis is adequately described by other authors. The critical factor in this prosthesis is that the outside structure be composed of a rigid material, such as polypropylene, laminated polyester, or acrylic resin. The internal portion of the structure may or may not be lined; patients tend to prefer internal lining, such as one half inch plastazote. The base of the prosthesis is made up of a polyurethane foam material and is set in the neutral position. The prosthesis is closed by Velcro straps. A newer modification that has been successful in two cases is a corset front to manage the pressure on the ostomies and prevent prolapse. The technique for donning and doffing the prothesis in a supine position is taught and can be independently managed by the patient (Fig. 15–8).

Before the patient is discharged, the occupational and physical therapists schedule a home visit to determine architectural barriers and wheelchair accessibility. Problem solving with the home health care therapists is ideally done at this time, and much information can be shared regarding the patient's treatment plan. The family is included in the discussion of construction of ramps and bathroom accessibility. Once the recommendations are implemented, the patient is ready for discharge. The patient and family members who will be transporting the patient are instructed in car transfer.

After the patient is discharged, the rehabilitation team maintains contact through outpatient visits, follow-up telephone calls, and reports from the home health agency. Weekly rehabilitation team meetings are an excellent way to maintain a high degree of communication and disseminate patient information. Concerns regarding ostomy care, medication usage, nutrition, functional activity level, family difficulties, psychosocial problems, and medical issues can be addressed during this meeting. The team can also address future issues, such as the appropriate timing of vocational rehabilitation counseling and a driver's training program.

In sumary, no one health professional can be all things to each patient. The use of a rehabilitation team relieves one person of this impossible responsibility. The rehabilitation team's goal is to ensure that patients and their families are taken care of physically as well as psychologically. The continued success of this team depends on the involvement of all the respective disciplines. Maintenance of a rehabilitation team requires time, hard work, and commitment but is well worth the effort when measured in improvement of quality in patients' lives.

CLINICAL EXPERIENCE

Between 1983 and 1985, four patients underwent translumbar amputation at the authors' insititution. The pertinent clinical information for each patient is summarized in Table 15–2.

Case Reports

CASE 1. This 33-year-old man had been treated in the previous 20 years with multiple procedures for recurrent chondroscarcoma of the pelvis; treatment included a right hemipelvectomy at the age of 13 and, with subsequent recurrences, resection of the rectum with an end colostomy, a right nephrectomy, an ileal conduit, and resection of the left sciatic plexus. On admission, the patient had recurrent tumor involving the remaining pelvis and edema with gangrene of the left lower extremity. A radionuclide bone scan and CAT scan of the abdomen and chest failed to demonstrate any tumor outside the pelvis. Although patients with sarcoma are not usually considered for this procedure, the long natural history of the tumor, the absence of distant metastases, and the persistence of a low-grade histological pattern in this chondrosarcoma throughout the many recurrences supported the recommendation for translumbar amputation.

From the patient's perspective, the procedure offered a possibility for complete removal of the tumor and a chance to regain physical independence. Within 3 months of surgery, the patient attained 95% of the rehabilitation goals. Nine months later, the patient developed hydrocephalus secondary to meningeal metastases, which required a ventriculovenous shunt. The patient retained the ability to care for himself and to move independently in a wheelchair until his last week of life, when he was admitted to the hospital, where he died from pulmonary failure secondary to extensive lung metastasis. This was 24 months after the translumbar amputation. The seeding of the meninges can be explained by the involvement of the sacral canal by the pelvic recurrence, and the lung me-

Table 15–2. SUMMARY OF CLINICAL DATA FOR PATIENTS UNDERGOING TRANSLUMBAR AMPUTATION (TLA)

	Case 1	Case 2	Case 3	Case 4
Age (years)/sex	33/M	17/F	59/M	29/M
Diagnosis	Chondrosarcoma	AV malformation	Chordoma	Chordoma
Duration of illness before TLA (years)	20	12	5	6
Duration of surgical procedure (hours)	5.3	11.0	10.0	13.4
Intraoperative blood loss (ml)	3000	5000	3500	3000
Fluid replacement (ml)				
Whole blood	2000	3500	2500	1500
Red blood cells	0	300	750	2000
Crystalloids	2000	5000	3500	5000
Colloids	0	2000	2000	1800
Hospital complications	None	Urinary fistula	Small bowel obstruction	Urinary fistula
Hospital stay (days)	50	100	65	40
Status at follow-up (months)	Dead with metastasis (24)	Alive and well (24)	Alive and well (15)	Alive and well (9)

AV = arteriovenous.

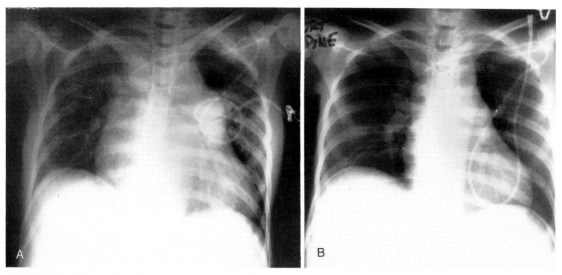

FIGURE 15–9. (Case 2.) *A,* Preoperative chest radiograph demonstrating marked enlargement of the cardiac silhouette, with prominent pulmonary vasculature. *B,* A chest radiograph 2 weeks after translumbar amputation shows a significant decrease in the size of the heart and disappearance of all prominent pulmonary vascular markings.

tastases are probably a result of the ventriculojugular shunt. The curative intent of this procedure was not accomplished, but the patient was able to be free of pain, to propel himself in a wheelchair, and to transfer with independence until his death.

CASE 2. This 17-year-old woman had a 12-year history of an arteriovenous malformation (AVM) involving the left lower extremity. Five years before her admission to City of Hope National Medical Center, the patient underwent a left hip disarticulation for pathological fracture of the femur and massive attempts at embolization of the pelvic arteriovenous (AV) communications with only temporary success.

At the time of the current admission, the patient had extensive necrosis of soft tissue and bone in the sacral region, associated with massive bleeding, sepsis, and congestive heart failure from the AV shunting (Fig. 15–9). She was malnourished, required continuous narcotic administration for pain control, and had a nonfunctional bladder and rectum. The translumbar amputation was considered as a measure of last resort, in light of the angiographic information that the source of the AV communications was limited to the pelvis (Fig. 15–10). Involvement of the spinal canal and proximal aorta was ruled out with selective angiograms of the pertinent vessels.

From the patient's and parents' perspective, this was an extremely difficult decision

to accept. They realized reluctantly the critical condition and the lack of any alternative form of treatment or temporizing measure. The patient tolerated the surgical procedure well but developed an unexplained fistula from the urinary ileal conduit that required surgical repair. The patient has gained 30 pounds and has fulfilled all the rehabilitation goals, including obtaining a driver's license, during the 4 years since surgery.

CASE 3. This patient had a 5-year history of sacral chordoma treated with two laminectomies, one transabdominal debulking, and radiotherapy (6500 rads) (Fig. 15–11). Unrelenting pain was the most significant clinical symptom. From the onset of his illness, the patient was consuming 30 tablets of oxycodone (Percodan) and 10 mg of hydromorphone (Dilaudid) each day. There was radiographic evidence of disease progression. There was a neurological deficit limited to a sense of burning on the left foot and absence of the left Achilles tendon reflex. The patient spent most of his time in a wheelchair but was able to drive to work. The extrasacral extension of the tumor precluded total sacral resection; therefore, translumbar amputation was suggested as the only alternative to control the disease. Because of the chronicity of the symptoms, the patient delayed his decision for 6 months.

The surgical procedure itself was uneventful. The immediate postoperative course was

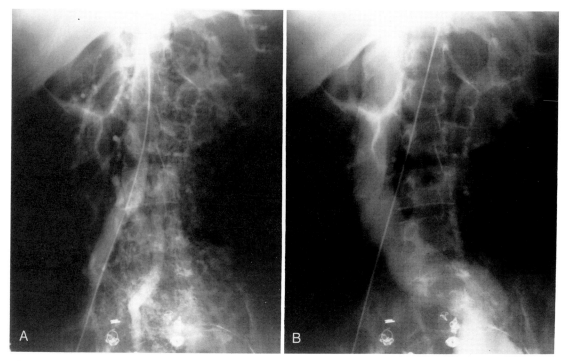

FIGURE 15–10. (Case 2.) Abdominal aortograms through the right femoral artery. *A,* Significant dilatation of the right common iliac, external iliac, and inferior mesenteric arteries. The arteriovenous malformation extends to both sides of the pelvis. *B,* Venous phase, with marked dilatation of the inferior vena cava and left common iliac vein.

complicated by 24 hours of anuria and a small bowel obstruction, both of which re-solved spontaneously without surgery. He also developed anemia, hypertension, and renal acidosis. The anemia was treated with several blood transfusions during the first 6 months, but thereafter, red blood cell counts returned to normal. This anemia could have

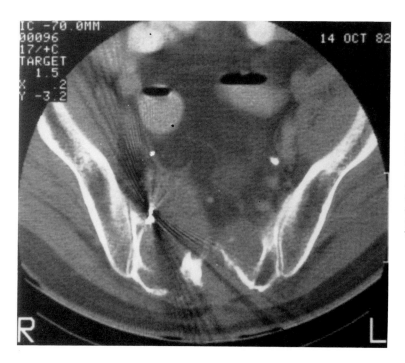

FIGURE 15–11. (Case 3.) Computed tomogram of the sacrum, dem-onstrating a large, centrally lo-cated sacral tumor mass that is expanding the central vertebral canal, with extensive bone dam-age posteriorly. The soft tissue mass extends anteriorly through the first sacral segment.

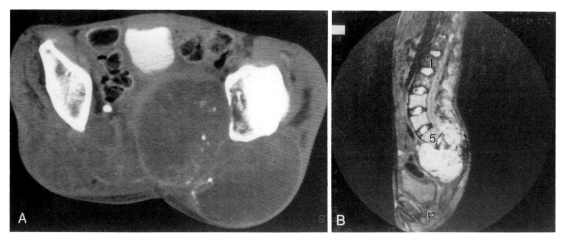

FIGURE 15–12. (Case 4.) *A,* December 1980: computed tomogram of the pelvis shows destruction of the cortex of the sacrum posteriorly, with extension into the soft tissue of the low back and buttocks. *B,* May 1985: magnetic resonance imaging demonstrates marked progression of the tumor mass, with bilateral destruction of the sacroiliac joints. The mass involves most of the true pelvis and obliterates the spinal canal at the fifth lumbar vertebra.

been explained by the acute loss of bone marrow that persisted until other sites developed their functioning marrow capacity. The hypertension eventually resolved. The patient became independent in transfer, and he spends 6 to 8 hours in his office. However, he continues to depend on 6 to 8 tablets of oxycodone daily to ameliorate significant phantom pain. The patient remains free of disease at 15 months after surgery, but his continued dependence on pain medication is disappointing. Of the authors' translumbar amputation patients, he is the only one who has continued to complain of pain severe enough to require medication.

CASE 4. This patient had a 5-year history of a sacral chordoma that had been treated 4 years previously with partial resection and fast neutron therapy, without response (Fig. 15–12*A*). At the time of admission, the patient was bedridden and was unable to sit upright or lie in the supine position (Fig. 15–12*B*). The bladder and rectum were not functional. Bilateral hydronephrosis secondary to intrapelvic extension of the chordoma was present; because of a septic episode, bilateral nephrostomies were performed before translumbar amputation. The tumor also extended posteriorly, involving the buttocks bilaterally. The patient appeared chronically ill and was heavily dependent on narcotics. The recommendation for translumbar amputation in this patient was based on the probability of cure and elimination of serious life-threatening conditions that developed because of tumor progression. He realized the significance of his current con-

dition and the limited time available to make a decision. The surgical resection was uneventful; however, the patient developed an ileal conduit fistula that closed spontaneously 3 months later. Two years after the operation, he no longer requires narcotics and has completed his physical rehabilitation.

RESULTS

Translumbar amputation was performed initially in patients with advanced localized neoplasms arising in the pelvic organs (rectum, bladder, vagina). However, the results from such a radical procedure did not prove rewarding, as most of these patients died from metastatic disease. On the other hand, this early experience demonstrated that the procedure was well tolerated physically and emotionally and that the patient could undergo successful physical rehabilitation.

Only two of the reported 20 patients who underwent translumbar amputation died as a result of the surgical procedure. Reported postoperative problems include wound problems, infection, pressure sores, surgical or phantom pain, acute hemodynamic changes, feelings of helplessness, lack of control, and functional limitations. None of the authors' four patients manifested any difficulties during anesthesia or in the postoperative period as a result of the acute loss of body mass. The two urinary fistulae from the ileal conduit in our patients are difficult to explain but are not considered to be related to the magnitude of the surgical procedure. Wound healing occurred without difficulties. Pain, a major component of the clinical symptoms in all four patients, disappeared completely in all but one patient (Case 3). This individual has continued to complain of severe phantom pain and cramps of the abdominal and truncal muscles.

The fitting of the prosthetic bucket and subsequent adjustment takes 2 to 4 months. Once this is accomplished, all patients adjust well and soon become independent in transfer, self-care, and transportation. A major element in the recovery process is strong family support and a high degree of visibility of all members of the rehabilitation team. Within this framework, patients and their families are able to overcome the preoperative apprehensions about the surgical procedure and the negative feelings of the early postoperative period. The eradication of the life-threatening condition and its associated pain and the expectation of a normal life span provide the patients with the incentive to accomplish the goals of the rehabilitation programs.

SUMMARY

Translumbar amputation is a lifesaving procedure that is well tolerated. Its use should be limited to persons with a life-threatening disease localized to the pelvis (bones or viscera) in whom a normal life span is expected if the disease is eliminated. In this category are patients with locally advanced sacral chordomas in whom local treatments have failed and paraplegics with intractable decubitus ulcers. A well-motivated patient with a good understanding of the significance of the procedure and a well-organized team integrated by surgical oncologists and rehabilitation personnel are essential for the success of this radical, therapeutic procedure.

REFERENCES

Hemipelvectomy

 1. Chretien PA, Sugarbaker PH: Surgical technique of hemipelvectomy in the lateral position. Surgery 90:900, 1981.

 2. Eilber FR, Grant TT, Sakai D, Morton DL: Internal hemipelvectomy—excision of the hemipelvis with limb preservation: An alternative to hemipelvectomy. Cancer 43:806, 1979.
 3. Karakousis CP, Vezeridis MP: Variants of hemipelvectomy. Am J Surg 145:273, 1983.
 4. Larson DL, Liang MD: The quadriceps musculocutaneous flap: A reliable, sensate flap for the hemipelvectomy defect. Plast Reconstr Surg 72:347, 1983.
 5. Lawrence W Jr, Neifeld JP, Terz JJ: Manual of Soft-Tissue Surgery, Operations for Sarcomas of the Lower Extremity. New York, Springer-Verlag, 1983, pp 75–113.
 6. Malawer MM, Zielinski CJ: Emergency hemipelvectomy in the control of life-threatening complications. Surgery 93:778, 1983.
 7. Nowroozi F, Salvanelli ML, Gerber LH: Energy expenditure in hip disarticulation and hemipelvectomy amputees. Arch Phys Med Rehabil 64:300, 1983.
 8. Steel HH: Resection of the hemipelvis for malignant disease: An alternative to hindquarter amputation for periacetabular chondrosarcoma of the pelvis. Semin Oncol 8:222, 1981.
 9. Sugarbaker PH, Barofsky I, Rosenberg SA, Gianola FJ: Quality of life assessment of patients in extremity sarcoma clinical trials. Surgery 91:17, 1982.
10. Temple WJ, Mnaymneh W, Ketcham AS: The total thigh and rectus abdominis myocutaneous flap for closure of extensive hemipelvectomy defects. Cancer 50:2524, 1982.
11. Weddington WW Jr, Segraves KB, Simon MA: Psychological outcome of extremity sarcoma survivors undergoing amputation of limb salvage. J Clin Oncol 3:1393, 1985.

Translumbar Amputation

12. Ariel IM, Verdu C: Chordoma: An analysis of twenty cases treated over a twenty-year span. J Surg Oncol 7:27, 1975.
13. Cummings BJ, Hodson DI, Bush RS: Chordoma: The results of megavoltage radiation therapy. Int J Radiat Oncol Biol Phys 9:633, 1983.
14. Davis SW, Chu DS, Yang CJ: Translumbar amputation for nonneoplastic cause: Rehabilitation and follow-up. Arch Phys Med Rehabil 56:359, 1975.
15. Easton JKM, Aust JB, Dawson WJ Jr, Kottke FJ: Fitting of a prosthesis on a patient after hemicorporectomy. Arch Phys Med Rehabil 64:335, 1983.
16. Frieden FH, Gertler M, Tosberg W, Rusk HA: Rehabilitation after hemicorporectomy. Arch Phys Med Rehabil 50:259, 1969.
17. Friedmann LW, Marin EL, Park YS: Hemicorporectomy for functional rehabilitation. Arch Phys Med Rehabil 62:83, 1981.
18. Miller TR: Translumbar amputation (hemicorporectomy). Prog Clin Cancer 8:227, 1982.
19. Miller TR, Mackenzie AR, Randall HT: Translumbar amputation for advanced cancer: Indications and physiologic alterations in four cases. Ann Surg 164:514, 1966.
20. Pearlman W, McShane RH, Jochimsen PR, Shirazi SS: Hemicorporectomy for intractable decubitus ulcers. Arch Surg 111:1139, 1976.

16

Immediate Postoperative Prostheses and Temporary Prosthetics

Joseph H. Zettl, C.P.

HISTORY OF EARLY PROSTHETIC FITTING

A review of the literature shows the use of early prosthetic fitting by the German surgeon von Bier. In 1893, he fitted patients with temporary prostheses within days of amputation and allowed them to stand and walk.[8] Wilson, a Boston surgeon, reported the use of a plaster-of-Paris socket, with special prosthetic components attached, in members of the American Expeditionary Force during 1917 and 1918 (Fig. 16–1). He experienced good results using the early prosthetic fitting technique during World War I (Fig. 16–2). Wilson credits Froehlich of Nancy and Spitzy of Vienna with being the first to use plaster-of-Paris sockets with simple pegs attached to allow early weight bearing.[24] Other advocates of this approach to amputee management were Little of Roehampton and several surgeons in European field hospitals during World War I and II who applied temporary plaster-of-Paris sockets to broomstick pylons at the time of suture removal.[20] In 1938, Verth reported the use

of early fitting with temporary prostheses after wound healing of the residual limb.[8]

In spite of these pioneers who recognized the advantages of early prosthetic fitting, these teachings and techniques did not enjoy a wide acceptance and were rapidly ignored and forgotten for several decades.

HISTORY OF IMMEDIATE POSTSURGICAL PROSTHETIC FITTING (IPPF)

The concept of fitting patients with prostheses immediately after amputation surgery and initiating gait training in 1 to 2 days originated with Berlemont in the late 1950s. He reported his results in 1961.[1, 2] Berlemont's procedure was investigated and modified by Weiss, who presented it in a lecture at the Sixth International Prosthetic Course in Copenhagen in July 1963. Later that year on a lecture visit to the United States, Weiss stimulated interest at the University of California Medical School in San Francisco and

177

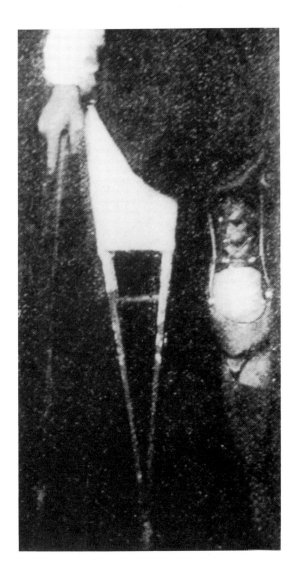

FIGURE 16–1. Wilson's Bone & Joint early prosthetic fitting (1922): an above-knee plaster socket terminates in a crutch pylon. (*From* Wilson PD: Early weight-bearing in the treatment of amputations of the lower limbs. J Bone Joint Surg 4:224, 1923.)

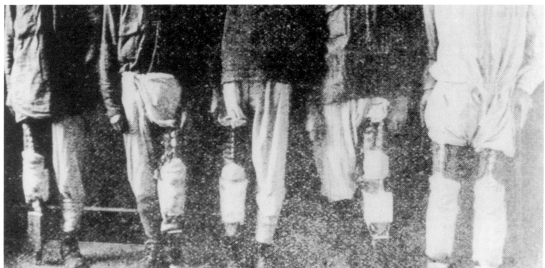

FIGURE 16–2. Wilson's Bone & Joint early prosthetic fitting (1922): a group of below-knee amputees with plaster sockets. (*From* Wilson PD: Early weight-bearing in the treatment of amputations of the lower limbs. J Bone Joint Surg 4:224, 1923.)

at the US Naval Hospital in Oakland, California.[5, 6, 21–23] The promising results obtained at these institutions prompted the Veterans Administration's Prosthetic and Sensory Aids Service to support a research and investigative program proposed by the Prosthetic Research Study (PRS) in Seattle, Washington, under the direction of Ernest M. Burgess. The techniques described in the following text are the fruits of this research and present, with few exceptions, the results and recommendations of the PRS.[5, 6]

Additional studies were instituted at Duke University, the University of Oregon, Rancho Los Amigos Hospital, the University of Miami, Marquette University, the Institute of Physical Medicine and Rehabilitation in New York, and the Hospital for Joint Diseases in New York.[6, 19] Because detailed published material on the subject was unavailable when the studies began, the various investigators approached IPPF with different techniques.

In November 1964, a PRS team visited Weiss in Poland to investigate his technique in detail. The basic principles learned were combined with technical improvements and refinements and have continued to be effective over the years.[5, 6] In 1966, at the Twelfth International Congress for Prosthetists at Copenhagen, Marquart of the University of Heidelberg reported the use of the technique on patients with upper extremity amputations.[13, 14] In 1968 and 1969, Sarmiento in Miami,[17, 18] Nigst in Basel,[16] Loughlin in Atlanta, Georgia,[10] and Childress in Chicago, Illinois,[7] followed with their reports.

By 1968, Burgess and Romano reported gratifying results in 160 consecutive unselected patients with IPPF. These cases were observed in the first 3 years of the continuing PRS study.[4] The same year, Goldbranson and colleagues,[9] from the Navy Prosthetic Research Laboratory in Oakland, reported good results with IPPF in 100 lower extremity amputees. However, these authors favored delay of immediate weight bearing in those patients who underwent amputation for peripheral vascular disease. Moore and associates,[15] in San Francisco, reported the results of 20 consecutive lower extremity amputations performed for ischemic gangrene. The investigators used the IPPF procedure described by Burgess and concluded that there was a definite advantage with this method of treatment. In 1971, Burgess[3] reported satisfactory results in 193 lower extremity amputations performed for peripheral arterial

insufficiency, and by 1978, he and his group had performed over 1500 consecutive unselected amputations with the IPPF approach.

Many individual professionals and study groups consisting of physicians and prosthetists from worldwide medical centers visited the PRS in Seattle to be instructed in the details of IPPF. Pilot courses were given to teams from major Veterans Administration Hospitals throughout the United States and to the teaching staffs of the Prosthetic Education Programs of Northwestern University, New York University, the University of California at Los Angeles, and the University of Washington at Seattle. Formal IPPF courses for physicians, surgeons, prosthetists, therapists, and rehabilitation personnel are still available in the major Prosthetic Education institutions. PRS staff members traveled worldwide to teach the principles of IPPF at conventions, professional seminars, and major medical centers.[28]

GENERAL PRINCIPLES OF IPPF

Application of the rigid plaster-of-Paris dressing or cast-socket after amputation must be considered as critical as the amputation itself. The sole purpose of IPPF is to assist in achieving rapid wound healing and residual limb maturation; it is not a cure for poor amputation surgery. The procedure, while precise, is not technically difficult but must result in a perfectly fitting cast-socket interface; there is no opportunity to check the residual limb for factors requiring socket adjustments or modifications. Attention and adherence to details are the prerequisites of any technique for creating an effective and protective residual limb environment. This includes immediate prosthetic replacement of an amputated extremity. Basic biochemical fitting practices and static and dynamic alignment principles familiar to the prosthetist are an integral part of the overall technique.

The application of the rigid dressings incorporates the total-contact prosthetic principles used to achieve tissue rest and immobilization. Lack of total-contact tissue support results in edema, skin blistering, and, in extreme cases, wound separation and residual limb breakdown. Proximal constriction by a too tightly applied plaster-of-Paris cast-socket must be avoided so as not to restrict circulation. For this reason, a patellar tendon shelf and popliteal compression are not incorporated into the below-knee rigid dressing. Similarly, in the above-knee cast-socket, ischial weight bearing is avoided until wound healing has been accomplished and the sutures have been removed. Adequate cast-socket suspension and rotational stability are provided by molding the plaster to the patient's anatomy wherever possible, and auxiliary suspension systems are provided by a waist belt or flexible hip spica. The cast-socket, suspension, prosthetic unit, pylon, and foot should be lightweight and functional and duplicate the action of a temporary or definitive prosthesis whenever possible.

The patient benefits from an effective immediate postsurgical prosthesis by accelerated wound healing and residual limb maturation. IPPF minimizes postsurgical edema and pain and produces profound psychological benefits from the time the patient awakens in the recovery room with the prosthesis in place. Phantom pain and the effects of inactivity have been reduced through controlled weight bearing and ambulation. Early hospital discharge and rapid rehabilitation of the patient yield appreciable economic benefits as compared with conventional amputation methods.[12]

PREOPERATIVE PROSTHETIC CONSIDERATIONS

IPPF is a team effort. Team members have overlapping responsibilities and communicate freely and effectively with the surgeon, who is the team leader. The team consists of a surgeon, prosthetist, therapist, nurse, and possibly a social worker. Other professionals may be required in special circumstances.

At this stage of IPPF's development, the materials and prosthetic components used are mostly standardized, but occasionally it is necessary to fabricate a special component for adaptations. For this reason, prosthetists should be notified as early as possible of the impending amputation and the proposed level so they may see the patient, explain their role, and secure pertinent information to make proper preparations.[27] This information gathering entails notations of the patient's physical size and general condition; evidence of flexion contracture; recent surgeries, such as attempted revascularization

procedures; the side of amputation; the level of amputation; the foot size, and any physical defects that might require special considerations in the application of the rigid dressing and temporary prosthesis.

All components, materials, and tools are organized in an instrument bag, or its equivalent, so that IPPF may proceed on short notice. In some cases, these preparations for IPPF must anticipate and include components and materials for a higher level of amputation than was originally planned.[25]

PROCEDURE FOR SPECIFIC LEVELS

Syme's Amputation

On completion of the amputation, the surgeon applies a sterile nonadherent dressing (Owen's silk, petrolatum or nitrofurazone [Furacin] gauze) over the suture line of the incision, followed by three to four layers of sterile, fluffy gauze placed over the distal end of the residual limb, covering the entire amputation site. A gas-sterilized Orlon-Lycra-Spandex sock of an appropriate size, usually 5 by 3½ by 14 inches, is carefully rolled up over the wound, proximal to the knee and is suspended by either an assistant or a temporary shoulder strap (Fig. 16–3). The Orlon-Lycra-Spandex socks are available in five sizes, which cover the residual limbs of all lower and upper extremity amputation levels.

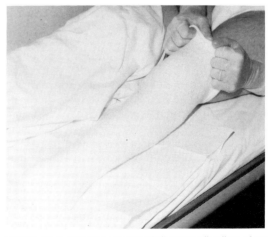

FIGURE 16–3. Left Syme's amputation: application of an Orlon-Lycra-Spandex sock.

Preformed polyurethane pressure-relief pads—available in prefabricated standard left and right sizes—are positioned, fitted, and trimmed to provide an adequate pressure-relief channel for the tibial crest. The medial relief pad has a posterior extension, the center of which is placed on the concave apex of the medial tibial condylar flare. The anterior distal extension is positioned one fourth of an inch from the tibial crest and extends distally to the formation level of the bulbous heel. Any trimlines required to achieve proper fit and placement should be beveled or skived to avoid ridges and indentations on the inside of the finished cast-socket. The lateral relief pad is placed one fourth of an inch from the tibial crest and is cut one half of an inch from the medial relief pad distally. A one half inch channel should thus be formed to protect the tibial crest from undue cast pressure (Fig. 16–4).

A strip of reticulated polyurethane sheeting—one half of an inch thick, 2 inches wide,

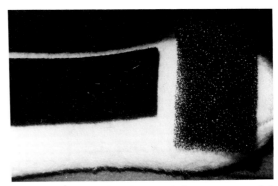

FIGURE 16–5. Left Syme's amputation: pressure-relief pads in place and reticulated polyurethane sheeting applied over the incision.

and approximately 7 inches long, with its edges beveled—is prepared to cover the surgical site of a classic Syme's amputation. The polyurethane strip is glued to the Orlon-Lycra-Spandex sock with Dow Corning Medical Adhesive, Type B (Fig. 16–5).

Elastic plaster-of-Paris bandages (4 inch Orthoflex*) are used for the initial plaster wrap. The elasticity of the bandage allows controlled tissue compression and conforms well to contours without being tugged; this provides a smooth inner cast. The wrap is always started on the distal lateral aspect of the residual limb. This covers the polyurethane sheeting, including the lower ends of the pressure-relief pads. One and three fourth circumferential turns anchor the elastic plaster bandage to itself at a point posterolaterally. Bringing the wrap anteriorly over the distal lateral portion of the heel flap with moderate tension supports the flap and reduces tension on the suture line. At the anterior margin, tension is reduced on the plaster bandage, and the wrap is directed medially then posteriorly, where the tension is increased again. The wrap is brought centrally to the anterior margin.

The direction is now altered to lateral, with reduced tension, and brought posterior then medially, where tension is increased as the wrap proceeds anteriorly (Fig. 16–6). This procedure is then repeated in reverse to ensure a double layer of elastic plaster coverage. The remaining plaster is wrapped circumferentially in a proximal direction, with decreasing tension and equally overlapping wraps. Care must be taken to maintain the

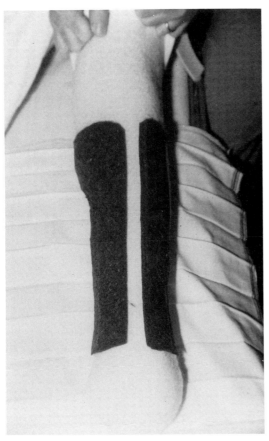

FIGURE 16–4. Left Syme's amputation: pressure-relief pads in place.

*Johnson & Johnson Inc., New Brunswick, New Jersey.

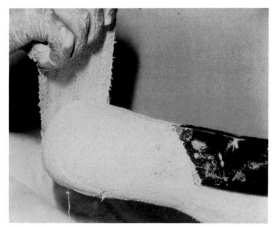

FIGURE 16–6. Left Syme's amputation: application of the initial elastic plaster wrap.

ventional plaster bandage is applied first at the distal bulbous portion of the cast and is wrapped in an even, smooth fashion with overlapping circumferential turns proximal to the level where the previous elastic plaster wrap terminated.

A 1 inch cotton webbing strap approximately 20 inches long is looped through a 1½ inch safety buckle. The safety buckle is located 2 inches proximal to the patella. The two ends of the webbing strap extend distally past the medial and lateral borders of the patella. Two turns of the remaining conventional plaster bandage are placed over the webbing straps to incorporate them into the plaster wrap. The protruding ends of the straps are folded back and anchored firmly in place with the remaining plaster bandage.

The tension on the suspended Orlon-Lycra-Spandex sock is now released; any excess is trimmed with bandage scissors to retain 2 inches of sock, which is folded back on the cast and secured with a double-layer 3 by 15 inch plaster splint. The suspension waist belt is applied and secured with safety buckles to the waist and cast.

The patient is now positioned so that the pelvis is parallel to the foot edge of the operating table, with the knees about 1½ inches apart (Fig. 16–8). The PRS adjustable prosthetic unit for a Syme's amputation, with all adjustments in neutral, is then fitted to the distal end of the cast-socket to achieve a one half inch foot inset when measured with an imaginary vertical line from the center of the proximal cast-socket brim (Fig. 16–9). The three stainless steel socket attachment straps are shaped to the contours of the cast-socket and are located so as not to block the drain, which will later be removed. The prosthetic unit is secured to the cast-socket with one 4 inch roll of conventional plaster bandage, and the cast is well smoothed by hand (Fig. 16–10). The prosthetic foot is aligned and secured to the prosthetic unit according to established prosthetic alignment principles. To discourage flexion contractures, do not place a pillow under the cast-socket, but retain the limb in a flat position in bed. The patient is now ready for transfer to the recovery room (Fig. 16–11).

heel flap in a position central to the cut end of the tibia and to avoid any mediolateral or anteroposterior displacement. A second elastic plaster bandage is usually needed to complete the initial wrap. The wrap is terminated at the level of the tibial tubercle. Before the initial elastic plaster wraps harden, a flat-surfaced board, or the equivalent, is pressed against the distal heel flap to effect a flat central weight-bearing surface (Fig. 16–7). Any displacement of the heel pad in any direction is to be avoided.

Owing to the structural weakness of elastic plaster-of-Paris bandages, the initial wrap must be reinforced with conventional plaster bandages and splints. Double layers of 4 by 15 inch plaster splints are applied over the distal portion of the cast anteroposteriorly and mediolaterally. One roll of 4 inch con-

Partial Foot Amputation

Transmetatarsal, Chopart's, Lisfranc's, and Pirogoff's amputations are treated with the

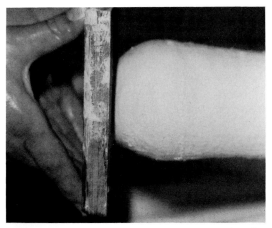

FIGURE 16–7. Left Syme's amputation: flattening the distal weight-bearing surface.

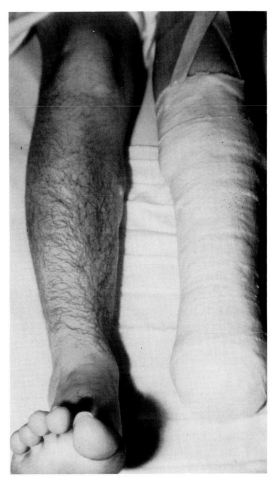

FIGURE 16–8. Left Syme's amputation: completed cast-socket.

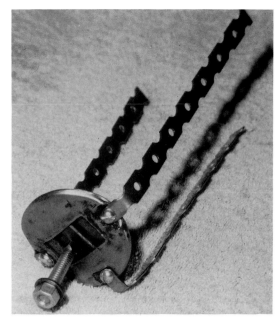

FIGURE 16–9. PRS adjustable prosthetic unit for a Syme's amputation.

Below-Knee Amputation

The application of surgical dressings and an Orlon-Lycra-Spandex residual sock of proper size, including the suspension, is performed as with a Syme's amputation. Likewise, the basic application principles of the prefabricated compressed reticulated polyurethane pressure-relief pads are the same except that the distal extension must extend past the cut end of the tibia. Pie-shaped pieces must be cut from the distal anterior relief pads to ensure a continuous one half inch relief channel. A prepatellar pad is ap-

same technique as described for the Syme's amputation with the following exceptions. The malleoli are protected with properly contoured reticulated polyurethane sheeting to prevent pressure points. The surgical incision is also covered with reticulated polyurethane sheeting or a preformed reticulated polyurethane distal pad of appropriate size. The additional bulk caused by the polyurethane distal pad is inconsequential, since a rubber walking heel or a plastic socket bottom is used for ambulation.

The remaining forefoot is held in a neutral position of 90° during casting and hardening of the plaster cast; this prevents equinus deformity complications. An auxiliary waist belt suspension is not required for partial foot amputations if the anatomical contours allow good cast-socket suspension and rotational stability.

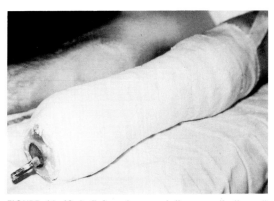

FIGURE 16–10. Left Syme's amputation: prosthetic unit attached to the cast-socket.

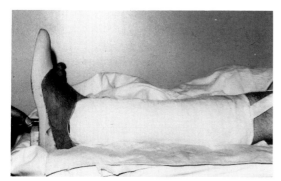

FIGURE 16–11. Left Syme's amputation: IPPF completed.

plied to cover the entire patella. A reticulated polyurethane distal pad of appropriate size, 4 or 5 inches in diameter, is applied over the distal end of the residual limb and extends proximally over the underlying pressure-relief pads (Fig. 16–12).[29]

The initial elastic plaster-of-Paris application is repeated as with a Syme's amputation. Emphasis is placed on supporting the posterior skin flap by lifting it up toward the anterior flap and relieving any tension on the suture line. During the plaster-of-Paris bandage application, the knee is maintained in 5 to 15° of flexion. To ensure maximal retention of the resulting cast-socket, the plaster wrap extends 4 to 5 inches past midthigh (Fig. 16–13). The initial elastic Orthoflex plaster wrap is reinforced with conventional plaster-of-Paris bandages and splints, as with a Syme's amputation (Fig. 16–14).

A 1½ inch cotton webbing suspension strap with a safety buckle is incorporated into the reinforced plaster wrap at the anterior proximal level with two turns of overlying conventional plaster-of-Paris bandage. The

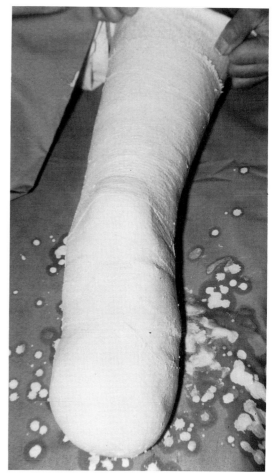

FIGURE 16–13. Left BKA: application of the initial elastic plaster wrap.

remaining distal portion of the webbing strap is folded back and anchored in place with the remaining plaster bandage wrap (Fig. 16–15).

Variation: For an obese patient with excessive soft tissue over the thigh, it is necessary to incorporate a second suspension strap with a safety buckle into the plaster-of-Paris reinforcement wrap at the proximal posterolateral level. This second strap is necessary for added suspension when the patient is flexing the hip, which makes the anterior suspension attachment ineffective. Also, for additional suspension, the Orlon-Lycra-Spandex sock is glued to the skin of the thigh from the knee up with Dow Corning Medical Adhesive, Type B.

While the plaster-of-Paris wrap is moist and moldable, the cast is gently compressed with the heel of each hand just proximal to the femoral condyles and slightly anterior from the lateral midline; this molding pro-

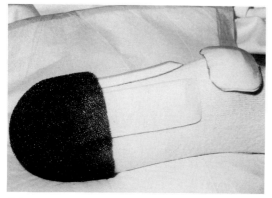

FIGURE 16–12. Left BKA: pressure-relief pads with the distal end pad in place.

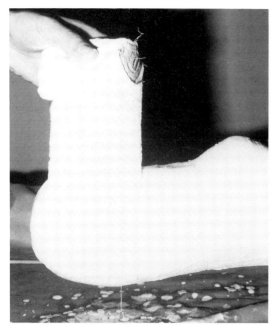

FIGURE 16–14. Left BKA: reinforcement wrap.

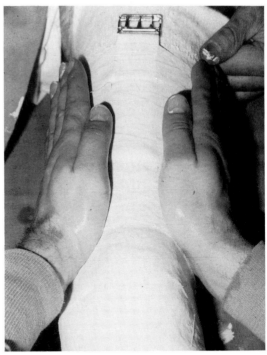

FIGURE 16–16. Left BKA: molding the cast-socket proximal to the femoral condyles.

vides an effective built-in suspension mechanism. Care must be taken that compression is applied proximal to the condyles and not directly on them, while the knee is maintained in 5 to 15° of flexion until the plaster has hardened sufficiently (Fig. 16–16). At this time, the sock suspension can be disconnected or released, and the waist suspension belt applied (Fig. 16–17).

For the application of the prosthetic unit, the patient is positioned with the pelvis parallel to the foot edge of the operating table and with the knees approximately 1½ inches apart (Fig. 16–18). The socket attachment straps are shaped to the exterior contours of

the plaster-of-Paris socket so that the socket attachment plate is located 90° from the table top when viewed laterally and is inset medially one half of an inch from an imaginary vertical line through the middle of the knee. The resulting position is marked on the plaster-of-Paris socket with an indelible pencil (Fig. 16–19).

A double layer of 4 by 15 inch conventional plaster splints is folded three times length-

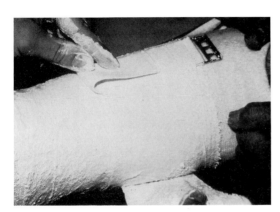

FIGURE 16–15. Left BKA: securing the suspension strap in the reinforcement wrap.

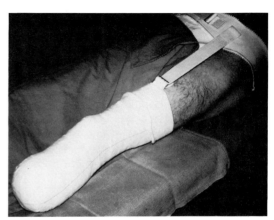

FIGURE 16–17. Left BKA: completed cast-socket and suspension system.

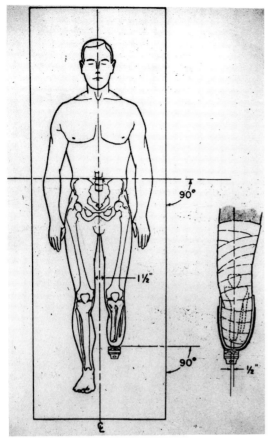

FIGURE 16–18. Left BKA: prosthesis alignment.

With a sharp plaster knife or scalpel, a round circle of plaster-of-Paris is smoothly cut in the corresponding area of the underlying prepatellar pressure-relief pad. The blade of the knife is held horizontally to avoid cutting the underlying Orlon-Lycra-Spandex sock. The cut is made smaller than the previously applied prepatellar pressure-relief pad (Fig. 16–21). After the plaster-of-Paris has been cut away, the polyurethane prepatellar pressure-relief pad is pulled through the resulting window. This creates flared plaster edges and avoids irritation from cast contact with the skin. To discourage flexion contractures, do not place a pillow under the cast-socket, but retain the residual limb flat in bed. The patient is now ready for transfer to the recovery room.

Above-Knee Amputation and Knee Disarticulation

Owing to the anatomy of the resulting, usually cone-shaped above-knee residual limb, the IPPF of this amputation level is

wise; when placed in the predetermined position between the distal end of the plaster-of-Paris socket and the socket attachment plate, it fills all hollows and voids. The socket attachment straps are secured to the cast with one roll of 4 or 5 inch conventional plaster-of-Paris bandage.

With all adjustments in neutral, the adjustable prosthetic unit is placed on the socket attachment plate. The pylon tube is bolted securely to the solid ankle, cushion heel (SACH) foot prosthesis. A standard lightweight SACH foot is used if the patient has a pair of shoes available. If the shoes are unavailable or unsuitable, a Kingsley immediate postsurgical SACH foot with built-in heel is used. The pylon tubing is cut to the appropriate length and secured with a hose clamp to the prosthetic unit, accommodating appropriate toe-out (Fig. 16–20). The prosthetic assembly, consisting of the adjustable prosthetic unit, pylon, and SACH foot, is disconnected from the socket attachment plate, to be reattached only when the patient is standing or ambulating.

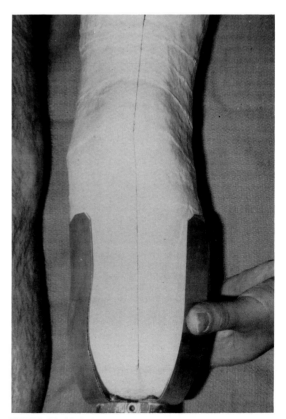

FIGURE 16–19. Left BKA: alignment of the socket attachment plate.

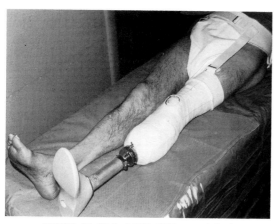

FIGURE 16–20. Left BKA: IPPF completed.

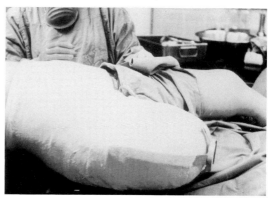

FIGURE 16–22. Right AKA: cast-socket with a rigid hip spica.

considered the most complex and difficult. Although a rigid plaster-of-Paris hip spica connected to the plaster-of-Paris socket provides secure retention, it restricts the patient to a supine position, which is uncomfortable (Fig. 16–22). Because of these and other simplifying considerations, the IPPF technique underwent several design changes and technical improvements that resulted in a dependable, secure IPPF that is effective and tolerated well by the patient.

Sterile dressings, including a properly sized Orlon-Lycra-Spandex sock and suspension, are applied as with the previous amputation levels. The patient is positioned on the operating table in a manner that extends the residual limb, including the buttock area, over the table edge. An alternative is to roll the patient partially onto the sound side. The excess sock is cut with bandage scissors lengthwise medially to the perineum and the level of the adductor longus. A second cut is

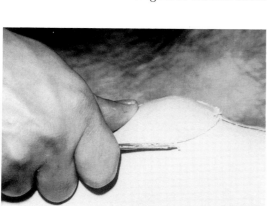

FIGURE 16–21. Left BKA: cutting the patellar pressure-relief window.

made 1 to 1½ inches posterior to the initial one. These cuts are correct when tissue bunching or adductor roll is avoided and all tissues, while under slight compression, are comfortably contained inside the sock. Compression is satisfactory when the medial distal tissues of the residual limb appear well supported and there are no noticeable wrinkles in the Orlon-Lycra-Spandex sock.

Suspension is temporarily released, and the sock is folded back on itself to midthigh, without exposure of the surgical site. The exposed skin of the upper thigh, including the waist and hip areas of the amputated side, are sprayed with Dow Corning Medical Adhesive, Type B. The corresponding area of sock is also sprayed with the glue (Figure 16–23). The adhesive becomes tacky in 5 seconds. Both hands are inserted between the folded-back portion of the sock, and the material is stretched in a proximal direction with even, firm pressure, avoiding wrinkles in the application. The suspension system is reattached, or an assistant holds the sock tightly suspended.

A perineal apron is fashioned from 25 by 6 inch bias-cut stockinette and glued circularly to the proximal portion of the Orlon-Lycra-Spandex sock to protect the perineum area and any skin from the plaster-of-Paris wrap (Fig. 16–24).

To achieve rotational stability, the plaster-of-Paris socket is contoured into a modified quadrilateral shape. The PRS above-knee casting fixture developed for this purpose is fitted while the residual limb is in an adducted and slightly flexed position.[26] The anteroposterior dimension is one half to three fourths of an inch larger than that

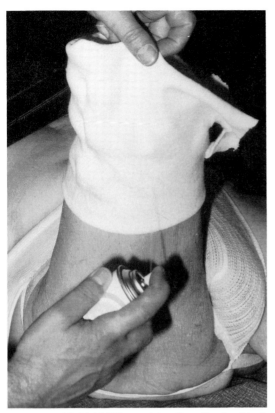

FIGURE 16–23. Right AKA: applying Dow Corning Medical Adhesive.

bandages are sufficient to achieve a minimal thickness of three layers of plaster-of-Paris bandage (Fig. 16–27). The elastic plaster wrap is extended proximally with decreasing tension to the level of the perineum; it includes Scarpa's triangle and extends 2 inches proximally over the gluteal fold and greater trochanter.

While the elastic plaster-of-Paris wrap is still moist, the PRS casting fixture, with the handle in the down and open position, is reapplied up to the level of the gluteal fold. The handle is brought upward into the closed position, and all adjustments are rechecked for proper positioning and fit. The anterior excess plaster wrap extending proximally over Scarpa's triangle of the casting fixture is rolled down and smoothed into a round edge (Fig. 16–28). The perineal apron is pulled distally to mold the medioproximal plaster wrap outward in a flare away from the skin. This procedure is repeated at the posterior gluteal area. While the initial elastic

normally used in fabrication of an ischial weight-bearing socket. This increased size places the ischial tuberosity inside the cast-socket, results in gluteal weight bearing only, prevents proximal constriction, and ensures positive continuous distal tissue support.

The mediolateral dimension of the PRS casting fixture is determined by pushing its lateral wall against the femur and adjusting the thumb screws to the femur's shape while providing a distal lateral relief area (Fig. 16–25). The anterior handle of the PRS casting fixture is pushed down into the open position, and the fixture is removed. Both anteroposterior and mediolateral dimensions are enlarged one half of an inch to compensate for the thickness of the plaster-of-Paris wrap.

A reticulated polyurethane distal pad of appropriate size, 5 or 6 inches in diameter, is placed over the distal residual limb. For the initial wrap, elastic plaster-of-Paris bandages, 5 inch Orthoflex, are used, and the wrapping technique is repeated as with a Syme's or below-knee amputation (Fig. 16–26). Two or three elastic plaster-of-Paris

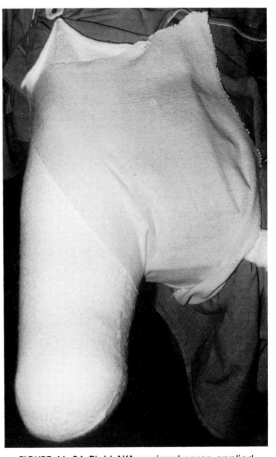

FIGURE 16–24. Right AKA: perineal apron applied.

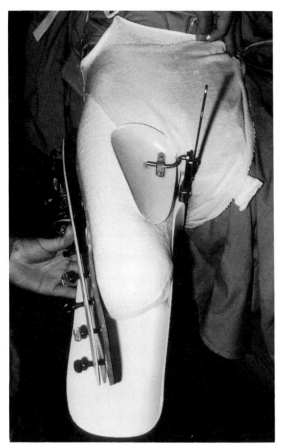

FIGURE 16–25. Right AKA: a PRS casting fixture is fitted.

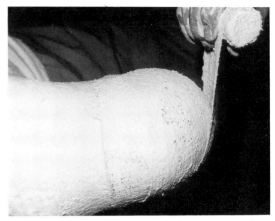

FIGURE 16–27. Right AKA: elastic plaster wrap supporting the posterior skin flap.

the casting fixture is opened and carefully removed (Fig. 16–29).

Variation: Prefabricated polyethelene quadrilateral socket brims have been used but have been found to be hot and to cause occasional blisters on the underlying skin. It is also difficult to make any meaningful adjustments to these brims while patients are wearing them. If a prefabricated socket brim is preferred, in the absence of the PRS casting fixture, it is recommended that the socket brim be fabricated from plaster-of-Paris bandages molded over a correspondingly sized above-knee plaster mold (Fig. 16–30).

The initial elastic plaster-of-Paris wrap is reinforced with two double layers of 4 by 15 inch conventional plaster-of-Paris splints placed anteroposteriorly and mediolaterally over the distal end. The areas of Scarpa's triangle and of the medial and posterior proximal cast brim are also reinforced with

plaster-of-Paris wrap hardens, the residual limb is kept in a properly adducted and flexed position. With a finger, the plaster is molded into a channel for the adductor longus muscle and to provide a generous reverse flare. Once the plaster wrap has hardened,

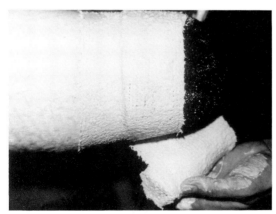

FIGURE 16–26. Right AKA: application of an elastic plaster wrap over the distal pad.

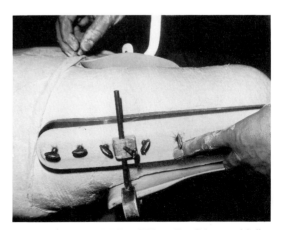

FIGURE 16–28. Right AKA: a PRS casting fixture molds the initial plaster wrap.

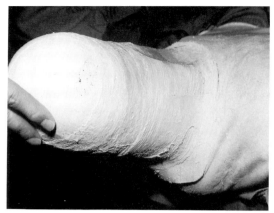

FIGURE 16–29. Right AKA: elastic plaster wrap with molding completed.

folded conventional plaster-of-Paris splints. All plaster splints are secured in place with one roll of 4 or 5 inch conventional plaster-of-Paris bandage, which starts at the proximal socket brim and winds distally with even, overlapping, circular wraps.

For application of the prosthetic unit, the patient is positioned with the pelvis level to the foot edge of the operating table. The residual limb is positioned in an adducted and slightly flexed position, with the sound extremity extended in a neutral anatomical position.

The socket attachment straps are shaped to the exterior contours of the plaster-of-Paris socket so the socket attachment plate is located 90° to the table top when viewed laterally and so an imaginary vertical line drawn from the ischial tuberosity bisects the medial border of the socket attachment plate. The resulting position is marked on the plaster-of-Paris socket with an indelible pencil and is secured to the cast-socket as with a below-knee amputation.

With all adjustments in neutral, the prosthetic unit is connected to the socket attachment plate. The pylon tube attached to the SACH foot is cut to the proper length and secured with a hose clamp to the base of the prosthetic unit, accommodating appropriate toe-out and external knee-bolt rotation (Fig. 16–31). For short above-knee amputations, it is necessary to size a pylon-thigh extension by placing it next to the prosthetic unit and knee joint; the pylon is cut to achieve a knee center height equal to that of the sound side (Fig. 16–32).[30]

The auxiliary suspension is provided by a flexible hip-waist spica, which is applied as follows: a folded surgical towel is placed as a

FIGURE 16–30. Right AKA: prefabricated plaster socket brim.

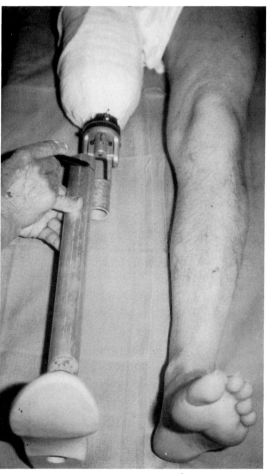

FIGURE 16–31. Right AKA: prosthesis assembly and pylon attachment.

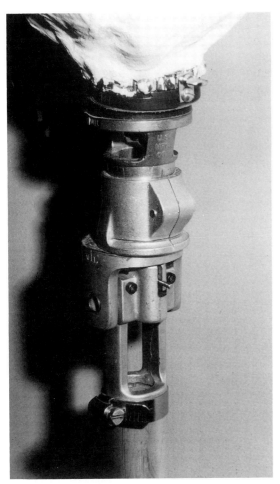

FIGURE 16–32. Right AKA: short residual limb pylon-thigh extension installed.

this wrap under the patient's back, it is necessary to roll the patient from side to side with the aid of an assistant.

A roll of 4 inch Elastoplast is wrapped in place over the previously applied bias-cut stockinette in the same sequence as previously described, reinforcing the junction between the waist suspension and cast-socket (Fig. 16–35). Both bias-cut cotton stockinette and Elastoplast have flexibility and stretch characteristics that contour well, and without wrinkles, to the irregular surfaces of the underlying anatomy. However, it must be reinforced with 2 inch surgical tape to establish a constant, secure connection between the flexible hip-waist spica and the cast-socket.

The bias-cut cotton stockinette extending from under the Orthoflex application is folded back and secured with 2 inch surgical tape, repeating the previous wrapping technique sequence; this provides a neat finished edge and further reinforces the positive connection between the hip-waist spica and the cast-socket (Fig. 16–36). On completion of the suspension system, the abdominal towel

spacer over the patient's abdomen. A roll of 6 inch by 6 yard bias-cut cotton stockinette is wrapped in three circular turns to the midportion of the cast-socket. The wrap is then slanted diagonally and proximally over the greater trochanter, to the sacral area of the lower back, to the contralateral junction of the iliac crest and the lower waist of the sound side. The wrap is continued over the abdominal towel toward and over the previous application, forming a second layer (Fig. 16–33). As the bias-cut stockinette wrap continues again over the abdominal towel, it is redirected distally to the middle of the socket where two additional circular wraps are applied. From there, the procedure is repeated twice until the entire roll of bias-cut cotton stockinette has been used to connect the waist and cast-socket (Fig. 16–34). This results in a minimum of three to four layers of bias-cut cotton stockinette. To pass

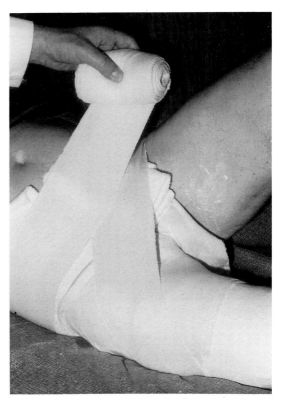

FIGURE 16–33. Right AKA: application of a bias-cut cotton stockinette hip spica. The wrap is continued over the abdominal towel.

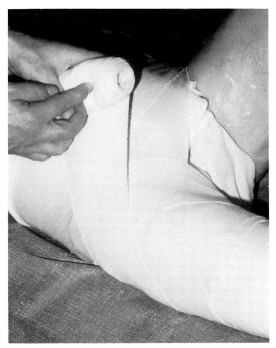

FIGURE 16–34. Right AKA: application of a bias-cut cotton stockinette hip spica. The procedure is repeated twice.

incision is located posteriorly, approximately 1½ inch proximal from the distal end of the residual limb. In this case, the initial elastic plaster-of-Paris wrap must be reversed so that the support of the skin flaps is achieved by wrapping from anterior to posterior.

Whenever the surgeon is forced, through the patient's lack of viable skin, to improvise on a skin closure, the initial elastic plaster-of-Paris wrap must be applied in such a manner as to support the skin flaps in relation to each other and to maintain the tissues at rest. The technique must always take this into consideration as the wrap is applied. The remaining casting principles and the application of the prosthetic components are the same as with above-knee IPPF. On occasion, when prominent femoral condyles are present, it is possible to compress the plaster cast-socket mediolaterally just proximal to the femoral condyles to achieve suspension and rotational control. This eliminates the need for the auxiliary hip-waist spica suspension. This should not be a routine procedure; it is applicable only in suitable, select cases.

is removed from under the spica. To discourage flexion contractures, do not place a pillow under the cast-socket, but retain the residual limb in a flat position in bed. The prosthetic assembly is disconnected from the socket attachment plate, to be reattached only for standing or ambulating. The patient is now ready for transfer to the recovery room.

Knee Disarticulation Retaining the Patella

For a knee disarticulation that maintains the patella in place, an appropriate pressure-relief pad is required. The relief pad is fashioned from one half inch thick reticulated polyurethane sheeting material in the general shape of a horseshoe. The inner arc of the pressure-relief pad is trimmed to fit around the border of the patella and is left at full thickness and about 1 inch wide. The outer arc is skived to a feathered edge so it will blend smoothly into the plaster wrap without leaving a ridge in the inner cast-socket (Fig. 16–37).

In the classic knee disarticulation, the skin

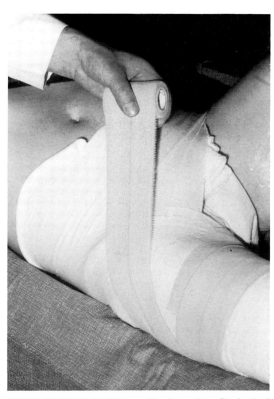

FIGURE 16–35. Right AKA: application of an Elastoplast hip spica.

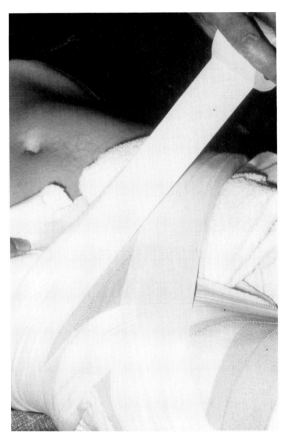

FIGURE 16–36. Right AKA: application of a surgical tape hip spica.

Hip Disarticulation

For the application of the hip disarticulation cast-socket, a fracture table is helpful but is not absolutely necessary. The patient can be rolled from side to side with assistance to facilitate the application.

Sterile, nonadherent dressings, including well-fluffed gauze, are applied to cover the entire skin incision area. A sterile hip disarticulation Orlon-Lycra-Spandex sock of a proper size is applied without displacing the surgical dressings. In the absence of a hip disarticulation sock, a large 9 by 7 by 18 inch Orlon-Lycra-Spandex sock can be substituted. The sock is unrolled completely and is cut lengthwise along its lateral aspect distal to the border of the box toe section. The uncut box toe section of the sock is placed over the fluffed gauze dressings and is firmly pulled diagonally in a proximal direction. The entire border of the sock and the corresponding skin area are sprayed about 4 inches wide with Dow Corning Medical Adhesive, Type B. The sock is glued to the skin in a proximal, diagonal direction, any wrinkling of the material is avoided. A folded surgical towel is placed over the lower stomach area as a spacer.

Depending on the patient's size, a 5 or 6 inch by 6 yard roll of bias-cut cotton stockinette is applied over the Orlon-Lycra-Spandex sock (Fig. 16–38). The wrap is started on the lateral distal portion of the amputated side and is wound diagonally across the towel on the abdomen toward the iliac crest and lower waist of the sound side. Alternating wraps are placed over the pelvis and lower waist, including the surgical incision. Firm tension to the bias-cut stockinette is applied when the wrap passes over the area of the buttock and skin incision. All areas of the skin incision, pelvis, and lower waist to be

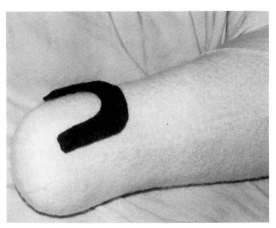

FIGURE 16–37. Left knee disarticulation: patellar pressure-relief pad.

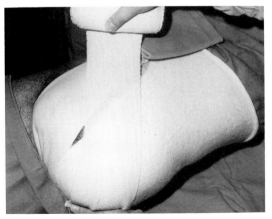

FIGURE 16–38. Left hip disarticulation: bias-cut cotton stockinette wrap over an Orlon-Lycra-Spandex sock.

included in the plaster wrap should be protected by three to four layers of bias-cut stockinette.

The surgical skin incision area is covered by appropriately sized one half inch reticulated polyurethane sheeting with the edges beveled and feathered thin. Any depressions or concave areas of the incision should be filled with an additional layer of reticulated polyurethane sheeting. These compression pads are glued in position against the bias-cut stockinette wrap with Dow Corning Medical Adhesive, Type B.

Prominent iliac crests are relieved with elongated horseshoe-shaped, one half inch thick, medium-hard felt relief pads or one half inch thick reticulated polyurethane sheeting. When the relief pads have been sized, the outer edges are beveled and skived to blend smoothly into the cast-socket. The inner arc remains at full thickness to create a bridging of the cast and to avoid pressure on the iliac crest (Fig. 16–39).

The initial plaster wrap consists of 5 inch Orthoflex elastic plaster-of-Paris bandages. The plaster wrap is started on the lateral-distal margin of the amputation and continues proximally and diagonally across the lower abdomen to the contralateral iliac crest and lower waist. This procedure is repeated twice then alternated, circumferentially covering the entire pelvis and lower waist region. Firm tension is applied to the buttock area and the distal soft tissues whenever the wrap is directed over the amputation side. The pelvic and lower waist area acts as the anchor point and suspension of the resulting cast-socket. The wrap is extended proximally to

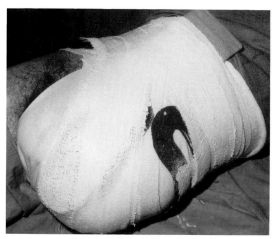

FIGURE 16–40. Left hip disarticulation: application of the initial elastic plaster wrap.

include the two lower ribs. By reducing the tension to the plaster wrap, the proximal edge is allowed to flare outward away from the body (Fig. 16–40). Sufficient elastic plaster-of-Paris bandages are used to form a three to four layer thickness of the initial wrap.

Approximately four to six double layers of 4 by 15 inch conventional plaster-of-Paris splints are applied over the distal portion of the initial plaster wrap anteroposteriorly, partially overlapping each previous layer. One roll of 5 inch conventional plaster-of-Paris bandage is applied over the plaster splints and is alternated in a diagonal and circumferential manner with even, overlapping wraps until the entire cast-socket has been covered. While the plaster is still moist, it can be molded slightly over the iliac crests to ensure adequate suspension and rotational stability.

At the anterior proximal level of the cast-socket, two 1 inch safety buckles sewn to 1 by 8 inch cotton webbing straps are located 4 inches apart. At the posterior proximal level of the cast-socket, two 1 inch by 5 foot cotton webbing shoulder suspension straps are located 4 inches apart and in a direction so that they will cross in the back when placed over both shoulders (Fig. 16–41). The cotton webbing straps are incorporated into the cast-socket with two circumferential turns of a 4 inch roll of conventional plaster-of-Paris bandage over the cotton webbing straps. The distal 2 inches are folded back and secured with the remaining plaster bandage. The excess bias-cut cotton stockinette and the Or-

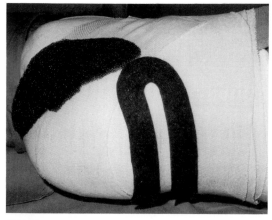

FIGURE 16–39. Left hip disarticulation: polyurethane sheeting and iliac crest pressure-relief pads.

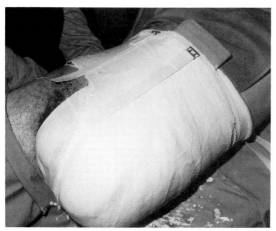

FIGURE 16–41. Left hip disarticulation: elastic plaster wrap completed, suspension buckles located.

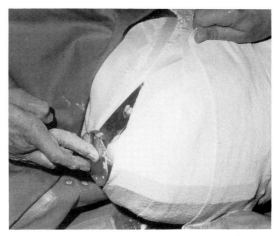

FIGURE 16–43. Left hip disarticulation: socket attachment plate secured to the cast-socket.

lon-Lycra-Spandex sock are rolled back onto the cast-socket brim and are secured with several 3 by 15 inch conventional plaster-of-Paris splints to form a smooth finished edge. The shoulder suspension straps are connected to the safety buckles and secured. The patient is now ready for transfer to the recovery room (Figs. 16–42, 16–43).

The prosthetic unit is not applied at this time, since it would interfere with the removal of the drains. Once the drains have been removed, 48 to 72 hours after surgery, the prosthetic unit can be applied to the cast-socket.

The patient is positioned supine with the pelvis parallel to the foot edge of the bed or casting table and with the sound leg in a neutral position. The three socket attachment straps are shaped to conform closely to the exterior contours of the cast-socket. The po-

sition of the socket attachment plate should be parallel to the foot edge of the table. It is located in the center of the cast-socket when viewed laterally, 90° to the table top, and outset so that an imaginary vertical line from the ischial tuberosity bisects the medial border of the socket attachment plate. The socket attachment straps are marked and secured to the cast-socket with a combination of 4 by 15 inch conventional plaster-of-Paris splints and 4 inch plaster bandages (Fig. 16–44). The pylon sections of the thigh and lower leg are cut to the correct lengths to ensure a compatible knee center location and rotational alignment of knee and foot components (Fig. 16–45). The plaster must be allowed to harden for 24 hours before weight bearing is attempted. The prosthetic assembly is disconnected from the socket attachment plate, to be reattached only for standing and ambulating.

Upper Extremity Amputations

Wrist Disarticulation and Below-Elbow Amputation

The principles of IPPF as applied to lower extremities are equally effective for upper extremities. For wrist disarticulation and below-elbow amputations, a small 5 by 3½ by 14 inch sterile Orlon-Lycra-Spandex sock is rolled over the surgical dressings, past the elbow to the axilla; it is suspended manually by an assistant or by a strap arrangement. The bony prominences of the olecranon and

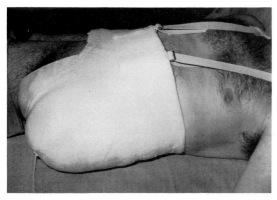

FIGURE 16–42. Left hip disarticulation: cast-socket and shoulder suspension completed.

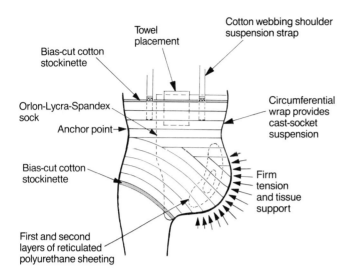

FIGURE 16–44. Left hip disarticulation: drawing of the cast-socket components.

epicondyles are padded with one half inch thick pieces of reticulated polyurethane sheeting with all edges beveled and skived to a thin, feathered edge. These pressure-relief pads are glued in place with Dow Corning Medical Adhesive, Type B. The distal end of the residual limb is covered with a small 3 inch preformed reticulated polyurethane distal pad.

For the initial plaster wrap, elastic plaster-of-Paris bandages are used. While the patient's elbow is flexed approximately 75°, the plaster wrap is extended past the elbow to 2 inches below the axilla. The elastic plaster-of-Paris wrap is reinforced with conventional 3 by 15 inch plaster-of-Paris splints and a 4 inch plaster bandage. The soft tissues just proximal to the epicondyles are slightly compressed mediolaterally before the plaster cast-socket has completely hardened. This enhances suspension and rotational stability.

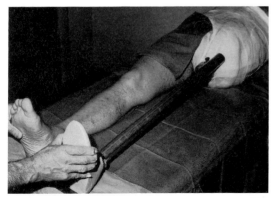

FIGURE 16–45. Left hip disarticulation: application of the foot pylon to the prosthetic unit.

An aluminum friction wrist unit of appropriate size, to which stainless steel attachment straps are fastened, is wrapped in proper alignment and length to the distal cast-socket with a roll of conventional 4 inch plaster-of-Paris bandage. Likewise, retainer plates for the activating cable and harness fasteners are located and secured to the cast-socket with conventional 2 inch plaster-of-Paris bandages. A lightweight aluminum terminal device, figure-eight harness, and Bowden control cable are fitted to complete the prosthetic assembly (Fig. 16–46).

Above-Elbow Amputation

The above-elbow IPPF requires that the upper one third of the Orlon-Lycra-Spandex sock be glued to the skin of the arm and shoulder to assist suspension. The bony prominence of the acromion is padded with one half inch thick reticulated polyurethane sheeting, and a reticulated polyurethane distal pad of appropriate size is applied over the surgical site.

The initial elastic plaster-of-Paris wrap is extended to the axilla and over the acromion in the shape of a standard above-elbow socket. The wrap is reinforced with conventional 3 by 15 inch plaster-of-Paris splints and a 4 inch plaster bandage. A conventional exoskeletal or endoskeletal forearm with a locking elbow, lightweight aluminum friction wrist unit, and stainless steel attachment straps located on the turntable is aligned and wrapped to the cast-socket with a roll of conventional 4 inch plaster-of-Paris bandage. Retainer plates and harness attachment

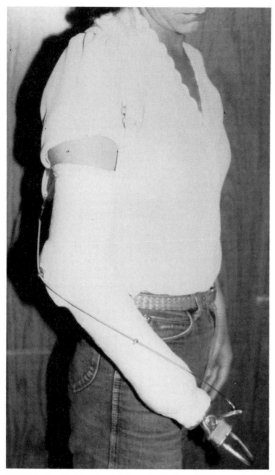

FIGURE 16–46. Right wrist disarticulation: IPPF completed.

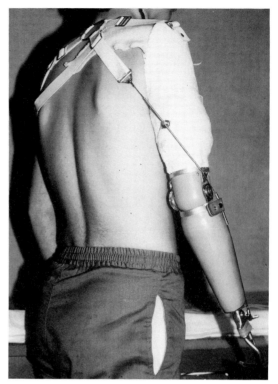

FIGURE 16–47. Right above-elbow amputation: IPPF completed.

until a satisfactory fit is obtained. The entire border of the sock and the corresponding skin area are sprayed about 4 inches wide with Dow Corning Medical Adhesive, Type

straps are located, aligned, and secured to the cast-socket with a 2 inch roll of conventional plaster-of-Paris bandage. An aluminum terminal device, a Bowden control cable, and a figure-eight or ring-type harness complete the prosthetic assembly (Figs. 16–47, 16–48).

Shoulder Disarticulation and Forequarter Amputation

Sterile, nonadherent dressings, including well-fluffed gauze, are applied as with the previous amputation levels and cover the entire skin incision area. A sterile 8 by 6 by 18 inch Orlon-Lycra-Spandex sock is unrolled completely and is cut lengthwise along its lateral aspect, distally to the border of the box toe section. The uncut box toe section is placed over the remaining shoulder. For the forequarter amputation, the box toe is reduced by extending the cut into the sock

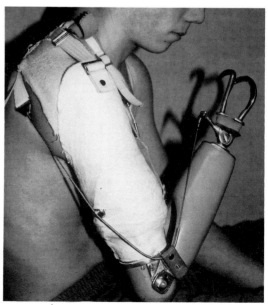

FIGURE 16–48. Right above-elbow amputation: after IPPF, the patient activates the terminal device.

B. While the sock is stretched, it is glued to the skin, and any wrinkling of the material is avoided. Bony prominences, such as the acromion, clavicle, spine of the scapula, and the area of the skin incision, are covered with one half inch thick reticulated polyurethane sheeting and are glued in place with Dow Corning Medical Adhesive, Type B.

A 4 inch by 4 yard roll of bias-cut cotton stockinette is applied over the Orlon-Lycra-Spandex sock. The wrap extends from the amputated shoulder across the chest, below the axilla of the sound side, crossing in back of the lower border of the scapula, back to the amputation site. The initial elastic plaster-of-Paris wrap repeats the same sequence to achieve a minimum of three layers of plaster bandages. The elastic plaster-of-Paris is reinforced with 4 by 15 inch conventional plaster-of-Paris splints and 4 inch plaster bandages. The excess bias-cut cotton stockinette is folded over the plaster edges and is secured with 2 by 15 inch conventional plaster splints to form a smooth finished edge.

Owing to the complexity and weight of the standard body-powered prosthetic components, fitting of the prosthesis is delayed until after suture removal. If immediate fitting is preferred, an endoskeletal prosthesis should be considered to minimize the weight of components acting on the surgical site. Alignment follows accepted prosthetic principles, and some function is sacrificed initially to maintain simplicity of design and lower weight. For economic reasons, IPPF of upper extremities has been restricted to conventional body-powered prosthetic systems and components. In 1984, Malone and associates reported their excellent results with upper extremity IPPF using myoelectric and externally powered prosthetic component systems.[11]

PATIENT MANAGEMENT

Good, precise patient management is an intricate part of effective and successful IPPF. Full weight bearing, or weight bearing up to the patient's tolerance, is excessive and counterproductive and can result, in extreme cases, in wound separation and tissue breakdown. All patient complaints of excessive discomfort or pain should be promptly investigated. A common complaint is a feeling of a hot steel band constricting the distal residual limb circumferentially. This is caused by the rigid cast-socket preventing formation of edema. It is not advisable to bivalve the cast, since the sensation reoccurs with additional edema formation. However, complaints of localized pressure over bony prominences should be promptly relieved.

On the first or second postoperative day, the patient is allowed static weight bearing, up to 20 pounds for 1 to 5 minutes at bedside with the assistance of a physical therapist. The prosthetist is also present to check the static alignment of the prosthesis. Bathroom scales or weight-bearing control devices installed in the prosthetic pylon can monitor exact compliance (Figs. 16–49, 16–50). If the patient is unable to stand or in the case of a bilateral amputation, a tilt table can be used (Fig. 16–51). Simulated weight bearing can be initiated manually if the patient is physically unable to stand; this is done by intermittently pushing against the distal end of the cast-socket. The patient can also be taught to place a towel over the distal end of the cast-socket and pull by hand on both ends of the towel to simulate intermittent weight bearing. The hip disarticulation patient can be brought to a seated position to accomplish weight bearing before the prosthesis is incorporated into the cast socket. The intermittent pressure to the amputation side has a beneficial pumping effect that reduces the tendency for postsurgical edema formation and increases patient comfort. Standing or simulated weight bearing activities can be increased to twice a day.

After 48 hours, the Penrose drain is removed with sterile instruments through a 2 by 2 inch window cut into the cast-socket

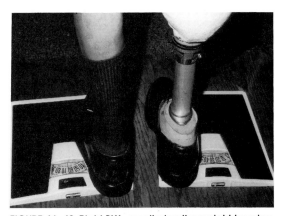

FIGURE 16–49. Right BKA: monitoring the weight-bearing potential.

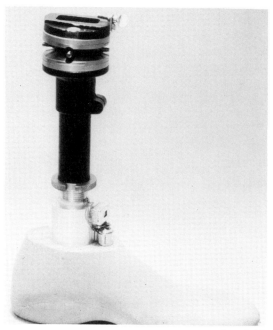

FIGURE 16–50. Left BKA: a Moore load cell weight-bearing control device.

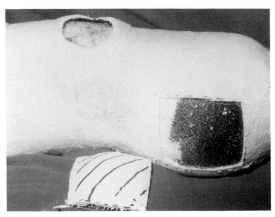

FIGURE 16–52. Right BKA: removal of the Penrose drain.

directly over the drain site (Fig. 16–52). The dressings are disturbed as little as possible. The window is replaced and secured with a conventional plaster-of-Paris bandage wrap. Adhesive tape alone is not sufficient and will allow window edema to develop. Suction drains can usually be pulled from the cast-socket without cutting a window.

On the third or fourth postoperative day, ambulation can be initiated between parallel bars or with a walkerette. The prosthetist should be present to check the dynamic align-

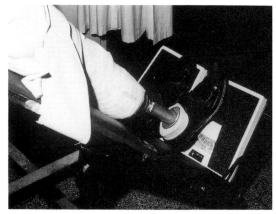

FIGURE 16–51. Bilateral BKA: monitoring the weight-bearing potential on a tilt table.

ment of the prosthesis and to adjust the knee friction control of the above-knee shank when the knee is unlocked. Daily observation is essential to ensure that excessive looseness of the cast does not develop. The auxiliary suspension straps must remain snug. If excessive pistoning, exceeding one half of an inch, is noted, the cast-socket should be changed immediately. Walking twice a day with up to 20 pounds of weight bearing is encouraged (Figs. 16–53 to 16–57). Unsupervised walking is not allowed, and the pylon prosthesis should be withheld from patients who do not comply with this request.

The cast-sockets for transmetatarsal, Pirogoff's, Syme's, below-knee, and below-elbow amputations and wrist disarticulation are ordinarily changed on the twelfth postoperative day. However, they may have to be changed earlier if excessive edema was present during surgery or if the patient is obese. Similarly, the above-knee, hip disarticulation, above-elbow, and shoulder disarticulation cast-sockets require changing on the tenth postoperative day, sooner if evidence indicates loosening of the residual limb in the cast-socket.

Partial or total suture removal may be indicated at the first or second cast change. Sterile adhesive strips can provide substitute wound reinforcement. Cast changes should be expedited to avoid formation of edema in a residual limb that has been exposed overly long. Static and dynamic prosthetic alignment must be re-established after each cast change. If the cast-socket comes off inadvertently, the residual limb should immediately be wrapped correctly with elastic bandages; a new cast is applied as soon as possible.

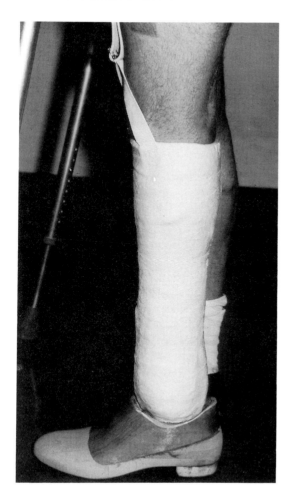

FIGURE 16–53. Left Syme's amputation: IPPF completed.

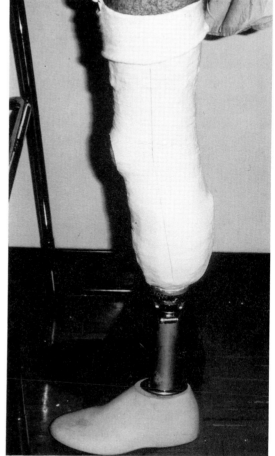

FIGURE 16–54. Left BKA: IPPF completed.

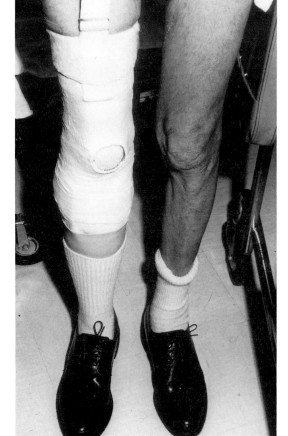

FIGURE 16–55. Right BKA: IPPF completed, with a cosmetic cover.

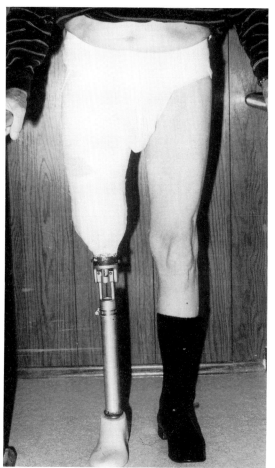

FIGURE 16–56. Right AKA: IPPF completed.

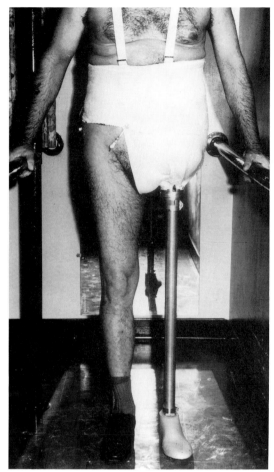

FIGURE 16–57. Left hip disarticulation: IPPF completed without a prosthetic knee joint.

Patients may be discharged before the first cast change if they are considered dependable. They can be seen for ambulation instruction and monitoring by the physical therapist and for regular follow-up by the surgeon before the initial cast-socket change. As progressive wound healing occurs, weight bearing can be increased slowly, but full weight bearing should not be allowed at any time in an immediate postsurgical prosthesis. Standard principles of gait training are followed, and the distance walked is increased slowly and steadily, though it should not exceed the point of the patient's fatigue or discomfort. Ambulation progresses from the parallel bars or a walkerette to crutches as the patient learns to handle these tasks safely and securely (Fig. 16–58). A confused or irresponsible patient should not be discharged on an outpatient basis but should be transferred to

an extended care facility where professional nursing care and physical therapy supervision are available.

TEMPORARY PROSTHESES, SOCKETS, AND MATERIALS

Temporary prostheses and sockets, also referred to as preparatory or intermediate prostheses, have a relatively short-term patient use, seldom exceeding 3 months. The terms definitive or permanent prostheses and sockets are actually misnomers describing long-term prostheses and sockets that are used for years but eventually require replacement if the patients enjoy a long enough active life. Temporary sockets are made from materials lending themselves to expedient working techniques that create an acceptable, economical product lasting a short time as compared with the so-called definitive or permanent prosthesis, which is the result of a more complex and expensive fabrication procedure.

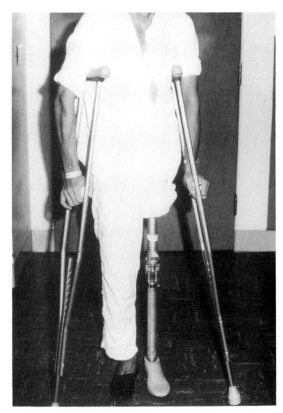

FIGURE 16–58. Left hip disarticulation: IPPF completed with a prosthetic knee joint.

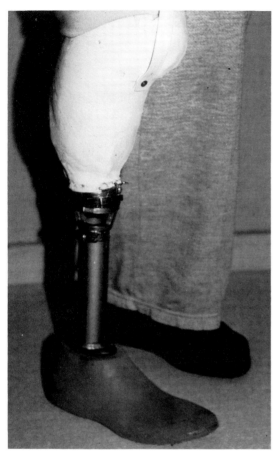

FIGURE 16–59. Right BKA: temporary suprapatellar Zoroc cast-socket on a pylon prosthesis.

As wound healing is completed and edema subsides after the second or third cast change, consideration is given to a temporary prosthesis if the volume of the residual limb is expected to decrease in the near future. Fabrication of this type of prosthesis must take into consideration the patient's social, vocational, recreational, and even psychological requirements. Patients require at least the ability to attain reasonable goals consistent with their physical capabilities if total independence is not possible.

At this stage of rehabilitation, the below-knee amputee has the knee joint mobilized to allow for a more natural gait. Suprapatellar cast-sockets have been fabricated with the same casting technique as is used for below-knee amputation but with the cast-socket terminating at the knee. A forked nylon webbing suspension strap is attached to a waist belt, and the adjustable prosthetic unit, py-

lon, and SACH foot fitted to a shoe are reused in this application (Fig. 16–59). Weight bearing is limited to approximately 50% of body weight at all times. This short cast-socket can be worn at night in bed or can be removed and replaced by a well-fitted elastic shrinker or a properly applied elastic bandage to control residual limb volume (Fig. 16–60). Wool socks of various plies can be added to compensate for additional atrophy. After wearing the short cast for 12 to 14 days, most patients can have their residual limbs casted and measured for the definitive prosthesis.

For the above-knee amputation patient, a removable ischial weight-bearing cast-socket, fitted with a wool sock and suspended with a modified silesian belt, can be mounted on the temporary pylon and SACH foot (Fig. 16–61). Whenever this cast-socket is removed, the residual limb is contained in a well-fitted elastic shrinker or a properly applied elastic bandage to control residual limb volume. Weight bearing is limited to 50% of the body weight at all times. A wool sock of appropriate ply can be added or minor socket adjustments performed to compensate for residual limb atrophy.

By the second or third cast change, most patients have a relatively mature residual limb with little, if any, residual edema. These patients are fitted with an elastic shrinker over which an elastic bandage is applied. The patients are provided with an instructional booklet and are shown how to rewrap the elastic shrinker and bandage once in the morning and once in the evening. After 8 to 10 days, the patients are ready for casting and measurements for the definitive pros-

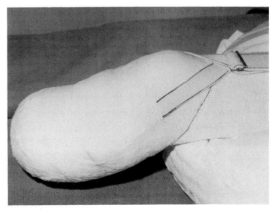

FIGURE 16–60. Left BKA: temporary short cast.

In the late 1960s, Polysar X414,* a thermoplastic material in extruded tubular forms, was used in the fabrication of temporary sockets by direct molding to the patient's residual limb. The resulting socket had to be kept from heat sources to prevent distortion and remolding. Polysar X414 is no longer used in prosthetics.

In the early 1970s, the National Aeronautics and Space Administration was instrumental in developing a product that was being marketed under the trade name of Lightcast. This fiberglass impregnated with unsaturated polyester resin had been treated to begin the first stage of polymerization. The polymerization was interrupted before it was completed, and the bandage material was packaged in an airtight wrap until application, when the curing process was completed with an ultraviolet lamp. This allowed for the speedy fabrication of economical porous sockets, and the material was also useful as a plaster-of-Paris bandage substitute (Fig. 16–62). The disadvantages of this material were

*Polymer Corporation, Ltd.

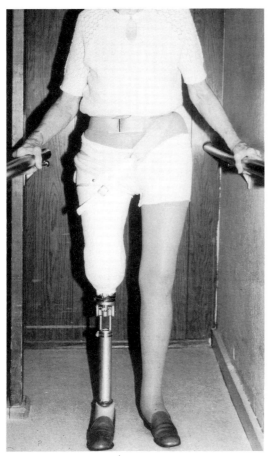

FIGURE 16–61. Right AKA: temporary Zoroc cast-socket with a silesian suspension and a manual locking pylon.

thesis. Of course, the obvious disadvantage of this procedure is that the patient is unable to ambulate while the definitive prosthesis is being fabricated. However, the patients are fitted early with their definitive prostheses, which allow gait training with full weight bearing, or at least up to tolerance, and save the cost of temporary prostheses. It might be argued that these patients do not escape this expense but simply incur it through premature socket replacement, and it is a fact that 95% of these patients require a socket replacement between 6 months and a year.

Fabrication of the inexpensive temporary socket has been aided by the continual developments in plastics, especially in the last 3 decades. As materials were developed and utilized, they were quickly abandoned in favor of improvements enabling the prosthetist to fabricate more quickly a better, lighter, and at times a more economical product.

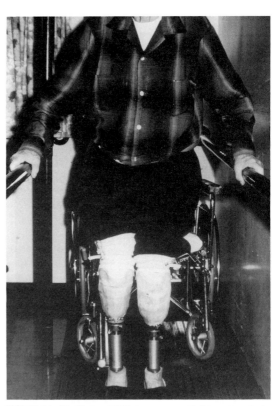

FIGURE 16–62. Bilateral BKA: temporary Light cast sockets mounted on pylon prostheses.

its need of the rather bulky lamp used for curing and its inability to control tissues during application, as is possible with elastic plaster-of-Paris. The product is no longer commercially available.

Zoroc (Johnson & Johnson Inc.), a resin-impregnated plaster bandage that hardens into a very rigid and durable cast, was an excellent material for fabrication of temporary sockets and for reinforcing elastic plaster-of-Paris (Fig. 16–63). The only contraindication was in individuals known to be sensitive to formaldehyde. Production of Zoroc has also been discontinued.

A more recent product, 3M Scotchcast, replaced by Scotchcast-2, is a knitted fiber glass fabric impregnated with polyurethane resin that produces very lightweight and durable temporary sockets. Other suitable synthetic fiber glass casting tapes commercially

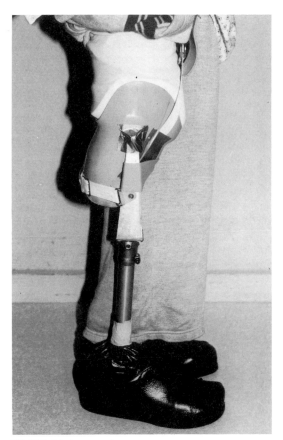

FIGURE 16–64. Right BKA: temporary laminated total-surface weight-bearing socket with a soft insert and dynamic socket pivot to reduce the 40° knee flexion contracture.

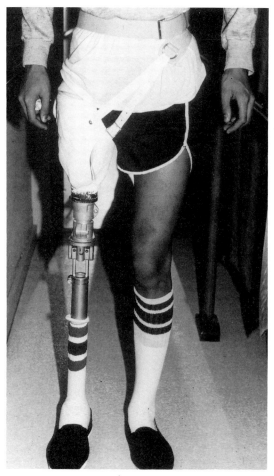

FIGURE 16–63. Right AKA: temporary Zoroc cast-socket with a silesian suspension, manual locking pylon, and pylon-thigh extension for a short residual limb.

available are Zim-Flex (Zimmer, Warshaw, Indiana) and Johnson & Johnson's Delta-Lite "S." Cast-sockets fabricated for synthetic fiber glass materials take 50% less drying time than regular plaster, are moisture resistant, result in porous sockets that allow air circulation, and do not decay. When synthetic casting tapes are used on an ischemic, diabetic amputee with neuropathy, care must be taken to pad the rough outer surface of the cured material adequately to prevent abrasion of the remaining extremities. Synthetic fiber glass casting tapes are also more difficult to handle for tissue control and support during application if used in place of elastic plaster-of-Paris Orthoflex in IPPF or temporary cast-sockets. Synthetic fiber glass casting tapes are best used for temporary sockets; it is molded over a modified positive residual limb replica or is used to reinforce the initial elastic plaster-of-Paris Orthoflex wrap. This reduces the resulting weight of a completed cast-socket to some extent. However, greater weight reduction is achieved by replacing the prosthetic assembly with carbon-fiber prosthetic components.

The new generation of IPPF involves the initial application of elastic plaster-of-Paris Orthoflex to provide controlled tissue support; it is reinforced by Scotchcast-2, and carbon-fiber prosthetic components complete the ultralightweight system. Improvements in prosthetic components are required in the form of scaled-down models for children and a quick-disconnect system for upper extremity prostheses. Continual technical improvements will emerge as new material de-

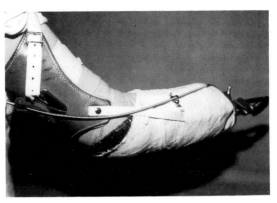

FIGURE 16–66. Right below-elbow amputation: temporary conventional plaster cast-socket, triceps pad, flexible elbow hinges, figure-eight harness, Bowden cable, and terminal device.

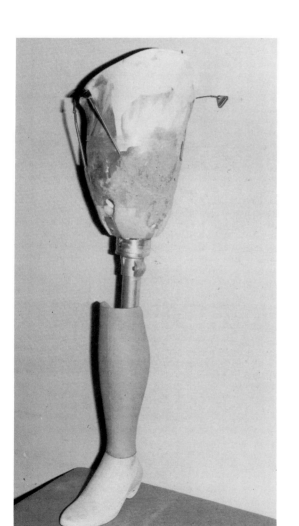

FIGURE 16–65. Left AKA: temporary laminated quadrilateral socket with a Bowden cable suspension, mounted on a pylon without a prosthetic knee joint.

velopments provide opportunities for advancement.

In most instances, when the IPPF is complete and the final cast is discontinued, the patient can soon be fitted with the definitive prosthesis. Such patients receive priority treatment to expedite delivery of the prosthesis and limit the time the patient is nonambulatory. If a temporary prosthesis and socket are indicated, the choice of materials and technique should be left to the individual prosthetist. Numerous options are available, and it is only a matter of individual choice and preference. The economics of the system must remain reasonable and affordable but meet the individual patient's requirements (Figs. 16–64 to 16–66).

REFERENCES

1. Berlemont M: Notre expérience de l'appareillage précoce des amputés des membres inférieurs aux establissements Hélio-Marins de Berck. Ann Med Phys 4:4, 1961.
2. Berlemont M, Weber R, Willot JP: Ten years of experience with the immediate application of prosthetic devices to amputees of the lower extremities on the operating table. Prosthet Orthot Int (Kbh) 3:8, 1969.
3. Burgess EM: Immediate postsurgical prosthetic fitting: A system of amputee management. Am J Phys Ther 51:139, 1971.
4. Burgess EM, Romano RL: The management of lower extremity amputees using immediate postsurgical prostheses. Clin Orthop 57:137, 1968.
5. Burgess EM, Romano RL, Zettl JH: The management of lower extremity amputations: Surgery, immediate postsurgical prosthetic fitting, rehabilitation. Bulletin TR 10–6. Washington, DC, US Government Printing Office, 1969.

6. Burgess EM, Traub JE, Wilson AB Jr: Immediate postsurgical prosthetics in the management of lower extremity amputees. Bulletin TR 10–5. Washington, DC, Veterans Administration, 1967.
7. Childress DS, Hampton FL, Lambert CN, et al: Myoelectric immediate postsurgical procedure. Artif Limbs 13:55, 1969.
8. Dederich R: Amputationen der unteren Extremität, Operationstechnik und prothetische Sofortversorgung. Stuttgart, Thieme, 1970.
9. Golbranson FL, Asbelle C, Strand D: Immediate postsurgical fitting and early ambulation: A new concept in amputee rehabilitation. Clin Orthop 56:119, 1968.
10. Loughlin E, Stanford J, Phelps M: Immediate postsurgical prosthetic fitting of a bilateral below-elbow amputee—a report. Artif Limbs 12:17, 1968.
11. Malone JM, Fleming LL, Roberson J, et al: Immediate, early, and late postsurgical management of upper-limb amputation. Rehabil Res Dev 21:33, 1984.
12. Malone JM, Moore WS, Goldstone J, Malone SJ: Therapeutic and economic impact of a modern amputation program. Bull Prosthet Res 16:1, 1979. Washington, DC, Veterans Administration.
13. Marquardt E: Frühversorgungen von amputationen der oberen extremität. Orthopädie Technik, Heft 7/1970.
14. Marquardt E: Prothetische Sofort und Frühversorgung; Rehabilitation, Band III. Herausgegeben von KA Jochheim und JF Scholz. Stuttgart, Thieme, 1975.
15. Moore WS, Hall AD, Wylie EJ: Below-knee amputation for vascular insufficiency. Arch Surg 97:886, 1968.
16. Nigst H: ≪Immediate fitting≫ nach amputationen wegen funktionsloser hand bei irreparablen plexuslähmungen. Handchirurgie, 3 Jg, S 126–128, 1969.
17. Sarmiento A, McCollough N, Williams E, Sinclair W: Immediate postoperative prosthetic fitting in the management of upper extremity amputees. Artif Limbs 12:14, 1968.
18. Sarmiento A, McCullough NC, Williams EM, Sinclair WF: Immediate postsurgical prosthetic fitting in the management of upper extremity amputees. Prosthet Orthot Int (Kbh) 3:45, 1969.
19. Tosberg W: Immediate postoperative prosthetic fitting. (Correspondence between William A Tosberg, CPO, and Dieter Mozer, CPO.) Orthop Prosth Appl J 19:30, 1965.
20. Vitali M, Robinson KP, Andrews BG, Harris EE: Amputations and Prostheses. London, Baillière Tindall, 1978.
21. Warren R, Kihn RB: A survey of lower extremity amputations for ischemia. Surgery 63:107, 1968.
22. Weiss M: Myoplasty, immediate fitting, ambulation. Presented at the World Commission on Research in Rehabilitation. Tenth World Congress of the International Society, Wiesbaden, Germany, 1966.
23. Weiss, M: The Prosthesis on the Operating Table from the Neurophysiological Point of View: Report of Workshop Panel on Lower Prosthetics Fitting. Washington, DC, National Academy of Sciences, 1966.
24. Wilson PD: Early weight-bearing in treatment of amputations of the lower limb. J Bone Joint Surg 4:224, 1922.
25. Zettl JH: Materials and equipment for immediate postsurgical prosthetics. Bull Prosthet Res 10–8:194. Washington, DC, Veterans Administration, 1967.
26. Zettl JH: The PRS above knee casting fixture. Artif Limbs 14:75, 1970.
27. Zettl JH: Immediate postsurgical prosthetic fitting: The role of the prosthetist. Am J Phys Ther 51:144, 1971.
28. Zettl JH: Mission to the Congo. Rehabil World 2:18, 1976.
29. Zettl JH, Burgess EM, Romano RL: The interface in the immediate postsurgical prosthesis. Bull Prosthet Res 10–12:8. Washington, DC, Veterans Administration, 1969.
30. Zettl JH, Van Zandt ML, Gardner J: The immediate postsurgical adjustable pylon prosthesis for the hip disarticulation and short above knee amputee. Bull Prosthet Res 10–13:64. Washington, DC, Veterans Administration, 1970.

17

Complications of Lower Extremity Amputation

James M. Malone, M.D.

There are approximately 50,000 to 60,000 new major lower extremity amputations performed in the United States each year. Two thirds of these amputations are required for complications of diabetes mellitus or peripheral vascular disease.

Not surprisingly, there is a high incidence of associated medical diseases in patients undergoing lower extremity amputation (Table 17–1). These coexistent diseases significantly increase the morbidity and mortality of amputation surgery. A review of the literature suggests that the mortality rates for above-knee and below-knee amputation are still 12 to 40% and 4 to 16%, respectively.[2, 3, 7, 13, 15, 18, 20, 29] Review of the causes of late mortality after successful amputation surgery suggests that two thirds of the patients die from cardiovascular diseases, approximately one half of whom die from myocardial infarction alone.[15] For those patients with diabetes mellitus, the risk of losing their second leg in the 5 years after amputation of the first leg approximates 3 to 7% per year. In addition, one third to one half of diabetic amputees die of complications of diabetes mellitus or other cardiovascular diseases within 5 years of their first limb amputation.[13, 17, 21, 27] If diabetic amputees do not die

of cardiovascular disease first, it can safely be said that they will become bilateral lower extremity amputees.

The major postoperative complications of lower extremity amputation, with ranges of frequency of occurrence, are listed in Tables 17–2 and 17–3. Each of the complications can be subdivided into the time of occurrence with respect to surgery (early versus late).

EARLY POSTOPERATIVE COMPLICATIONS

Operative Mortality

The overall incidence of death after major lower extremity amputation ranges from 0 to 35%.[3, 5, 6, 12, 13, 15–18, 27, 28] An overall average mortality rate of 6 to 10% is probably to be expected even in centers treating large numbers of amputees.[12, 13] The overall mortality rate at the Tucson Veterans Administration (VA) Medical Center in 1986 was one death in 137 consecutive lower extremity amputations (0.7%). Data from the Tucson VA Medical Center/University of Arizona, as well as other reports in the literature, support a

Table 17–1. CONDITIONS PRESENT BEFORE MAJOR LOWER EXTREMITY AMPUTATION

	Incidence (%)
Smoking	50–100
Diabetes mellitus	62–82
Cardiovascular disease	26–77
Hypertension	15–70
Cerebrovascular disease	20–25
Pulmonary disease	5–20
Renal insufficiency	1–10

three- to fourfold increase in mortality for patients undergoing above-knee amputation as compared with below-knee amputation.[6, 11–13, 15, 27, 28] The incidence of death after lower extremity amputation is also related to patient age, and most series report a two- to threefold increase in mortality for patients over 70 years of age.[6, 9, 19] As might be expected, two thirds of all postoperative deaths are due to cardiovascular complications, including myocardial infarction, stroke, and congestive heart failure, and approximately one third to one half of all early postoperative deaths are due to myocardial infarction alone.

Failure to Heal

The incidence of failure to heal after major lower extremity amputation ranges from 3 to 29%.[3, 10, 11, 13–16, 18, 27, 28] Failure to heal is a major complication, since it almost always results in an amputation at a higher level. The conversion rate of a below-knee amputation to an above-knee amputation for complications due to failure to heal or infection ranges from 0 to 29%.[3, 10, 13, 27] In general,

Table 17–2. EARLY POSTOPERATIVE COMPLICATIONS

	Incidence (%)
Residual limb pain/phantom pain	5–85
Revision to higher level	0–29
Death	0–35
Failure to heal	3–29
Pulmonary embolus	4–38
Pulmonary complications	8–30
Residual limb infection	0–28
Cardiovascular complications	2–25
Stroke	3–14
Deep venous thrombosis	1–5
Flexion contracture	1–3
Renal insufficiency	1–3

Table 17–3. LATE POSTOPERATIVE COMPLICATIONS

	Incidence (%)
Contralateral limb loss (5 yr)	15–66
Failure of rehabilitation	0–71
Death (5 yr)	25–70
Local residual limb revision	3

failure to heal represents a complication due to inadequate blood supply at the level selected for amputation, traumatic intraoperative handling, prolonged ischemia of marginally vascularized tissue, a residual limb hematoma with or without secondary infection, or primary residual limb infection. Noninvasive amputation level selection techniques suggest that the failure rate after lower extremity amputation should approximate 9%; therefore, a higher failure rate can most probably be related to the methods used for amputation level selection or to surgical technique.[12, 13] At the worst, the failure rate for below-knee amputation should not exceed 17%, since, as reported by Lim and associates,[10] 83% of all patients heal a below-knee amputation. At the Tucson VA Medical Center, the early wound-healing failure rate after lower extremity amputation in 1986 was 1 in 137 (0.7%). Such a high level of primary amputation healing is directly correlated with careful preoperative objective amputation level selection. Reviews of various level selection techniques are discussed extensively in other chapters, and the interested reader is referred to those chapters for more detailed information on the type and accuracy of the various techniques available for objective preoperative amputation level selection.

The incidence of major lower extremity amputation in patients who have undergone prior attempts at arterial reconstruction ranges from 12.5 to 45%.[4, 9, 13, 21, 22] The literature suggests that lower extremity revascularization before lower extremity amputation does not adversely affect the ultimate level at which the amputation is performed.[4] However, data published by the vascular surgery group at Northwestern University suggest that prior performance of a distal bypass may adversely affect amputation healing.[22] In that series, patients who underwent primary amputation without a prior distal bypass had an incidence of healing problems of 14.3% (14/98), whereas the rate of healing problems in patients who underwent bypass before amputation was 35% (31/89) (p < 0.0005).[22]

Residual Limb Infection

The incidence of residual limb infection after lower extremity amputation ranges from 0 to 28%[1, 3, 8, 13, 18, 22] and is directly related to the reason for performing the amputation. This complication can be reduced by appropriate management of pre-existing ipsilateral distal extremity infections, including the use of perioperative antibiotics and wide debridement or drainage of the infection before definitive amputation.[11, 28]

There have been five residual limb infections in the last 137 consecutive lower extremity amputations (3.6%) at the Tucson VA Medical Center. Many factors are important in achieving a low rate of residual limb infection, but the most important factors are proper drainage of ipsilateral distal extremity infections before amputation, good wound hemostasis and avoidance of residual limb hematomas, perioperative antibiotic therapy, and objective preoperative amputation level selection to validate satisfactory blood flow for primary wound healing. Studies by both Tripses and Pollak[28] and Berardi and Keonin[3] have suggested that the use of drains in patients undergoing amputations for peripheral vascular disease significantly increases the risk of infection. If drains are to be used, especially in residual limbs that are being closed "wet," closed suction drainage systems appear to be superior to open latex drains.

Rubin and coworkers[22] have suggested that infection in a thrombosed below-knee prosthetic graft after lower extremity amputation is a highly morbid and potentially lethal complication. That group reported an overall incidence of graft infection of 1.4% (10/711) in patients undergoing lower extremity revascularization but an incidence of 16% (14/31) in patients undergoing major lower extremity amputation who had a *prior* infrapopliteal bypass.[22] In that series, local care of the residual limb without graft removal resulted in a high rate of recurrent residual limb infection and significant patient mortality. Similar problems in four of ten patients were reported by Johansen and Zorn.[8] The best management of a noninfected retained distal bypass graft in a patient undergoing a major lower extremity amputation is unknown; however, simple transection of the graft high in the operative field is probably not appropriate.[8, 22] Whether removal of most of the graft (leaving the femoral portion of the graft in place) or removal of the entire graft (with an autogenous vein or artery patch on the femoral arteriotomy) is best is unclear at the present time. A reasonable approach appears to be to cut down on the graft in an easily accessible place in the midthigh. If the graft appears to be well incorporated and noninfected, it can be transected, its proximal portion can be obliterated in soft tissue, and its distal portion can be excised with the amputation. If, however, the graft is not well incorporated or there is a question of infection when the graft is exposed in the midthigh, the entire graft should be removed concomitantly with or before amputation.

Pain

The incidence of disabling residual limb pain and phantom limb pain after major lower extremity amputation ranges from 5 to 30%.[13] Both the experience of the author and the surgical literature, however, may underestimate the real incidence of phantom pain problems in lower extremity amputees. Sherman and colleagues,[25] in a retrospective random review of 5000 VA amputees, found that 85% of the amputees responding to their survey noted significant phantom pain. Of greater concern was the fact that only a few of the 68 treatment methods used for phantom pain gave satisfactory results.[23–26]

The issue of pain after lower extremity amputation is extensively addressed in Chapter 18, to which the interested reader is referred.

Renal Insufficiency

The incidence of renal insufficiency is 1 to 3% after major lower extremity amputation.[11, 13–16, 18] If proper attention is paid to perioperative hydration and antibiotic dosage, especially in patients with diabetes mellitus or recognized renal insufficiency, this complication, for the most part, is avoidable. In an occasional patient with unexplained renal insufficiency, the presence of renal arterial stenosis or renal arterial thrombosis should be considered, since renal arterial reconstruction for renal salvage may be appropriate.

Flexion Contracture

The incidence of flexion contracture of the knee or hip joint after major lower extremity amputation ranges from 1 to 3%.[11, 13–16] The incidence of flexion contracture is increased in elderly patients (over 80 years of age) and in patients undergoing amputation on the side of a prior stroke.[13] Flexion contractures greater than 20° prohibit successful fitting of a prosthesis, and their presence often necessitates amputation at a higher level, which may further diminish the prospect for successful patient rehabilitation. Rigid postoperative dressings, with or without the use of an immediate postoperative pylon, and agressive physical therapy decrease the incidence of postoperative flexion contractures. Ideally, a physical therapist should evaluate a prospective amputee before amputation, and the patient should be started on a course of range of motion and upper and lower extremity strengthening exercises before surgery. If preoperative physical therapy is not possible, the patient should be referred to the rehabilitation medicine department as soon as possible after amputation.

Pulmonary Complications

The incidence of pulmonary complications, including pneumonia, atelectasis, and sepsis, is variable after lower extremity amputation but probably averages 8%.[13] It is clear, however, that the rate of pulmonary complications is significantly increased in patients undergoing above-knee amputation.[7] Active exercise, physical therapy, and agressive pulmonary toilet are all valuable treatments for decreasing the incidence of pulmonary complications after lower extremity amputation. Since most prospective amputees have significant smoking histories, pulmonary function testing and perioperative respiratory therapy are also important in diminishing the rate of postoperative pulmonary complications.

Thromboembolic Complications

The reported incidence of pulmonary embolism and deep venous thrombosis following major lower extremity amputation ranges from 4 to 38% and from 1 to 5%, respectively.[13, 30] In addition to the significant morbidity and mortality due to major venous thromboembolic complications, the additional impairment of pulmonary function and blood oxygenation may further compromise the healing of ischemic tissue in the residual limb.

Williams and associates[30] have suggested that low-dose heparin therapy may not be effective in preventing thromboembolic complications in patients undergoing above-knee amputation. However, patients undergoing elective major lower extremity amputation in whom there are major risk factors for venous thromboembolic complications probably should receive subcutaneous heparin prophylaxis (5000 units every 12 hours). The use of a closed-suction drainage system is advisable in patients undergoing heparin prophylaxis, since there may be an increase in hematoma formation. However, the most important factors in preventing postoperative thromboembolic complications are the avoidance of prolonged periods of preoperative or postoperative bed confinement and the use of adequate perioperative hydration. Aggressive physical therapy is another useful adjunct in avoiding thromboembolic complications. The use of thromboembolic elastic stockings on the nonamputated extremity is recommended. Strict attention to the details of perioperative management, particularly as they relate to patient hydration and activity, should result in a low incidence of thromboembolic complications. In the author's experience, the incidence of pulmonary embolism and deep venous thrombosis is less than 1% in patients undergoing lower extremity amputation.

Local Revisions

The actual incidence of early local revision after major lower extremity amputation is unknown. Factors that lead to early local revisions are errors in surgical technique at the time of amputation (such as failure to bevel the anterior edge of the tibia during below-knee amputation) or skin breakdown due to prosthetic fitting problems. At the Tucson VA Medical Center, the incidence of early local revisions has been 0.7% (one patient) in 137 consecutive lower extremity amputations. Careful attention to surgical detail and prosthetic management during the postoperative period is important in preventing what is almost certainly an avoidable postoperative complication.

LATE COMPLICATIONS

Late Death

In their review of the fate of geriatric amputees in England and Wales, Harris and colleagues[6] found that although the patients' expected 3-year survival rate was 90%, only 30% of 75 patients undergoing lower extremity amputation survived 3 years. Similar data were found by Mazet and coworkers[17] in a 10-year follow-up of 1770 geriatric patients from the VA and County Hospitals in Los Angeles. They reported a 1-year postamputation mortality rate of 33 and 45% for VA and County patients, respectively. However, the continued mortality curve from the Mazet study for years 1 through 9 demonstrated that late death was not much lower than that for the general population (age and sex matched).[17] Roon and associates[21] reported a 45% overall 5-year survival rate after lower extremity amputation compared with an expected 85% 5-year survival rate for the age-adjusted normal population. Most important, however, was their analysis of the projected 5-year survival rate for diabetic versus nondiabetic amputees. The projected 5-year survival rate for nondiabetic amputees was almost normal (75%), whereas it was only 39% for patients with diabetes mellitus.[21] Smith reported similar 5-year survival data for diabetic patients (41%) in his review of lower extremity amputations in diabetic geriatric patients.[27]

The reported incidence of late causes of death in patients after major lower extremity amputation are listed in Table 17–4. Approximately one half of patients dying from cardiovascular disease die because of acute myocardial infarction alone. The literature suggests that cardiac complications may be increased in patients with diabetes mellitus[5] and that the incidence of death due to pul-

Table 17–4. LATE CAUSES OF DEATH

	Incidence (%)
Cardiovascular complications	60
Acute myocardial infarction	30
Pulmonary complications	6–34
Cancer	8
Gastrointestinal bleeding	1

monary complications may be age-dependent.[3, 6, 13]

Contralateral Limb Loss

The incidence of contralateral limb loss ranges from 5 to 13% per year and 15 to 66% over 5 years after major lower extremity amputation.[13, 17, 27] In Mazet and colleagues'[17] study of geriatric patients from the VA and County Hospitals, 18 to 28% of the patients had lost their opposite limb within 2 years, with little difference between diabetic and nondiabetic patients. However, by 5 years after amputation, significantly more diabetics than nondiabetics had lost their opposite limb in both the VA series (66 versus 28%) and the County series (42 versus 28%).[17] If diabetic amputees live long enough, it is likely that they will become bilateral lower extremity amputees; however, in all probability, diabetic amputees are most likely to die of cardiac disease before contralateral limb loss occurs. Owing to the high risk of contralateral limb loss in diabetic patients, care and attention should be paid to regular examination of the contralateral limb as well as to patient education in appropriate skin and foot care. Preliminary data from the Tucson VA Medical Center suggest that a diabetic foot care patient education program significantly decreases the incidence of contralateral lower extremity amputation in high-risk patients (Table 17–5).

Residual Limb Revision

In a previous report by Malone and coworkers[16] in which there was a 97% rate of primary healing after major lower extremity amputation, 88% of the lower extremity amputees were without residual limb revision up to 18 months after surgery. In that group of patients, the incidence of prosthesis use was 100%. Roon and associates[21] reported

Table 17–5. THE EFFECT OF PATIENT EDUCATION ON THE RATE OF CONTRALATERAL LIMB LOSS*

Group	Patients	Limbs	Amputations	Percentage
Control	85	156	19	12†
Education	91	179	7	3.9†

*100% diabetic patients, prospective and randomized.
†p ≤ 0.01.

similar information, wherein 91% of their patients were ambulatory on prostheses for an average of 44 months after amputation. In a prior review of 351 patients who underwent major lower extremity amputation at the Tucson VA Medical Center/University of Arizona, the late incidence of local residual limb revision was 2.3% (8/351).[12] Not surprisingly, the Tucson VA Medical Center/University of Arizona series documented that most late revisions occurred in patients who were ambulatory on their prostheses. The incidence of late revisions is most probably directly related to the quality of prosthesis fit and careful long-term postoperative follow-up.

REHABILITATION AFTER LOWER EXTREMITY AMPUTATION

Successful ambulation after major lower extremity amputation is dependent on the age of the patient, activity before amputation, and level of amputation. The incidence of successful rehabilitation after lower extremity amputation ranges from 29 to 98%.[9–18] The rates of successful ambulation and rehabilitation after lower extremity amputation should be greater than 90% for the unilateral below-knee amputee, greater than 80% for the bilateral below-knee amputee, probably less than 50% for the unilateral above-knee amputee, and less than 20% for the bilateral amputee with one amputation at the above-knee level.[11, 13–16]

The reported length of hospital stay after major lower extremity amputation (including rehabilitation) ranges from 14 to 384 days.[3, 11, 13–16] Malone and associates[15, 16] have reported that the average length of stay for postoperative rehabilitation with and without the use of immediate and early postoperative fitting is 32 and 125 days, respectively. It is important to recognize that the projected length of stay for lower extremity amputation (including preoperative days in hospital and rehabilitation) under Diagnosis-Related Groups (DRG) guidelines is only 25 days.

SUMMARY

The average mortality rate after lower extremity amputation approximates 8 to 10% even in centers with a large volume of amputation surgery. The incidence of postoperative morbidity ranges considerably but, once again, is significant even in centers treating large numbers of amputees. Careful attention to selecting an optimal level of amputation that will heal primarily, offering the patient immediate or early postoperative prosthetic rehabilitation, educating high-risk patients on both the risk of and avoidance of contralateral limb loss, and careful long-term follow-up can significantly decrease both the early and late postoperative complications of major lower extremity amputation.

The author believes that amputation surgery should not be relegated to a junior surgeon with minimal experience; rather, it should be performed or supervised by a senior surgeon who is willing to provide the attention to detail required to achieve maximum primary amputation healing and successful prosthetic rehabilitation. Furthermore, it is the obligation of amputation surgeons to participate in the postoperative rehabilitation process in order to ensure the highest degree of success in returning their patients to bipedal ambulation.

REFERENCES

1. Bailey MJ, Johnston CLW, Yates CJP, et al: Preoperative haemoglobin as predictor of outcome of diabetic amputations. Lancet 2:168, 1979.
2. Bauer GM, Porter JM, Axthelm S, et al: Lower, extremity amputation for ischemia. Am Surg 44:472, 1978.

3. Berardi RS, Keonin Y: Amputations in peripheral vascular occlusive disease. Am J Surg 135:231, 1978.
4. Burgess EM, Marsden FW: Major lower extremity amputations following arterial reconstruction. Arch Surg 108:655, 1974.
5. Cranley JJ, Krause RJ, Strasser ES, Hafner CD: Below-the-knee amputation for arteriosclerosis obliterans with and without diabetes mellitus. JAMA 98:77, 1969.
6. Harris PL, Read F, Eardley A, et al: The fate of elderly amputees. Br J Surg 61:665, 1974.
7. Huston CC, Bivins BA, Ernst CB, Griffen WO Jr: Morbid implications of above-knee amputation. Report of a series and review of the literature. Arch Surg 115:165, 1980.
8. Johansen K, Zorn R: Amputation stump infection in patients with retained thrombosed prosthetic vascular grafts. Am Surg 47:228, 1981.
9. Kihn RB, Warren R, Beebe GW: The "geriatric" amputee. Ann Surg 176:305, 1972.
10. Lim RC Jr, Blaisdell FW, Hall AD, et al: Below knee amputation for ischemic gangrene. Surg Gynecol Obstet 125:493, 1967.
11. McIntyre KE, Bailey SA, Malone JM, Goldstone J: Guillotine amputation in the treatment of nonsalvageable lower-extremity infections. Arch Surg 119:450, 1984.
12. Malone JM: Complications of amputation surgery. *In* Bernhard VM, Towne J (eds): Complications of Vascular Surgery, 2nd Ed. New York, Grune & Stratton, 1984, pp 455–470.
13. Malone JM, Goldstone J: Lower extremity amputation. *In* Moore WS (ed): Vascular Surgery, A Comprehensive Review. New York, Grune & Stratton, 1983, pp 909–976.
14. Malone JM, Leal JM, Moore WS, et al: The "gold standard" for amputation level selection: Xenon-133 clearance. J Surg Res 30:449, 1981.
15. Malone JM, Moore WS, Goldstone J, Malone SJ: Therapeutic and economic impact of a modern amputation program. Ann Surg 189:798, 1979.
16. Malone JM, Moore WS, Leal JM, Childers SJ: Rehabilitation after lower extremity amputation. Arch Surg 116:93, 1981.
17. Mazet R Jr, Schiller FJ, Dunn OJ, Alonzo NJ: The influence of prosthesis wearing on the health of the geriatric patient. Project 431, Department of Health, Education, and Welfare, Office of Vocational Rehabilitation, Washington, DC, (unpublished), March 1963.
18. Moore WS, Hall AD, Lim RC Jr: Below the knee amputation for ischemic gangrene. Am J Surg 124:127, 1972.
19. Plecha FR, Bertin VJ, Plecha EJ, et al: The early results of vascular surgery in patients 75 years of age and older: An analysis of 3259 cases. J Vasc Surg 2:769, 1985.
20. Porter JM, Bauer GM, Taylor LM Jr: Lower-extremity amputation for ischemia. Arch Surg 116:89, 1981.
21. Roon AJ, Moore WS, Goldstone J: Below-knee amputation. A modern approach. Am J Surg 134:153, 1977.
22. Rubin JR, Yao JST, Thompson RG, Bergan JJ: Management of infection of major amputation stumps after failed femorodistal grafts. Surgery 98:810, 1985.
23. Sherman RA: Published treatment of phantom pain. Am J Phys Med 59:232, 1980.
24. Sherman RA, Sherman CJ, Gall NG: A survey of current phantom limb pain treatment in the United States. Pain 8:85, 1980.
25. Sherman RA, Sherman CJ, Parker L: Chronic phantom and stump pain among American veterans: Results of a survey. Pain 18:83, 1984.
26. Sherman RA, Tippens JK: Suggested guidelines for treatment of phantom limb pain. Orthopedics 5:1595, 1982.
27. Smith RJ: Amputations in geriatric patients. J Natl Med Assoc 66:108, 1974.
28. Tripses D, Pollak EW: Risk factors in healing of below knee amputation. Appraisal of 64 amputations in patients with vascular disease. Am J Surg 141:718, 1981.
29. Towne J, Condon RE: Lower extremity amputation for ischemic disease. Adv Surg 13:199, 1979.
30. Williams JW, Eikman EA, Greenberg SH, et al: Failure of low dose heparin to prevent pulmonary embolism after hip surgery or above the knee amputation. Ann Surg 188:468, 1978.

18

Pain Management after Lower Extremity Amputation

Robert P. Iacono, M.D.
Jennifer Linford, Pharm.D.

Phantom and residual limb pain after amputation is a multifaceted problem involving all spheres of patients' medical problems from their emotional states to the fitting of prostheses. Theoretical models are inadequate to explain phantom limb pain's pathogenesis and pathophysiology, but it appears to involve all levels of the neuraxis: peripheral nerves, spinal cord, and brain. Furthermore, no consensus concerning any aspect of this problem is to be found in the literature; many reports are contradictory, paradoxical, vague, or simply inadequate. The authors will attempt to describe and define postamputation pain objectively, analyze its incidence and the factors affecting its development, and outline both medical and surgical therapy and explore their theoretical implications. Although no one therapy can be universally applied or relied on to be effective, certain innovative neurosurgical procedures have shown promise for controlling refractory cases of phantom pain.

DEFINITION AND DESCRIPTION

Phantom sensations after amputation usually begin immediately and are almost uni-

versally experienced as a vivid illusion of the limb accompanied by paresthesias. Phantom pain appears as an exaggeration of these phantom sensations, characterized by four major properties:

1. It is persistent.
2. It can be triggered by either proximal or remote stimuli.
3. It is more likely to develop if preamputation pain was present—and may resemble it.
4. It can be temporarily or permanently abolished by transient changes of somatic input.[1, 49]

Two kinds of phantom pain are usually described by the patient: either an intense burning or the sensation of an agonizing abnormal or cramped posture. Residual limb pain may also be burning or paroxysmal and lancinating in quality, or both. Patients describe cramping, pressing, crushing, or burning sensations and note that the phantom fingers or thumb assume awkward positions, often as if the phantom extremity is in forced flexion.[62] In almost all cases, the pain is referred to the missing hand or foot, and little difference in the character of the pain is noted between upper and lower extremity amputations.

However, the phantom sensation is not

simply a reproduction of the amputated limb:[5] in the upper extremity, the palmar surfaces of the fingers are the most prominently noted, and the wrist and dorsum of the hand, as well as more proximal parts of the amputated limb, are not felt. Thus, the patients infer the presence of the phantom limb from specific impressions of small distal portions of the extremity. In lower extremity amputations, similar phantom patterning is found.[41] However, lower limb amputees less frequently experience pain than upper extremity amputees.[74] The pain may be continuous or intermittent and may be triggered by autonomic functions, such as urination or ejaculation, or by other body pains or sensations, such as those of disc herniation, angina, or prostatitis. Phantom pain appears very early and often simultaneously with the onset of phantom sensations. In one study which specifically addressed the issue, the average onset of phantom pain was 9 days after amputation.[33, 67]

The reports of the incidence of phantom limb pain show great discrepancy in the literature. Older, more frequently quoted figures place the incidence in the range of 5 to 10% for severe, disabling pain. In other more recent studies, in which responses from patients were sought concerning mild symptoms, 85% of patients indicated mild, infrequent pain or worse.[67, 69] In one of these studies, patients with pain one day a month constituted 14% of the 1200 veterans who responded. Jensen reported on 58 patients, 56 of whom had lower limb amputations due to arterial insufficiency. The incidence of phantom pain was 72% at 8 days and 67% at 6 months.[33] For residual limb pain, the incidence was 57 and 22%, respectively. Fifty percent of patients, however, reported that the intensity of their pain decreased during this 6-month period of observation.

The severity and incidence of phantom limb pain is correlated with a number of factors, including the level of amputation. Phantom limb pain is reported as 70 and 88% in those receiving hemipelvectomy and hip disarticulation, respectively, for cancer.[75] In 36% of the latter group, pain was reported as severe. There may also be a relationship between rehabilitation time and pain incidence. Steinbach and associates noted pain in 13% of traumatic amputees fitted with a prosthesis within 2 months of surgery, but this almost tripled to 33% for those required to wait up to 2 years to obtain a prosthesis.

The phantom limb is reported to "telescope" (draw closer to or be incorporated into the residual limb) in approximately 30% of patients. Pain is more frequent in those reporting the perceived phantom as short and fixed.[74] Patients are also likely to report lancinating or knifelike pains soon after amputation but squeezing, burning, or cramping pains later.

An interesting aspect of phantom pain is that it occurs more frequently in patients experiencing preamputation pain and can resemble this pain.[33, 81] Traumatic amputation may "freeze" the phantom fingers or toes in the exact position in which they were at the time of injury, resulting in a phantom pain having an agonizing cramp as its major character.[5, 82] In Jensen and colleagues' series, which includes 56 cases of lower limb amputation, 80% of those who had pain the day before surgery developed phantom pain thereafter.[33] A more recent study, also by Jensen and colleagues, confirms that preoperative pain is closely correlated with early phantom pain but possibly not late, persistent phantom pain—which may explain earlier contradictions in the literature.[34] The similarity with pre-existing pain may be as specific as in one patient whose phantom complaint was of an "ingrown toenail." In addition, patients in whom amputation is performed for trauma may have an increased incidence of phantom pain over those in whom amputation was done on a more elective basis; Carlen reported a 67% incidence of early phantom pain in the former group.[18]

The incidence of severe phantom pain may be linked to residual limb pain caused by suboptimal surgical results[74] and is increased to 40% in patients with brachial plexus or lumbosacral plexus avulsion.[9, 56]

THEORETICAL ASPECTS OF ETIOLOGY AND PATHOPHYSIOLOGY

It has been stated that "in many cases the pain associated with phantom limbs appears to be secondary to unresolved grief about the loss of the limb."[4] Although emotional factors can certainly play a role in phantom limb pain, this phenomenon does not originate at any one level of the neuraxis.[17] Search for a single mechanism or anatomic location responsible for phantom pain as "the whole explanation" has led only to frustration. A complex multifactorial interaction between the peripheral nerves, the central nervous system, and the sympathetic nerves, as well as psychological input, is likely.[60] Certainly, the patient's personality modifies the perception of the quality of phantom sensations. Innocuous sensations may be reinterpreted as painful when amplified by anxiety, stress, or expectation; reciprocally, the pain may enhance anxiety and stress.[69]

One cannot assume, however, that the pathogenesis of phantom limb pain is based on the same mechanism as painless phantom limb phenomena. Phantom illusions occur after loss of other body parts, especially the breast, and with congenital agenesis of a limb.[46] The phantom illusion disappears after creation of a parietal cortical lesion (topectomy), but parietal ablation does not abolish phantom pain.[68, 82] Thalamic stimulation causes such pain to abate and changes the position, size, or topography of the phantom limb. Therapeutic spinal (dorsal root entry zone [DREZ], discussed later) lesions can alleviate the pain while preserving the phantom illusion—although it may be altered. It is possible that spinal generators and brainstem integration are responsible for the subcortical awareness of pain, whereas parietal visual-spatial illusions are phenomena separate from the pain component.[40]

It has been demonstrated that abnormal sensory input is generated from damaged nerves remaining in a residual limb. After nerve division, large fibers degenerate, and small fibers spontaneously activate in volleys. Later, activity from sprouting and from neuromas occurs. Early exacerbation of phantom pain occurs at the time of nerve sprouting and may contribute to the initiation of central mechanisms assisting in the development of chronic pain.

However, peripheral input cannot be the cause of phantom pain. Surgical section of peripheral nerves usually fails to arrest the pain (extensive dorsal root section is also ineffective for pain relief).[66, 82] Phantom pain associated with complete brachial plexus or lumbosacral plexus avulsion, in which there is isolation of the extremity from the spinal cord (flail arm), is identical to the pain of those extremities with intact roots. Also, short-acting, local blocks of the nerves may give long-lasting relief, ruling out peripheral neuromas or irritable residual limbs as sole causes. Reamputation at a higher level and residual limb revision are notoriously ineffective in eliminating phantom pain. Moreover, the configuration or topography of the phantom limb frequently fails to change after residual limb revision or reamputation. After distal anesthetic nerve block, intraneural microelectrode recordings have shown abolition of mechanically induced afferent discharges; yet, spontaneous pain is still perceived, and spontaneous activity in the nerve remains.[58] Thus, this activity, as well as the pain, may be attributable to generators in proximal (central) sites.

Removal of normal afferent nerves initiates abnormal firing patterns in the spinal sensory areas (dorsal horn). These abnormal discharges may become self-sustaining, and it follows that any peripheral contributions may assume less importance. Coincident with these abnormal discharges of dorsal horn neurons are morphological changes in fine afferent terminals in the cord and changes in the receptive fields of these deafferented dorsal horn cells.[49]

Changes in the chemical milieu within the dorsal horn also occur with deafferentation. After rhizotomy, interneurons become depleted of, but supersensitive to, substance P, and methionine-enkephalin terminals all but disappear. Loss of these and other neuropeptide modulators of nociception may in part be responsible for denervation hypersensitivity.[13, 36] Large myelinated nerve fibers in the dorsal horn and dorsal columns show degenerative atrophy;[36] these changes, combined with the loss of normal afferent stimuli, lead to a decreased input to brainstem reticular areas that normally exert reciprocal centrifugal inhibitory influence on sensory transmission.[15] This may result in decreased thresholds and the observed abnormal bursting discharges of dorsal horn neurons. In this setting, facilitated conformations, or "memory," of prior pain at spinal levels may become more self-sustaining and are thought to cause recruitment of adjacent neurons (enhanced by decreased suprasegmental inhibition). This mechanism could also be responsible for the production of autonomic abnormalities, such as sweating or spontaneous movements of the residual limbs, noted in some patients.[31, 58] From the standpoint of a model, the autonomous activity of dorsal horn neurons may be likened to sensory epileptic discharges, and the analogy can be extended, since anticonvulsants are often effective in reducing phantom pain.[78] Furthermore, as will be discussed, lesions placed in the dorsal horn's substantia gelatinosa can also effectively treat phantom pain.

Further evidence against a purely peripheral pathogenic mechanism for phantom pain is the fact that total spinal anesthesia may fail to relieve such pain and, credibly, has been documented to unmask and exacerbate phantom pain. *This is because spinal anesthetics act primarily on nerve fibers and not on the cord itself, thus producing further deafferentation.* These findings, however, have been largely misinterpreted.[51, 54] Less convincing evidence is the failure of cordotomy or, in the case of phantom limb sensations in paraplegics (which may have a different origin), cordectomy to relieve phantom pain permanently or consistently.[50] These data point to other than purely spinal mechanisms; however, sympathectomy rarely produces relief, nor does high spinal anesthesia, which also blocks sympathetic nerves. The cerebral cortex is not the source, either, since postcentral gyrectomy or parietal lobectomy is ineffective. The brainstem, however, is thought to play a key role.

Several researchers have suggested a central biasing mechanism to explain the phenomenon of phantom limb pain.[17, 50] The model proposes the brainstem reticular formation acts to inhibit tonically or modulate all afferent somatic transmission.[50] The key is that input generates reciprocal inhibition, but this input is based on and maintained by normal skin sensory afferent nerves. Thus, the deafferentation after amputation leads to diminished inhibitory tone to the already hyperexcitable neuronal pools in the spinal dorsal horn.

An interesting twist to this theory arises from observations made during treatment of phantom pain by injections of local anesthetics or by application of acupuncture to points on the contralateral, normal extremity corresponding to painful areas in the perceived phantom.[28, 52] These points on the intact extremity are found to be tender and to have lowered electrical resistances. When these areas are blocked or stimulated by the high-intensity, low-frequency inputs of acupuncture, phantom pain can be relieved. Reticular neurons (which are known to have some ipsilateral projections and to have bilateral receptive fields) may be balanced or recalibrated by these maneuvers or by ipsilateral stimulation, such as that from transcutaneous or peripheral nerve stimulators.[30] Alternatively, pain relief from residual limb or peripheral nerve stimulation (as well as from dorsal column stimulation) is thought to produce patterned, temporally dispersed input that is out of phase with rhythmically firing neuron pools, disrupting their activity and, therefore, the pain signal. Dorsal column stimulation is also thought to induce descending inhibition by stimulation of large-fiber afferent nerves, as are the proprioceptive inputs supplied by functional use of a prosthetic limb. These factors will be explored further during the discussion of treatment.

MEDICAL MANAGEMENT OF LOWER EXTREMITY AMPUTATION PAIN

A myriad of medical treatments have been employed in the management of phantom and residual limb pain, with many primary case reports[2, 3, 23, 42, 45, 59] and small open trials being found in the literature.[10, 25, 39, 66, 67, 76, 78] Most treatments have been based on anecdotal reports of success with single agents, whereas little scientifically generated information has been reported. Follow-up and long-term evaluations are lacking. Methods of evaluation have generally been purely subjective. They have rarely included assessment of physical activity; the number, frequency, or intensity of pain episodes; the use of other analgesics and changes in usage during treatments; or other concurrent therapy. Frequently, the site of amputation has not been stated, nor the reason for amputation. The time of onset of pain relief and the duration of symptoms before initiation of therapy have commonly not been reported. Thus, little has been done to establish a scientific basis for treatment.

Medical treatment of phantom and residual limb pain should be geared toward the possible mechanism for pain. As noted in previous discussions, phantom limb pain is a complex phenomenon that may be both peripherally and centrally mediated. *The patient's description of the pain is the most important determinant of therapy and should not be overlooked.* The search for a simple pharmacologic treatment has been uniformly unsuccessful and may be related to the multifactorial pathogenesis of phantom pain.

Pharmacologic Therapy

Narcotics

Although narcotics are commonly used for moderate to severe pain, they are of little benefit in the long-term treatment of phantom limb pain. These agents do not relieve central pain of any form and simply add insult to injury by sedating the patient without removing pain sensations. Furthermore, opioids do not alter the threshold or responsiveness of afferent nerve endings to noxious stimulation, nor do they impair the conduction of the nerve impulses along the peripheral nerves.[32] These agents should be reserved for acute postamputation pain, and their use should be limited to the immediate postoperative period.

Placebos

Placebo use in pain management has shown a success rate of approximately 36%.[24] Effects are postulated to be due to a stimulatory effect on endorphins and enkephalins through psychological mediation.[14] The placebo effect is, however, short-lived and unreliable.

Beta-Blockers

One of the first agents reported to be successful for the treatment of phantom limb pain was propranolol.[2, 3, 45, 59] Oille first reported complete relief of the pain with 120 mg per day in an 86-year-old man who had been suffering from this phenomenon for 71 years. The response to propranolol was incidental, the drug having been employed for the treatment of paroxysmal atrial tachycardia.[59] Ahmad also observed similar effects in two phantom limb pain patients initially treated for angina and hypertension and in six additional patients suffering from phantom pain.[2, 3] He reported pain relief after 3 days in all patients, whereas Oille alluded to a 2-month period necessary for full effect.

Marsland and colleagues also evaluated three patients who were relieved of pain after receiving beta-blockers.[45] They employed propranolol in two patients and metoprolol in a third. They hypothesized that since the response to metoprolol was not complete, the patient continuing to complain of shooting and thumping pain at the 6-month follow-up, then β_2-adrenergic blockade was necessary for full response.[45] However, metoprolol was given in a dosage of 100 mg three times daily, which exceeds the dose for β selectivity.[6] Thus, the patient probably was receiving full benefit of β_1 and β_2 effects. Propranolol is more lipophilic than metoprolol, and since beta-blockers have been shown to have central activity, it is possible that this patient's pain relief was centrally mediated.[63, 72] This suggests that higher central nervous system levels of the drug were achieved in the patients who received propranolol than in those who received metoprolol.

Scadding and coworkers evaluated propranolol in post-traumatic neuralgia patients in an open trial and in a double-blind, randomized crossover comparison with a placebo.[65] Propranolol was effective in only three patients, none of whom were amputees.[1] Their trial lasted only 2 weeks, and the authors' experience has shown that it may take longer than this for the drug to take full effect (perhaps as long as 6 to 12 weeks).[3] The reason for this delay is not known, but it may be due to patient variability in achievement of adequate levels in the cerebrospinal fluid/central nervous system. A more extensive evaluation and a longer trial are warranted.

Beta-blockers are thought to increase serotonin levels and have effects similar to benzodiazepines and tricyclic antidepressants on electroencephalograph studies.[63, 65] Propranolol, oxprenolol, and atenolol have all produced impaired performance on psychomotor tests as well.[63, 72] These facts again imply that the action of beta-blockers is not simply peripheral but central. Consequently, agents with increased lipophilia probably produce the best response but are patient-dependent owing to various factors affecting central nervous system concentrations, such as fat stores. This concept deserves further investigation.

Anticonvulsants

Another group of agents commonly used in phantom limb pain are anticonvulsants. The most extensively evaluated have been carbamazepine and phenytoin, although reports of valproic acid and clonazepam efficacy can also be found.[23, 76–78] All these agents have been effective in treating neurogenic pain that resembles trigeminal neuralgia. The clinical features of trigeminal neuralgia are usually clear-cut, so treatment of this pain may serve as the prototype for drug therapy with anticonvulsants. Trigeminal neuralgia is paroxysmal and of a shooting or electric shock nature, a description also commonly presented by phantom limb pain patients.[23, 77] Elliot and associates used carbamazepine at average doses of 400 to 600 mg per day and found it effective in five patients who experienced phantom pain of a lancinating quality.[23] Only one patient in this group was a lower limb amputee. Unfortunately, the follow-up period was reported only as "6 months or longer," and it is unknown what the long-term efficacy of this therapy was.

Swerdlow and Cundill evaluated 22 patients with postamputation pain and found that 77% achieved relief on one of four anticonvulsants—carbamazepine, phenytoin, valproic acid, or clonazepam.[78] Therapy was initiated sequentially with one of the four agents, and the dosage was titrated to "therapeutic levels." No exact dosages were reported, and patients were switched to another agent if they did not experience "appreciable pain relief" at "therapeutic levels." (However, "therapeutic levels" have not been clearly established for the treatment of neuralgias, as they have for seizure disorders.[19]) With an average value of 3.9 mcg/ml, the levels of phenytoin achieved were lower than those generally accepted for seizure control. Despite this, response rates to phenytoin were similar to those of the other agents used in the trial. Thus, a mechanism separate from a strict anticonvulsant action has been suggested and is further supported by the relatively unsuccessful use of phenobarbital in phantom limb pain and neuralgias.[77] The effective drugs probably diminish abnormal neuronal hyperexcitability, suppress paroxysmal discharges, or inhibit transsynaptic spread.[19, 77]

Another agent that has central activity and may prove to be useful is baclofen, a derivative of the neurotransmitter gamma-aminobutyric acid (GABA). However, its efficacy is not related to activation of GABA receptors in the spinal cord. In fact, baclofen hyperpolarizes primary afferent fiber terminals, whereas GABA depolarizes them.[11] A GABA-modulated effect on other neurotransmitters may be involved.[77]

According to Carlen and associates, many phantom limb patients experience tremors or spastic movements of the residual or phantom limb; in some cases these are controllable, but in others they occur spontaneously.[18]

Baclofen has been used primarily in the treatment of spasticity associated with multiple sclerosis but may have some utility in phantom limb patients. It has been successfully used alone and in combination with carbamazepine for the treatment of trigeminal neuralgia.[7, 26] The authors' experience indicates that it was useful in combination with propranolol and phenytoin in two patients with autonomous residual limb movements and phantom limb pain.[31] The dosage, if baclofen is used, is generally 30 to 60 mg per day, to a maximal daily dose of 80 mg. If ineffective, the dose should be tapered gradually over several weeks, because seizures and hallucinations have been associated with abrupt discontinuation of this drug.

Tricyclic Antidepressants

The use of tricyclic antidepressants has become fairly commonplace in the treatment of many pain disorders. The rationale for their use is the discovery that increased serotonin levels in the brain tissue occur owing to a decreased re-uptake of serotonin.[22] Serotonin causes inhibition of transmitter output from nerve endings and inhibition of neurons receiving tryptaminergic input.[22] Descending pain-inhibiting neurons are thought to be activated by serotonin and to suppress afferent pain impulses in the segmental dorsal horn cells.[39] Tricyclic antidepressants also affect dopamine and norepinephrine concentrations and thereby affect depression.[22] Chronic pain often involves elements of depression and insomnia.[37] Tricyclic antidepressants affect sleep by a serotonergic mechanism of rapid eye movement (REM) sleep induction through the locus ceruleus. Therefore, these agents improve mood and alleviate insomnia.

The most commonly employed tricyclic antidepressants are amitriptyline, doxepin, imipramine, trazodone, and an agent available in Europe, clomipramine. Clomipramine has been reported to be effective in patients experiencing painful mono- and polyneuropathies. Twenty-two patients with residual and phantom limb pain were treated by Langohr and coworkers as part of an open trial evaluating the use of clomipramine with neuroleptics or of neuroleptics alone in a total of 82 patients.[39] Ten of the patients received neuroleptics alone, with a response rate of 40%, whereas 12 patients also treated with clomipramine achieved a response rate of

58%. This difference is not statistically significant (p = 0.5). Response was stratified as complete, good, partial, no relief, or discontinued secondary to intolerance. A breakdown of the pain relief for amputees was not presented, but overall response rates for the 82 patients were 92% for clomipramine-treated patients versus 68% for patients using neuroleptics. This difference was statistically significant by chi-squared analysis (p = 0.01).

The same researchers also compared clomipramine with aspirin for chronic pain relief in 48 patients, but none of these patients were identified as having residual or phantom limb pain. Clomipramine and aspirin were crossed over in a double-blind fashion at 2-week intervals. Overall response rates for clomipramine were 71 to 74%, as compared with those for aspirin of 33 to 63%. The differences were statistically significant. The group of patients receiving clomipramine before aspirin had the higher rate of relief, perhaps suggesting an inadequate washout period between therapies. Follow-up of a small number of patients for an average of 14 months after the 4-week trial showed a partial to complete response rate of 82%. Although other tricyclic agents have not been studied on an individual basis, Sherman and associates reported their widespread use in surveys of therapy.[66, 68]

Neuroleptics

The neuroleptics used have included the butyrophenones, phenothiazines, and benzamides.[10, 42, 66, 68] Neuroleptic use for pain control has been fraught with controversy. In general, data have been lacking that prove analgesic activity in patients with chronic pain.[48] Most phenothiazines may actually be antianalgesic in their action, with the only agent shown in a controlled trial to have analgesic activity being methotrimeprazine.[48] Most studies were conducted in postoperative patients. However, studies comparing this drug with morphine for chronic pain showed comparable efficacy in a small number of patients.[48] This efficacy has been attributed to sedation and not actual analgesia, but the use of neuroleptics in phantom limb pain has been reported to produce overall response rates of 40 to 100%. In these reports, these agents are thought to alter interpretation of pain stimuli centrally; however, they may also be acting peripherally to stabilize membranes, as do local anesthetics.[8] Logan re-

ported an interesting case of a patient with a 30-year history of phantom limb pain, which was partially controlled with carbamazepine at 800 mg per day.[42] Addition of chlorpromazine, 150 mg per day, abolished his residual pain. Follow-up at 2 years showed the patient's pain remained well controlled.

Benezet and Cochet reported an open trial[10] of tiapride (a benzamide neuroleptic) that, although it acts as a dopamine receptor antagonist, does not block dopamine stimulation of cerebral adenylate cyclase activity.[61] Tiapride was found to relieve pain in 90% of 20 patients who experienced phantom pain within the first few months after amputation for vascular insufficiency, gangrene, rhabdomyosarcoma, or trauma. The nontraumatic amputees in this trial appeared to have slightly better response rates than did amputees who underwent a traumatic event. Of 15 nontraumatic amputees, 47% had complete response; 13%, good; 33%, partial; 7%, no relief. Of the five patients who had traumatic events necessitating amputation, one had complete relief, one had good relief, and two experienced partial relief; one patient showed no response. Larger patient populations are necessary to evaluate the significance of trauma before amputation and its effect on postamputation pain. The study was of short duration, but based on the high response rates, long-term therapy deserves evaluation.

Miscellaneous Agents

In a single study, lysergic acid diethylamide (LSD-25) was tried at subhallucinogenic doses of 25 to 50 mcg per day. Fanciullacci and colleagues reported a placebo controlled crossover trial in seven patients.[25] Patients received placebo one week before the institution of LSD-25 at initial doses of 25 mcg per day for one week. The dose was then increased to 50 mcg per day for 2 weeks. This was again followed by placebo therapy for 4 weeks. Analgesic use by these patients was decreased by one half and was totally discontinued in 71% of the patients treated. Two patients (29%) did not respond to this therapy. Perceptive distortion occurred in four patients during the first 2 days of therapy, but the reaction disappeared with continued drug use. The long-term effects of LSD-25 were not evaluated, but this would be required before therapy could be initiated in a large population of patients.

LSD-25 and other lysergic acid derivatives are similar in structure to serotonin, all being substituted tryptamine moieties.[22, 25] LSD-25 can antagonize or potentiate serotonin activity. Like tricyclic antidepressants, it inhibits membrane re-uptake of serotonin, as well as reduces turnover and alters retention of serotonin.[22]

Sherman and associates have also reported usage of other agents such as reserpine.[66, 68] Reserpine inhibits serotonin granule uptake and storage, and it could be hypothesized that it would be effective for short-term therapy; however, once serotonin stores are depleted, its efficacy would be minimal.

Summary

The approach to the treatment of phantom limb pain should be similar to that of all pain therapy, with consideration given primarily to the type of pain and potential drug activity. Patients complaining of a constant dull, burning ache should be started on tricyclic antidepressants or beta-blockers. Those who report lancinating pain are better managed with anticonvulsants. Spasm may be controlled by baclofen, with or without a beta-blocker. Patients who do not respond to a single agent may respond to a combination of agents, as did the patients in Langohr and coworkers' study and the case report of Logan.[39, 42] Patients exhibiting several types of pain most certainly require combination therapy. The first step should probably be a single agent, with other agents added gradually after the response to the first drug dose is maximized; Table 18–1 details dosage and monitoring. Medical therapy should be instituted and maintained at optimal dosages for an adequate duration (6 to 12 weeks) before the use of surgical methods.

Neurosurgical Treatment

The possibility of neurosurgical intervention in the treatment of phantom and residual limb pain should be considered for those patients with severe symptoms in whom exhaustive pharmacologic trials have proved ineffective. Several new neurosurgical techniques have been employed with good results, and others hold promise. These include the placement of spinal dorsal root entry zone (DREZ) lesions, deep brain stimulation

(DBS), spinal cord stimulation (SCS, formerly dorsal column stimulation), and direct peripheral nerve stimulation. Conventional procedures, such as stereotaxic mesencephalotomy, cordotomy, parietal topectomy, dorsal rhizotomy, and peripheral nerve section, have very limited utility, are generally ill-advised, and, indeed, are rarely used.[57, 66, 68, 82]

Spinal Dorsal Root Entry Zone Lesions

An entirely new approach to phantom and residual limb pain has been developed by Nashold and involves radiofrequency thermocontrolled coagulation of the (spinal) substantia gelatinosa.[55, 56] Because histological confirmation of the lesion is lacking in humans, the target is referred to simply as the dorsal root entry zone; DREZ has become acronymic for this surgical procedure. The DREZ lesioned area is believed to comprise the substantia gelatinosa of the dorsal horn, including Rexed's lamina V and the overlying tract of Lissauer.[55] It is believed that here there is a convergence and integration of sensory input from many spinal levels and that partially disconnected and disinhibited neurons in this area generate aberrant signals experienced as pain (see the previous discussion). The segments of the spinal cord corresponding to the phantom-referenced dermatomes are surgically exposed; intraoperative somatosensory evoked potentials and direct cord recording aid in localization. With the operating microscope and a 0.25 mm diameter thermocoupled electrode, radiofrequency thermal lesions are then placed contiguously into the DREZ of the involved ipsilateral spinal segments.[55, 56, 64]

Nashold and Ostdahl originally reported 21 patients so treated for phantom limb pain associated with brachial plexus avulsion, with 67% obtaining good relief on follow-up.[55] A second series of 22 patients included nine lower extremity amputees suffering postamputation pain and has been published.[64] Amputations were performed because of trauma, vascular insufficiency, and cancer. Successful alleviation of pain was obtained in 33% of this group, with follow-up of 6 months to 4 years. Within the overall group, those patients undergoing a more refined technique achieved good results in 60% of cases. Thus, DREZ may be employed with some selectivity. It holds promise of gaining

Table 18–1. PHARMACOLOGIC TREATMENT OF PHANTOM LIMB PAIN

Drug	Dosage	Monitoring Parameters/Adverse Reactions
Beta-blockers		
Propranolol	40–240 mg per day.	Hypotension, AV nodal block or bradycardia, nightmares, fatigue, bronchospasm in asthma patients, exacerbation of congestive heart failure, mask of hypoglycemic symptoms in diabetics, and decreased GFR in renal dysfunction.
Metropolol	100–300 mg per day.	
Anticonvulsants		
Carbamazepine	Initiate at 100–200 mg 2–3 times per day. Average dose: 400–600 mg per day. Titrate up to 1800 mg per day. When pain is relieved, the dosage should be decreased to the lowest effective dose. Drug withdrawal should be attempted, as some patients do not have recurrence.	Drowsiness, ataxia, confusion, hematopoietic disorders (monitor weekly for 1 month, then monthly), aplastic anemia, agranulocytes, thrombocytopenia, and pancytopenia.
Phenytoin	300–600 mg per day; levels greater than 20 mcg/m associated with increased toxicity.	Ataxia, nystagmus, hematopoietic disorders, and gingival hyperplasia. Drug serum levels are useful in determining toxicity and may be helpful in determining how high doses may be titrated. Levels are decreased with hypoalbuminemia.
Baclofen	Initiate at 5 mg 3 times per day. Dosage may be increased by 5 mg per dose every 3 days. Maximum of 80 mg per day. Discontinuance of the drug should be done over several weeks, decreasing by 5 mg per dose every 3–7 days. Decrease dose in renal failure.	Drowsiness, insomnia, dizziness, weakness, and mental confusion. Sudden withdrawal after chronic administration can cause auditory and visual hallucinations, anxiety, and tachycardia. Seizures have also been reported in abrupt withdrawal, and the threshold is lowered in seizure patients.
Neuroleptics		
Chlorpromazine	50–500 mg per day. Initiate at 50 mg per day, and tirate to lack of pain. Give dose at bedtime.	Sedation and postural hypotension are major side effects; anticholinergic and extrapyramidal side effects are moderate when compared with other phenothiazines. Monitor for tardive dyskinesia in long-term usage.
Antidepressants		
Amitriptyline	Initiate therapy at 25–50 mg per day, and titrate to lack of pain. Maximum of 300 mg per day. Give dose at bedtime.	Sedation and anticholinergic side effects are high; serotonin effects are high. Monitor for cardiac effects in elderly or arrhythmia patients.
Doxepin	Initiate dose at 50 mg per day, and titrate to lack of pain. Maximum of 300 mg per day. Give dose at bedtime.	
Imipramine	Initiate at 50 mg per day, and titrate to lack of pain. Maximum of 300 mg per day.	
Trazodone	Initiate at 200 mg per day, and titrate to lack of pain. Generally, maximum of 600 mg per day.	Increased antianxiety activity. Lower anticholinergic, cardiotoxic, and sedative effects. Efficacy may be lower than other agents, and dosage may be very cautiously advanced to 1200 mg per day.
Benzodiazepines		
Clonazepam	Initiate at 0.5 mg orally given daily at bedtime. Increase by 0.5 mg increments weekly to 2.5–4.0 mg orally given daily at bedtime.	Nonlancinating pain persists. Drowsiness, lethargy, and, occasionally, changes in bladder control.

AV = atrioventricular, GFR = glomerular filtration rate.

a definite place in the treatment of postamputation pain, as it is based on appealing theoretical grounds.[29, 55]

Deep Brain Stimulation

DBS via stereotaxically implanted electrodes has undergone restricted use for the most severe cases of intractable postamputation pain. With the sensory nucleus of the thalamus, the periventricular gray, or the internal capsule as the target of DBS, a European cooperative study reported that 86% of 30 patients gained significant relief. Mundinger and Neumuller reported on ten patients receiving medial lemniscal or thalamic centrum median DBS for phantom limb, residual limb, or avulsion pain, with all achieving significant relief.[53] A number of theories have been proposed to explain these results. Mundinger and Neumuller consider that stimulation of the mesencephalic medial lemniscus or the thalamic ventroposterolateral (VPL) nucleus acts as a substitute for absent proprioceptive stimuli.[53] To support this contention, they reported a case of phantom limb pain controlled by DBS in which previous dorsal column stimulation had failed. They thus deduced that DBS control of pain is not due to downstream stimuli reaching the so-called spinal gate via the dorsal columns. Also, they point out that DBS is ineffective in painful states in which increased nociceptive (afferent) stimuli are present. Success with DBS is achieved in cases of chronic deafferentation, in which a disinhibition of central pain-generating mechanisms associated with a paucity of proprioceptive input or a lesion of integration centers occurs. Mazars and associates reported results of VPL stimulation that summarize and support these points: "Thalamic stimulation rubs off the pain for 2 to 6 hours, and *the phantom is reduced in size and its shape modified.* Although diffuse pain in the stump is well controlled, shoulder periarthritis is responsible for pain on mobilization."[47]

Stimulation of the mesencephalic periaqueductal gray matter, on the other hand, gives poor results for alleviation of phantom limb pain. This stimulation has been shown to result in an endorphin-mediated control mechanism (and is indeed blocked by naloxone). It is felt to activate a downstream inhibitory pain network based on an endorphin-serotonergic linked brainstem mechanism. Thus, its ineffectiveness is consistent with the uselessness of narcotics for this problem. However, a major theoretical paradox is that pharmacologic agents known to increase serotonin and putatively activate this same system have been reported to be effective.

Spinal Cord Stimulation

SCS for phantom and residual limb pain relief is generally effective in more than 50% of cases. This method was introduced as "dorsal column stimulation," based on the well-known gate-control theory of Melzack and Wall.[49, 80] (The mechanism of pain relief by spinal stimulation is not well understood, and experimental results are sometimes contradictory. Fibers of the dorsolateral funiculus, responsible for descending supraspinal pain suppression, are stimulated. Consistently, spinal stimulation can be effective after anterolateral cordotomy; it may also interfere with afferent impulses at the thalamic level.) It is now believed other spinal cord systems are important in the mechanism of pain relief. Originally, flat electrodes were placed over the spinal cord after laminectomy. Currently, these are used, or flexible wire electrodes are inserted percutaneously with the patient under local anesthesia. The electrodes are connected to the stimulating system, trials are carried out, and the electrode position is adjusted until paresthesias are felt in the painful area of the residual limb or are referred to the painful region of the phantom limb. The paresthesias should overlap the distribution of pain. The patient may report an immediate effect on the pain, but electrodes may be percutaneously stimulated for many days' trial before consideration of subcutaneous receiver implantation.

Krainick and Thoden have recently reported results of long-term SCS in 64 amputees. Good results were obtained in 52.4% after 2 years but decreased to 39% after 5 years. At the 5-year follow-up, 42.6% of 61 patients reported more than 25% relief for pure phantom pain as well as residual limb pain. It was noted by these authors, however, that painful throbbing of the residual limb associated with attacks of severe phantom pain was not affected by otherwise successful SCS.[38] Thus, patients report that "background pain" is usually controlled, whereas attacks of severe pain are not suppressed. Krainick and Thoden used this phenomenon to explain why decreased use of pharmacologic agents occurred in a higher percentage of patients than reported pain relief. Arm and leg amputees had similar benefits; however, all patients with brachial plexus avulsion in this series had poor results.[38]

Siegfried and Cetinalp compiled a series containing 150 patients with phantom limb pain treated by SCS.[70] Overall results for 25 to 100% pain relief ranged from 55 to 80%; long-term results averaged 55 to 67%. Because these neurostimulation techniques are not destructive and produce good results, they should be preferred methods of treatment. Failure to obtain lasting relief usually follows the inability to achieve stimulation referred to the painful area.

Transcutaneous Nerve Stimulation

Transcutaneous nerve stimulation (TNS) is an easily applied yet powerful method of dealing with postamputation pain. Many series have documented consistent response rates in the 45 to 65% range. More sophisticated TNS units with programmable stimulation parameters are being employed in some centers. TNS is the main line of defense against this pain syndrome and continues to evolve and provide reliable relief.[12, 35, 53, 79]

Krainick and Thoden reported a series of 124 amputees treated with TNS; 57% of the patients discontinued or took less medication. About 50% of patients with phantom or residual limb pain, or both, responded significantly to TNS.[38] These patients were characteristic in that "attacks" of pain were poorly controlled, whereas background pain was relieved. Follow-up showed unchanged results from 1 to 32 months; thus, a good initial response implied continued control. Gessler and colleagues reviewed nine lower extremity and six upper extremity patients with phantom limb pain that had persisted from 6 months to 40 years.[27] Phantom leg pain was noted to respond significantly better than phantom arm pain, and application of TNS to the residual limb was more effective than to other sites. Stimulation in this group was more successful at 100 Hz than at 2 Hz was also compared with placebo and subthreshold trials. Klinger and Kepplinger reported 25 patients treated with different TNS devices using simple or variable frequencies, with no difference found. Sixteen patients (64%) responded, with seven obtaining complete relief. The investigators noted failure of TNS in the presence of addiction and in patients not receiving continued instruction and

care.[35] Mundinger and Neumuller have used programmable units delivering a frequency of 40 to 450 Hz, in 3 to 17 impulse trains, with a 5 to 180 ms pause and a 0.2 to 0.4 ms impulse duration. This yielded a 50% relief rate. They suggest that regular action potential sequences of "pain" volleys are replaced by the varied and intermittent stimulation. Besides the elimination of pain, they suggest that its replacement with a pleasant warm sensation may have a secondary central effect on the affective (limbic–suffering) component of pain.[53]

In treating 11 lower extremity amputees experiencing pain, Winnem and Amundsen applied TNS (100 Hz) to the residual limb for 15 minutes, twice daily; treatment continued for 5 consecutive days.[83] Overall, there was a 63% response, but two patients obtained complete and lasting relief, with follow-up at 3 to 12 months. They theorized that TNS "breaks up the pain memory circuits" that "the CNS remembers even though the peripheral noxious stimulus has been removed." TNS is thought to activate large-diameter primary afferent fibers selectively within the nerve. These large myelinated fibers may activate inhibitory interneurons and evoke centrifugal inhibitory activity from the brainstem. Analgesia produced by TNS (or SCS) does not involve enkephalinergic interneurons and is not naloxone-reversible.

Guide to Rational Therapy

Therapy of postamputation pain must be begun as soon as the possibility of amputation is foreseen. Psychological preparation should be initiated early, before amputation is inevitable. The surgery should be viewed positively, as reconstructive. Psychological reactions including grief, which is universal, should be anticipated and dealt with.[16, 20] Preoperative somatic pain due to associated pathology should be controlled aggressively because it is believed to predispose the patient to the more frequent occurrence of phantom limb pain. For the same reason, surgery should not be so long delayed as to allow for prolonged preoperative pain and suffering. Technical aspects of residual limb fashioning, including the use of a rigid dressing and control of edema, are important to minimize residual limb pain, since complications may facilitate the development of delayed pain syndromes.[41, 44, 74, 84] However, different techniques for nerve transection have not been shown to be significantly helpful in preventing such pain.

The early use of a prosthesis has been associated with a reduced incidence of neurogenic pain syndromes; this, combined with early and intense rehabilitation therapy, is recommended. The continuing proprioceptive afferent stimuli that are generated by the use of a prosthesis may preclude the development of unopposed, or the incorporation of, facilitated pain conformations in the central nervous system.

When patients do develop phantom and residual limb pain, the elements of their complaints must be delineated. The patient's pain may include burning, cramping, lancinating, or abnormal movement components. Each component syndrome may require a specific therapy. Some patients have exacerbation of their pain at night, correlated with reduced afferent stimuli at these times. Thus, both combination medical therapy and physical measures such as stimulation are often necessary.

Neurogenic pain never yields to narcotics. Therefore, combined therapy with anticonvulsants and tricyclic antidepressants is the usual regimen for phantom and residual limb pain; these drugs treat the lancinating pain and background burning pain, respectively, with some overlap. Carbamazepine is probably the anticonvulsant of choice, but valproic acid, phenytoin, or clonazepam may also be used (see Table 18–1 for dose recommendations). Drug serum levels are required for determination of toxicity; no therapeutic levels for pain control have been established. Tricyclic antidepressants are also useful; however, pain control may be achieved with doses lower than those needed for depression. Propranolol may also be employed as a first-line drug for control of phantom limb pain. For cramping pain, flexor spasticity, or residual limb movement disorders, baclofen may be useful.

Unfortunately, partial relief or treatment failure is often the result of even the most diligent medical management. The clinician should then turn to TNS. The possibility of acupuncture, local anesthetic blocks, or other techniques, such as electromyogram-assisted biofeedback and relaxation, ultrasound, and injection of the residual limb with local anesthetic, should be considered.[14, 21, 43, 71]

When more conservative measures fail, SCS for phantom limb pain and peripheral nerve stimulation for residual limb pain should next be attempted. In patients with suspected lumbosacral nerve root avulsion (or brachial plexus avulsion), DREZ spinal lesioning may be the treatment of choice. This operation can also be effective in those patients without this additional pathological finding. Finally, DBS could be attempted for the most severe and recalcitrant cases.

As a further example of management strategy, TNS or SCS may provide for suppression of so-called background pain, whereas anticonvulsants may simultaneously eliminate lancinating pains. The use of tricyclic antidepressants in the same patient may improve overall pain control while benefiting mood and eliminating nighttime exacerbation (in the absence of SCS or TNS or with reduced endogenous afferent activity). The addition of propranolol could boost partial relief, whereas baclofen could also be instituted to control abnormal movement of the residual limb. In short, many approaches may be necessary. Constant vigilance of the therapeutic management scheme will almost certainly be required.

Other measures, such as residual limb revision, neuroma resection, cordotomy, mesencephalotomy, and dorsal rhizotomy, cannot be generally recommended.[70] Certainly, a surgical procedure should never be considered before exhaustion of medical and all other available, more conservative measures. Referral to multidisciplinary pain clinics may obviate unnecessary operations.[69]

SUMMARY

The problem of postamputation pain is unfortunately complex and often extremely difficult to manage. This condition is not uncommon and should be accepted when recognized: complaints of postamputation pain should be sought from patients—who often have many reasons to be reticent.[73, 81] In tumor patients, the association of such pain with tumor recurrence should not be forgotten.[75] Aggressive, early, and, when possible, preoperative treatment should be instituted, with the use of all available modalities in a rational sequence or combination. Patience is necessary to obtain pharmacologic action, which may be delayed. Definitive treatment in many patients awaits future understanding of neurophysiological and neurochemical mechanisms.

REFERENCES

1. Abramson AS, Feibel A: The phantom phenomenon: Its use and disuse. Bull NY Acad Med 57:99, 1981.
2. Ahmad S: Phantom limb pain. South Med J 77:804, 1984.
3. Ahmad S: Phantom limb pain and propranolol. Br Med J 1:415, 1979.
4. Aldrich CK: Phantom limb pain. Am Fam Physician 25:50, 1982.
5. Anani A, Korner L: Discrimination of phantom hand sensations elicited by afferent electrical nerve stimulation in below-elbow amputees. Med Prog Technol 6:131, 1979.
6. Arnold CL, Fischer JM: Critical evaluation of beta blockers. Hosp Form 18:299, 1983.
7. Baker KA, Taylor JE, Lilly GE: Treatment of trigeminal neuralgia: Use of baclofen in combination with carbamazepine. Clin Pharm 4:93, 1985.
8. Baldessarini RJ: Drugs and the treatment of psychiatric disorders. In Gilman A, Goodman LS, Rall TW, Murad F (eds): The Pharmacological Basis of Therapeutics, 7th Ed. New York, Macmillan, 1985, pp 394–398.
9. Barnett HG, Connolly ES: Lumbosacral nerve root avulsion. Report of a case and review of the literature. J Trauma 15:532, 1975.
10. Benezet P, Cochet C: Tiapride et douleur chez l'ampauté. Semin Hôp Paris 58:2203, 1982.
11. Bianchine JR: Drugs for Parkinson's disease: Centrally acting muscle relaxants. In Gilman A, Goodman LS, Rall TW, Murad F (eds): The Pharmacological Basis of Therapeutics, 7th Ed. New York, Macmillan, 1985, pp 486–489.
12. Birkhan J, Carmon A, Meretsky P, et al: Clinical effects of a new TENS using multiple electrodes and constant energy. Belgian Congress of Anesthesiology Proceedings, 1982, pp 239–245.
13. Blumenkopf B: Neuropharmacology of the dorsal root entry zone. Neurosurg 15:900, 1984.
14. Bonnica JJ: Management of pain with regional analgesia. Postgrad Med J 60:897, 1984.
15. Bowsher D: Pain mechanisms in man. Resident Staff Physician 29:26, 1983.
16. Bradway JK, Malone JM, Racy J, et al: Psychological adaption to amputation: An overview. Orthotics and Prosthetics, 38:46, Autumn 1984.
17. Brunette DD: The nature of phantom limb. J Tenn Med Assoc 73:712, 1980.
18. Carlen PL, Wall PD, Nadvorna H, et al: Phantom limb and related phenomena in recent traumatic amputations. Neurology 28:211, 1978.
19. Dalessio DJ: Trigeminal neuralgia, a practical approach to treatment. Drugs 24:248, 1982.
20. Dawson L, Arnold P: Persistent phantom limb pain. Percept Mot Skills 53:135, 1981.
21. Doughtery J: Relief of phantom limb pain after EMG biofeedback assisted relaxation: A case report. Behav Res Ther 18:355, 1979.
22. Douglas WW: Histamine and 5-hydroxytryptamine (serotonin) and their antagonists. In Gilman A, Goodman LS, Rall TW, Murad F (eds): The Pharmacological Basis of Therapeutics, 7th Ed. New York, Macmillan, 1985, pp 626–633.
23. Elliot F, Little A, Milbrandt W: Carbamazepine for phantom-limb phenomena. N Engl J Med 295:678, 1976.
24. Evans FJ: The placebo response in pain reduction. Adv Neurol 4:289, 1974.
25. Fanciullaci M, Del Bene E, Franchi G, et al: Phantom limb pain: Sub-hallucinogenic treatment with lysergic acid diethylamide (LSD-25). Headache 17:118, 1977.
26. Fromm GH, Terrence CF, Chaltha AS: Baclofen in the treatment of neuralgia: A double-blind study and long term follow-up. Ann Neurol 15:240, 1984.
27. Gessler M, Struppler A, Oettinger B: Treatment of phantom pain by transcutaneous stimulation (TNS) of the stump, the limb contralateral to the stump, and the other extremities. In Siegfried J, Zimmermann M (eds): Phantom and Stump Pain. New York, Springer-Verlag, 1982, pp 93–98.
28. Gross D: Contralateral local anesthesia in the treatment of phantom limb and stump pain. Pain 13:313, 1982.
29. Iacono RP: New neurosurgical techniques in the treatment of intractable pain. AZ Med 42:300, 1985.
30. Iacono RP, Nashold BS Jr: Mental and behavioral effects of brain stem and hypothalmic stimulation in man. Hum Neurobiol 1:273, 1982.
31. Tourian A, Iacono RP: Involuntary movements of the lower extremity in a man following DREZ for phantom pain. Appl Neurophysiol 51:212, 1988.
32. Jaffe JH, Martin WR: Opiod analgesics and antagonists. In Gilman A, Goodman LS, Rall TW, Murad F (eds): The Pharmacological Basis of Therapeutics, 7th Ed. New York, Macmillan, 1985, p 499.
33. Jensen TS, Krebs B, Nielsen J, et al: Phantom limb, phantom pain and stump pain in amputees during the first 6 months following limb amputation. Pain 17:243, 1983.
34. Jensen TS, Krebs B, Nielsen J, et al: Immediate and long-term phantom limb pain in amputees: Incidence, clinical characteristics and relationship to pre-amputation limb pain. Pain 21:267, 1985.
35. Klinger D, Kepplinger B: Transcutaneous electrical nerve stimulation (TNS) in the treatment of chronic pain after peripheral nerve lesions. In Siegfried J, Zimmermann M (eds): Phantom and Stump Pain. New York, Springer-Verlag, 1982, pp 103–106.
36. Knyihár E, Csillik B: Effect of peripheral axotomy on the fine structure and histochemistry of the Rolando substance: Degenerative atrophy of central processes of pseudounipolar cells. Exp Brain Res 26:73, 1976.
37. Kocher U, Siegfried J, Perret E: Age and personality profiles of patients with chronic pain. Appl Neurophysiol 45:523, 1982.
38. Krainick JU, Thoden U: Spinal cord stimulation in post-amputation pain. In Siegfried J, Zimmermann M (eds): Phantom and Stump Pain. New York, Springer-Verlag, 1982, pp 163–166.
39. Langohr HD, Stohr M, Petruch F: An open and double-blind crossover study on the efficacy of clomipramine (anafranil) in patients with painful mono- and polyneuropathies. Eur Neurol 21:309, 1982.
40. Levitt M, Heybach JP: The deafferentation syndrome in genetically blind rats: A model of the painful phantom limb. Pain 10:67, 1981.
41. Livingston KE: The phantom limb syndrome: A discussion of the role of major peripheral nerve neuromas. J Neurosurg 2:251, 1945.
42. Logan TP: Persistent phantom limb pain: A dramatic response to chlorpromazine. South Med J 76:1585, 1983.

43. Mackenzie N: Phantom limb pain during spinal anesthesia. Anaesthesia 38:886, 1983.

44. Malone JM: Complications of lower extremity amputation. *In* Bernhard VM, Towne JB (eds): Complications in Vascular Surgery, 2nd Ed. Orlando, Grune & Stratton, 1985, pp 455–470.

45. Marsland AR, Weekes JWN, Atkinson RL, et al: Phantom limb pain: A case for beta blockers? Pain 12:295, 1982.

46. Mayeux R, Benson DF: Phantom limb and multiple sclerosis. Neurology 29:724, 1979.

47. Mazars GJ, Merienne L, Cioloca C: Contribution of thalamic stimulation to the physiology of pain. *In* Bonica JJ, Albe-Fessard D (eds): Advances in Pain Research and Therapy, Vol 1. New York, Raven Press, 1976.

48. McGee JL, Alexander MR: Phenothiazine analgesia—fact or fantasy? Am J Hosp Pharm 36:633, 1979.

49. Melzack R: Central neural mechanisms in phantom limb pain. Adv Neurol 4:319, 1974.

50. Melzack R, Loeser JD: Phantom body pain in paraplegics: Evidence for a central ""pattern generating mechanism" for pain. Pain 4:195, 1978.

51. Mihic DN, Pinker E: Phantom limb pain during peridural anesthesia. Pain 11:269, 1981.

52. Monga TN, Jaksic T: Acupuncture in phantom limb pain. Arch Phys Med Rehabil 62:229, 1981.

53. Mundinger F, Neumuller H: Programmed transcutaneous (TNS) and central (DBS) stimulation for control of phantom limb pain and causalgia: A new method for treatment. *In* Siegfried J, Zimmermann M (eds): Phantom and Stump Pain. New York, Springer-Verlag, 1982, pp 164–178.

54. Murphy JP, Anandaciva S: Phantom limb pain and spinal anesthesia. Anaesthesia 39:188, 1984.

55. Nashold BS Jr, Ostdahl RH: Dorsal root entry zone lesions for pain relief. J Neurosurg 51:59, 1979.

56. Nashold BS Jr, Urban B, Zorub DS: Phantom pain relief by focal destruction of the substantia gelatinosa of Rolando. *In* Bonica JJ, Albe-Fessard D (eds): Advances in Pain Research and Therapy, Vol 1. New York, Raven Press, 1976, pp 959–963.

57. Nashold BS Jr, Wilson WP, Slaughter DG: Stereotaxic midbrain lesions for central dysesthesia and phantom pain. J Neurosurg 30:116, 1969.

58. Nystrom B, Hagbarth KE: Microelectrode recordings from transected nerves in amputees with phantom limb pain. Neurosci Lett 27:211, 1981.

59. Oille WA: Beta adrenergic blockade and the phantom limb pain. Ann Intern Med 73:1044, 1970.

60. Parkes JD: Diseases of the central nervous system—relief of pain: Headache, facial neuralgia, migraine, and phantom limb. Br Med J 4:90, 1975.

61. Price P, Parkes JD, Marsden CD: Tiapride in Parkinson's disease. Lancet 2:1106, 1978.

62. Roth YF, Sugarbaker PH: Pains and sensations after amputation: Character and clinical significance. Arch Phys Med Rehabil 61:490, 1980.

63. Salem SA, McDevitt DG: Central effects of beta-adrenoreceptor antagonists. Clin Pharmacol Ther 33:52, 1983.

64. Saris SC, Iacono RP, Nashold BS: Dorsal root entry zone lesions for post-amputation pain. J Neurosurg 62:72, 1985.

65. Scadding JW, Wall PD, Wynn Parry CB, et al: Clinical trial of propranolol in post-traumatic neuralgia. Pain 14:283, 1982.

66. Sherman RA: Published treatments of phantom limb pain. Am J Phys Med 59:232, 1980.

67. Sherman RA, Sherman CJ: Prevalence and characteristics of chronic phantom limb pain among American veterans—results of a trial survey. Am J Phys Med 62:227, 1983.

68. Sherman RA, Sherman CJ, Gall NG: A survey of current phantom limb pain treatment in the United States. Pain 8:85, 1980.

69. Sherman RA, Sherman CJ, Parker L: Chronic phantom and stump pain among American veterans: Results of a survey. Pain 18:83, 1984.

70. Siegfried J, Cetinalp E: Neurosurgical treatment of phantom limb pain: A survey of methods. *In* Siegfried J, Zimmermann M (eds): Phantom and Stump Pain. New York, Springer-Verlag, 1982, pp 148–155.

71. Siegfried J, Hood T: Current status of functional neurosurgery. *In* Krayenbuhl H (ed): Advances and Technical Standards in Neurosurgery, Vol 10. New York, Springer-Verlag, 1983, pp 296–342.

72. Sklar SJ, Huck LA: Possible association of nonlipophilic beta-blockers and acute psychosis. Clin Pharm 2:274, 1983.

73. Stein JM, Warfield CA: Phantom limb pain. Hosp Pract 17:166, 1982.

74. Steinbach TV, Nadvorna H, Arazi D: A five year follow-up study of phantom limb pain in post-traumatic amputees. Scand J Rehabil Med 14:203, 1982.

75. Sugarbaker PH, Weiss CM, Davidson DD, et al: Increasing phantom limb pain as a symptom of cancer recurrence. Cancer 54:373, 1984.

76. Swerdlow M: The treatment of "shooting" pain. Postgrad Med J 56:159, 1980.

77. Swerdlow M: Anticonvulsant drugs and chronic pain. Clin Neuropharmacol 7:51, 1984.

78. Swerdlow M, Cundill JG: Anticonvulsant drugs used in the treatment of lancinating pain. A comparison. Anaesthesia 36:1129, 1981.

79. Tamsen A, Hartvig P, Fagerlund C, et al: Patient controlled analgesia: Clinical experience. Acta Anaesthesiol Scand (Suppl) 74:157, 1982.

80. Wall PD: The gate control theory of pain mechanisms—a re-examination and re-statement. Brain 101:1, 1978.

81. Wall R, Novotny-Joseph P, McNamara TE: Does preamputation pain influence phantom limb pain in cancer patients? South Med J 78:34, 1985.

82. White JC, Sweet WH: Pain and the Neurosurgeon. Springfield, Illinois, Charles C Thomas, 1969, pp 68–86.

83. Winnem MF, Amundsen T: Treatment of phantom limb pain with TENS (letter). Pain 12:299, 1982.

84. Wynn Parry CB, Withrington RH: Painful disorders of peripheral nerves. Postgrad Med J 60:869, 1984.

19

Physical Management and Functional Restoration of the Lower Extremity Amputee

Zane Grimm, M.S., C.C.T.

Considerable advances have been made in the construction of the lower extremity prosthesis. Materials, techniques, and a greater understanding of anatomical, kinesiological, and physiological principles have made the lower extremity prosthesis a more comfortable, functional, and cosmetically acceptable appendage. These advances in prosthetic development were primarily brought about by the National Academy of Sciences-National Research Council, which organized a committee on prosthetic research and development. Congress appropriated funds for research and the training of physicians, prosthetists, and therapists. Surgeons became aware of the importance of the level of amputation and the muscle attachments so necessary for prosthesis use. Engineering principles were adapted and applied to the design of substitute limbs for patients undergoing definitive amputations. Prostheses have developed in the past 40 years from the cumbersome, highly inefficient systems of the past to the lightweight, efficiently engineered systems of the present. These new systems are designed to approximate normal human locomotion. These advancing techniques in prosthetics have been accompanied by increasing prices of the scientifically prescribed and constructed prosthesis; with the increased cost of hospitalization and postoperative care, the amputee is faced with financial problems unheard of 40 years ago. Although the amputee's future is bright regarding functional independence and employment, the present financial uncertainties complicate the psychological problems of changed self-image and feelings of dependency harbored by the recent amputee.

The National Center for Health Statistics claims that approximately 43,000 major amputations are performed yearly in the United States and that 68% involve lower extremities. With so many lower extremity amputations performed each year, the rationale behind the physical management and functional restoration of the amputees becomes of paramount concern. The amputation, the postoperative care, the fabrication and fitting of a prosthesis, and the functional training are all interdependent activities; none is complete without the others. The cost of hospitalization is high. The price of individually tailoring the prosthesis continues to increase the cost of the finished product. The time out of work drains the amputee's economic reserve. No matter how perfectly the specialists perform their individual tasks, the net result will be unsatisfactory to both the amputee and the surgeon unless these tasks are perfectly coordinated. Such a team effort can shorten the rehabilitation period and significantly reduce the expense of prosthetic repair. The focus of the entire procedure is to increase or improve the quality of the lower extremity amputee's life (Fig. 19–1).

Lower extremity amputation in the geriatric population has long been associated with a high mortality rate or a prolonged period of hospitalization. Because of these two complications, the amputees' physical restoration and functional independence are significantly reduced, and the patients may become burdens to their families. The major causes of increased hospitalization are pulmonary embolus and pneumonia resulting from postoperative confinement. By the time the ger-

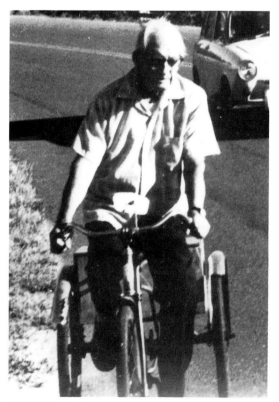

FIGURE 19–1. A 93-year-old patient who has suffered a right hemiparesis and a right below-knee amputation. He participated in the author's functional restoration program and today enjoys a relatively active life.

iatric lower extremity amputee has stabilized and the wound has healed, planning for hospital discharge should be well advanced. Nursing care and rehabilitation arrangements are then made. Because of these complications, prosthetic rehabilitation is less than ideal in geriatric amputees, and the patient may be restricted to a wheelchair for life. Prosthetic rehabilitation for the geriatric patient should start as soon as is medically feasible. Early ambulation is as important to the amputee as it is to any other patient who has undergone a major surgical procedure. Early ambulation for the lower extremity amputee necessitates the fitting of a prosthesis of some type. It is understood that ambulation without a prosthesis is in many cases practical with a three-point gait but not immediately after amputation. The ultimate objectives of a physical management and functional restoration program are to decrease the length of hospitalization by preventing postsurgical complications, to increase functional capacities by developing amputees' tolerance for work, to reduce the economic and emotional strains on amputees by eliminating their dependence, and to improve amputees' quality of life by increasing their physical and mental participation.

The physical restoration of the lower extremity amputee should be as important to the surgeon as is saving the patient's life. At one time, amputation was considered destructive surgery. However, with modern surgical techniques and an understanding of anatomical, kinesiological, and physiological principles, an amputation is no longer looked upon as merely the loss of a body part. With the developing art and science of prosthetic fabrication and with the reconstruction of viable tissue, the amputee is offered an opportunity for a meaningful life. The objectives of reconstructive lower extremity amputation are to prepare the residual limb for future prosthetic use and the amputee for a life of activity and relative independence.

Physical restoration attempts to use the patient's intact functioning neuromuscular system to accomplish the objective of reconstructive amputation. The challenge is to prepare the amputee for a productive life with a well-conditioned residual limb capable of withstanding the trauma of "reasonable work." For amputees to perform reasonable work, they must learn skills and techniques that allow them to function with an aesthetic grace that expends the least amount of energy. Therefore, the amputee must develop an efficient gait with a residual limb fit to a prosthesis that is comfortable, functional, and cosmetically attractive.

PREOPERATIVE CARE

The involvement of prospective lower extremity amputees and their families in prosthetic planning can be an asset in the successful transition from hospital care to independent ambulation. The patient who is faced with the prospect of losing a lower extremity fears uncertainty. The psychological assimilation of an amputation into the body image and self-concept understandably takes time. Geriatric patients facing amputation, in many instances, fear they will never leave the hospital. Preoperative care is directed toward helping the patient acknowledge and deal with these feelings. The motivation for rehabilitation comes from within the individual, and creating an atmosphere designed to produce constructive movement and activity can facilitate this motivation (Fig. 19–2).

As soon as an amputation is planned, the therapist establishes a relationship with the patient. Before the orientation, an evaluation of the patient's physical needs is made. Questions are answered as to the site or level of amputation: are contractures present? Does the patient have a disturbed proprioceptive sense? Is there a strength deficit? What kind of activities did the patient participate in before hospitalization? This information and the planned surgical procedure are used as guidelines in establishing the initial phase of physical management. If possible, the patient should be scheduled to work in the gymnasium; this gets the patient out of bed and into an area of physical activity. The information obtained from the initial evaluation provides a basis for prescribing strengthening exercises. The patient is placed on a positive course of program planning, which progresses from the simple exercises to the more difficult ones, depending on the patient's ability.

POSTSURGICAL CARE

The surgeon has several options in selecting postsurgical care for the patient. The surgeon may elect to apply a soft or rigid dressing. A soft dressing might be selected in the operating room, with a rigid dressing applied later. A rigid dressing might be used as part of an immediate postoperative prosthesis. The prime concern of dressing selection is wound healing.

In the physical management of the amputee, the prime concern is to complement the surgical procedure and enhance the healing process, but such management is more dependent on the surgeon's initial selection of the type of residual limb compression used. The type of program is then outlined in

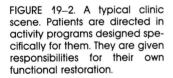
FIGURE 19–2. A typical clinic scene. Patients are directed in activity programs designed specifically for them. They are given responsibilities for their own functional restoration.

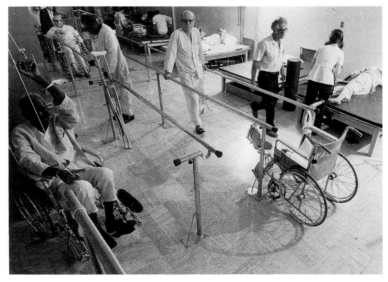

consultation with the surgeon. For example, if the amputee is placed in an immediate postsurgical prosthesis, ambulation will begin the day after surgery, with minimal weight on the residual limb. With a rigid dressing, a three-point gait will be used. With a soft dressing, ambulation will not begin immediately after surgery.

General Conditioning

After the amputation, the patient spends most of the time in bed and short periods in a wheelchair. The greatest concern at this time is the prevention of joint contracture and the subsequent pain, expenditure of money, and lost time. The prevention of contractures helps maintain the body symmetry and posture necessary for proper body mechanics during prosthesis use.

In addition to prevention of contracture during rehabilitation, careful attention is also paid to skin nutrition with respect to arterial perfusion and venous drainage. Bony prominences and potential pressure areas must be continually observed for trauma and impending ulceration.

To prepare the recent amputee for the transition from inactivity to a rigorous program of prosthetic training requires a progressive program of general therapeutic exercises designed to improve physical fitness (Fig. 19–3). Since amputees initially spend most of their time in bed, they are instructed in a series of progressively difficult bed activ-

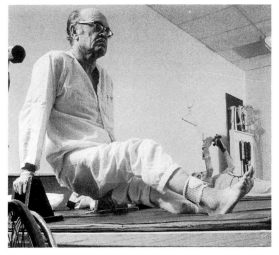

FIGURE 19–3. A recent below-knee amputee developing his shoulder depressors and elbow extensors, which are so necessary for crutch ambulation.

ities, starting with simple nursing care, such as attending to toilet needs and shifting body position. They advance to transfer activities, such as moving from the supine to the sitting position and transferring from bed to wheelchair. These simple self-care activities are usually mastered in a relatively short period and tend to build confidence by increasing the amputee's independence. If necessary, corrective splinting and assisting devices, such as sandbags, footboards, and trapezes, are used.

When the residual limb is in a soft dressing, the first three postsurgical days are usually uncomfortable. The amputee will probably not be able to tolerate range of motion exercises of the residual limb; therefore, exercises designed to maintain strength and muscle tone are applied only to the upper extremities. A trapeze is attached to the bed, and the amputee is instructed in methods of changing body position. During this time, the points where pressure is applied to soft tissue—specifically the heel and medial and lateral malleoli—are observed, since the possibility of tissue breakdown must be eliminated.

As soon as the pain in the residual limb starts to subside, measures are taken to prevent contractures. Range of motion exercises are given to increase or maintain adduction, extension, and internal rotation at the hip joint. If the amputation is below the knee joint, knee extension exercises are included. During this time when amputees are confined to bed or limited to short periods in wheelchairs, they are instructed to lie flat, with no pillows under the residual limb or between the thighs. They are also taught to lie in the prone position with the face down and the hips level for part of the day. If the below-knee amputee spends time in a wheelchair, a leg extension device should be used. An above-knee amputee should spend very little time in a wheelchair for the first 10 days after surgery. As soon as the amputee is allowed to be transferred from bed to the gymnasium in a wheelchair, transfer activities are taught—how to get in and out of bed and how to get on and off the toilet. The amputee also learns how to wheel through doors.

Preprosthetic Training

If the traditional soft dressing is used, general therapeutic exercises are usually

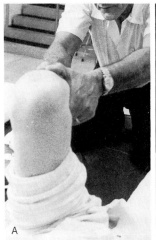 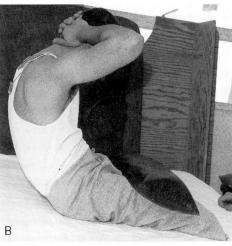 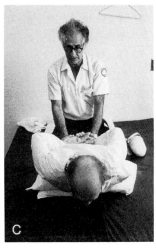

FIGURE 19–4. *A,* Manual resistance applied to the residual limb of a below-knee amputee. The patient is attempting to extend his leg at the hip and knee joints against resistance offered by the therapist. *B,* A patient, with an above-knee amputation on one side and a below-knee amputation on the other, doing sit-ups, using his body weight as resistance. *C,* Back arches are performed to strengthen the extensors of the back and stretch the hip flexors.

started between 3 and 5 days after surgery. Mat and postural exercises are started as soon as possible and are probably the most important part of preprosthetic training. These exercises incorporate the principles of body resistance and manual resistance while developing neuromuscular skills.

Body and manual resistance exercises are performed on the residual limb to create gross movements of the antigravity muscles, which tend to enhance proprioception (Fig. 19–4). The principal muscle groups involved are the hip extensors, adductors, and internal rotators. In the below-knee amputee, the quadriceps and especially the hamstring muscle groups are also exercised. The benefits of these exercises involve strengthening the muscle groups that surround and support the hip and knee joints. The exercises maintain or increase mobility of those joints and in some cases help to desensitize the residual limb and to coordinate body movements.

Standard postural exercises, including Williams' flexion exercises, are started as soon as the amputee is able to exercise in the gymnasium and are designed specifically to eliminate the possibility of lower back pain. If there is a marked deviation in the amputee's posture, specific exercises are employed. The mat exercises include push-ups, sit-ups, back arching, and rolling and are used to increase trunk mobility and improve the amputee's physical fitness.

Balancing in the standing or upright position is a prerequisite to crutch walking and begins with simple activities such as standing by the wheelchair and walking between the parallel bars. The patients progress to the more complicated activities necessary for self-care, such as hopping, squatting, and shifting the body position by pivoting from heel to toe in both right and left directions. When this balancing is mastered, the amputee is ready for crutches.

Crutch walking, using axillary crutches, is started as soon as is feasible. The amputee is instructed in the use of the crutches and warned about resting on the axillary bridge.

Residual Limb Bandaging

As soon as the sutures are removed and the residual limb is not draining, bandaging is started and continued until the amputee receives a prosthesis. Elastic compression bandages are used to shape and shrink the residual limb. For the above-knee amputee, two or sometimes three 6 inch elastic bandages secured together are used. The technique most frequently used is that described by the University of California, Los Angeles, Prosthetic School. This technique uses two recurrent bandages and two hip spicas with a posterior to anterior pull. The pressure is greatest at the distal end of the residual limb and decreases toward the proximal end. Three safety pins are used to secure the wraps—two for the anterior side of the thigh and one to secure the hip spicas (Fig. 19–5).

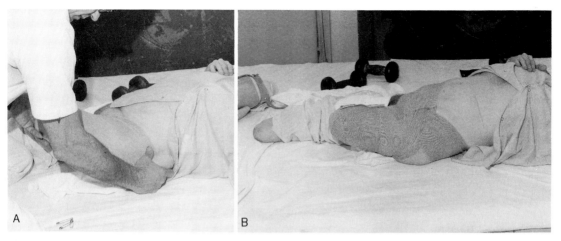

FIGURE 19–5. *A*, The elastic wrap is used to press the tissue in at the groin during application of the hip spica, preventing the bulge of tissue called the adductor roll. *B*, The completed above-knee compression bandage, secured by three safety pins: one holding the spica and two holding the wrap on the anterior side of the residual limb. (*From* Grimm Z: Physical management and rehabilitation of the lower extremity amputee. *In* Rutherford RB (ed): Vascular Surgery, 2nd Ed. Philadelphia, WB Saunders Co, 1984, pp 1521–1522.)

The below-knee compression bandage consists of two or three 4 inch elastic bandages secured together. Two recurrent bandages are applied with sweeping diagonal figure-eights extending up the thigh, leaving the patella uncovered. Here again, the greatest pressure is applied at the distal end and decreases toward the proximal end. The wrap is secured with paper tape (Fig. 19–6).

The Syme's amputation bandage is the same as that described for the below-knee amputation except that it goes no higher than the lower pole of the patella (Fig. 19–7).

The Rigid Dressing

A surgeon's rationale for selecting the elastic plaster wrap for residual limb compression is that edema prevention will enhance wound healing and residual limb maturation. Limiting postsurgical edema improves circulation and promotes wound healing. The therapist working with the amputee should constantly check the soft tissue at the proximal rim of the rigid dressing and also at the patellar pressure-relief window of the below-knee amputation dressing. If the tissue bulges at the rim, the surgeon should be notified, and the rigid dressing may need to be removed. After the first 10 to 15 days, the rigid dressing is usually removed and may be replaced, or elastic residual limb bandages may be applied.

Immediate Postsurgical Prosthetic Management

The background and rationale for the immediate postsurgical prosthetic management of the lower extremity amputee are well covered in the manual *The Management of the Lower-Extremity Amputation—Surgery—Immediate Postsurgical Prosthetic Fitting—Patient Care.** In the 1950s, the French surgeon, Berlemont, introduced the concept of using a rigid dressing for ambulation during the secondary healing phase of traumatic amputation. Weiss, a Polish orthopedic surgeon, adopted Berlemont's technique, applied it to primary closed amputation, and reported accelerated healing and rehabilitation. This concept of amputation with immediate ambulation has revolutionized the physical management and rehabilitation of the amputee. For many years, those who trained the amputee to function on a prosthetic device were challenged by the prosthetic engineers to devise ways of accelerating gait training and to improve rehabilitative techniques. What those engineers did not understand is that the surgeon dictates the course of action imposed on those who train the amputee.

Early ambulation is an integral part of the physical management of the amputee with

*Prosthetic and Sensory Aids Service, Department of Medicine and Surgery, Veterans Administration, Washington, DC. TR10-6, August 1969.

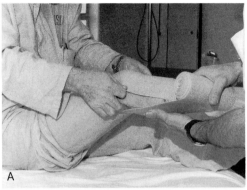
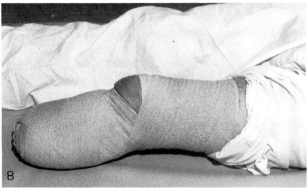

FIGURE 19–6. *A,* Application of the below-knee compression bandage starts with two recurrences, followed by sweeping figure eights. *B,* The finished appearance of a compression bandage on a below-knee amputated residual limb. This has been applied so that the greatest tension is exerted on the distal portion of the residual limb. The tension decreases as the wrap advances proximally.

an immediate postsurgical prosthesis. Early ambulation establishes an amputee's awareness of pressure and tension forces through the prosthesis to the body, which maintains an intact proprioceptive sense. The elevated posture tends to decrease the incidence of pulmonary complications.

In addition to early ambulation, self-care activities and general conditioning exercises are started simultaneously the day after surgery. Specific exercises are used to deal with specific problems. Even if ambulation is not possible the day after surgery, the amputee

can at least assume the upright posture. In rare cases in which the amputee is disoriented or so severely debilitated that standing is contraindicated, a tilt table is used, and intermittent pressure is' applied manually by the therapist.

The Above-Knee Amputee

The above-knee amputee who has been fitted with an immediate postsurgical prosthesis starts gait training as soon after surgery as is physically feasible. The above-knee im-

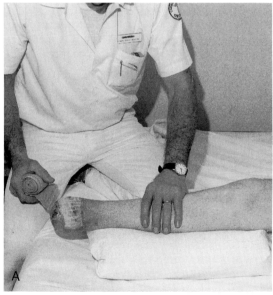
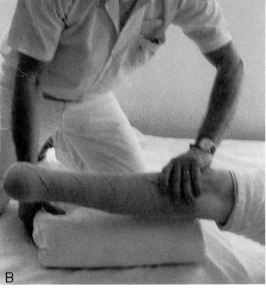

FIGURE 19–7. *A,* Two elastic wraps, 4 inches wide, are used for bandaging the residual limb of a Syme's amputation. *B,* The final appearance of the compression bandage. Note that it does not extend higher than the lower pole of the patella. (*From* Grimm Z: Physical management and rehabilitation of the lower extremity amputee. *In* Rutherford RB (ed): Vascular Surgery, 2nd Ed. Philadelphia, WB Saunders Co, 1984, pp 1522–1523.)

mediate postsurgical prosthesis approximates a permanent prosthesis in that it has a quadrilateral socket; waist band for suspension; single-axis constant-friction knee joint; and solid ankle, cushion heel (SACH) foot. The knee joint also incorporates a manual knee lock.

Early gait training of the above-knee amputee reduces hip flexion contractures by requiring the amputee to extend the residual limb at the hip joint while stepping over the prosthesis in forward movement. Since the rigid dressing is quadrilateral in shape, it is a total-contact socket, with the weight-bearing surface being the gluteal-ischial rim (Fig. 19–8); this configuration reduces the possibility of excessive pressure on the residual limb, which might compromise wound healing. The knee joint mechanism is used as soon as proprioception is established. Usually on the first day after surgery, above-knee amputees stand between the parallel bars and are asked to shift their weight from side to side, controlling the amount of pressure applied to the immediate postsurgical prosthesis. If a

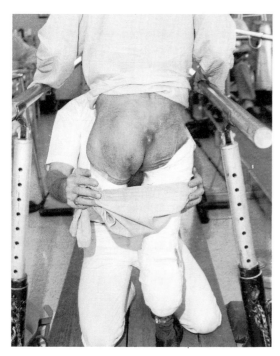

FIGURE 19–8. A patient with an above-knee amputation who was fitted with a rigid dressing and pylon attachment. It is a total-contact plaster-of-Paris quadrilateral dressing that supports weight bearing on the gluteal-ischial rim. (*From* Grimm Z: Physical management and rehabilitation of the lower extremity amputee. *In* Rutherford RB (ed): Vascular Surgery, 2nd Ed. Philadelphia, WB Saunders Co, 1984, p 1523.)

vertical load of between 20 and 25 pounds of pressure can be tolerated on the prosthesis, gait training is started; however, because the greatest weight bearing is on the gluteal-ischial rim, an inability to tolerate the 20 to 25 pounds does not necessarily preclude ambulation.

Ambulation begins with the knee locked. The prosthesis is aligned with a length one half of an inch shorter than that of the contralateral limb; this reduces the need for hiking the hip or circumducting the residual limb in the swing phase of the gait and also helps eliminate severe vertical loading. The three-point partial weight-bearing gait pattern is used. When the foot of the prosthesis is flat on the ground in the standing position, the major portion of body weight is supported by the arms. The rationale for the use of the immediate postsurgical prosthesis in above-knee amputations is that it aids in shrinking, shaping, and seasoning the residual limb and in teaching balancing, muscle function, and control in ambulation with tactile stimulation to the residual limb.

The length of time spent ambulating depends on the amputee's general condition. Much of the time in the gymnasium is used for ambulating between the parallel bars, with frequent rest periods. The first immediate postsurgical prosthesis is usually changed after 10 to 15 days.

When the second immediate postsurgical prosthesis is applied, alignment becomes important. The knee lock mechanism is no longer used, and gait training using the moveable joint is started. The amputee still controls the amount of weight bearing applied to the prosthesis during the stance phase of gait but now works with a moveable collapsible knee joint. Weight bearing increases to between 40 and 50 pounds of pressure. The length of time spent ambulating is progressively increased, and the length of the prosthesis is made equal to that of the contralateral limb, resulting in a dynamic alignment. Any fundamental defects in the prosthesis that interfere with gait training are brought to the attention of the prosthetist for correction. The amputee is then instructed in the technique of forward locomotion, which uses complete cycles in the swing and stance phases of gait.

The second immediate postsurgical prosthesis is removed after another 10 days, approximately 25 days after surgery. If wound healing is uneventful, the amputee is ready

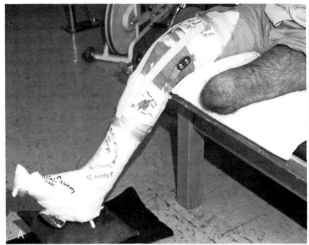
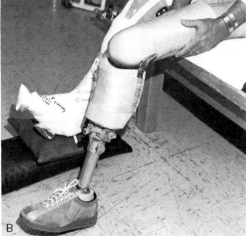
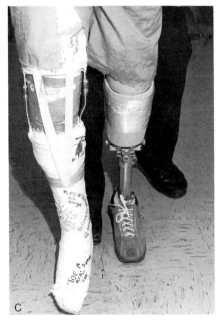

FIGURE 19–9. *A,* This patient has a left through-knee amputation and a fractured right femur. On the right leg, he is fitted with a fracture cast, an ischial weight-bearing rim, polycentric side joints, and a walking heel. *B,* The same patient donning his intermediate through-knee prosthesis. It is a double-walled, slip socket prosthesis with end-bearing side joints, and a SACH foot. *C,* While the patient's right leg is protected by the fracture cast, gait training is reversed to the extent that controlled weight bearing is on the fractured side and the prosthetic side assumes full weight.

for an intermediate prosthesis. The component parts of the intermediate prosthesis are a plastic quadrilateral socket, pelvic belt, single-axis constant-friction knee joint, and SACH foot (Fig. 19–9). The amputee uses this prosthesis while waiting for a permanent one to be prescribed, fabricated, and delivered (Fig. 19–10). All the fundamental skills of gait are now taught; they include balancing on the prosthesis, walking mediolaterally, walking outside the parallel bars, making turns, kneeling, stooping down and getting up, going up and down inclines, ascending and descending stairs, getting in and out of a car, sitting down and standing up, and falling down and getting up. The last is not

taught until amputees have developed confidence in their ability to ambulate. One must be careful not to instill a fear of falling while making it clear that this is a possibility.

The technique used to ascend and descend stairs is that one riser is taken at a time, with the prosthetic leg reaching the step after the nonamputated leg is extended, lifting to that step. Descending is just the reverse, with the prosthetic leg being lowered first. However, with the below-knee amputation, as weight-bearing tolerance increases on the amputated side, alternating steps can and, in most cases, will be used (Fig. 19–11). The above-knee amputee will probably prefer the single-step method of ascending and descending stairs.

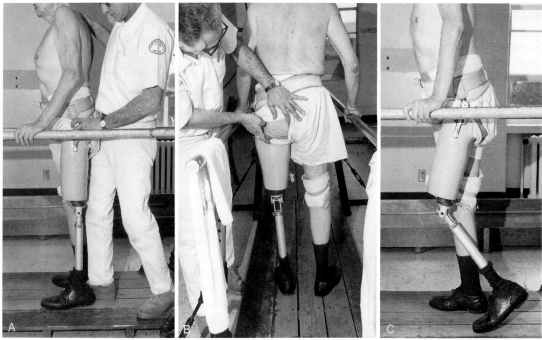

FIGURE 19–10. *A,* A patient with a right below-knee amputation and a left above-knee amputation. He has a definitive PTB prosthesis on his right side and an intermediate prosthesis on his left side. The intermediate prosthesis consists of a pelvic belt with a side joint, total-contact quadrilateral socket, single-axis constant-friction knee joint, and SACH foot. *B,* The therapist checks the socket fit, making sure that the patient's residual limb is properly in the socket of the prosthesis. Weight bearing is on the gluteal-ischial rim of the socket. *C,* After all variables are checked, the patient begins learning to control the prosthesis by using the muscles of the hip and residual limb.

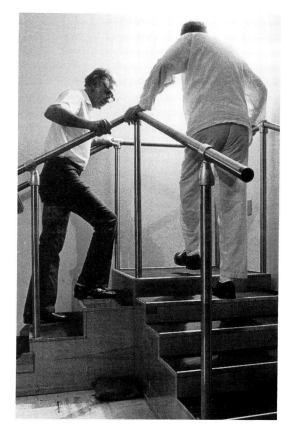

FIGURE 19–11. This patient is alternately ascending a flight of stairs with risers of 3½ inches. His residual limb is well healed, and he is awaiting hospital discharge. He is wearing an intermediate prosthesis, and a definitive prosthesis will be prescribed at a later date.

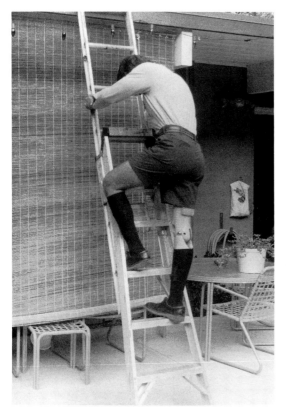

FIGURE 19–12. Climbing a ladder is almost comparable with stair climbing. The above-knee amputee makes sure that the foot of the prosthesis is secure on the rung before ascending with the nonamputated leg.

The younger above-knee amputee is taught a method of alternating steps when ascending and descending stairs (Fig. 19–12).

The Below-Knee Amputee

The below-knee amputee using the immediate postsurgical prosthesis also starts ambulating the day after surgery. With advanced technology and rehabilitation, almost all lower extremity amputees successfully become ambulatory. A surgical procedure that takes the future prosthetic fit into consideration and a meticulous application of the rigid dressing are the ingredients for successful immediate postsurgical prosthetic management. Basically, the rigid dressing extends high on the thigh and assumes a portion of the vertical load during weight bearing. Together with a waist band that is attached anteriorly to the rigid dressing, the prosthesis is attached to the residual limb. A length of tubing assembled with a SACH foot

fits in an alignment unit incorporated in the rigid dressing.

The below-knee amputee with an immediate postsurgical prosthesis routinely starts elevation and ambulation the day after surgery. The control of weight bearing is crucial because all of the weight on the amputated side is supported by the thigh, the tibial condyles, and the distal end of the residual limb. As shrinkage takes place, less weight is borne by the thigh and more by the tibial condyles and the distal end of the residual limb. Therefore, the amputee must learn how to control the amount of body weight placed on the prosthesis. Most of the time, weight bearing on the amputated side gives the amputee pain relief, and consequently there is a tendency to overload the residual limb. The weight-bearing tolerance of the residual limb of a recently amputated leg is between 5 and 15 pounds of pressure.

When ambulation commences, the prosthesis is designed to be one half of an inch shorter than the contralateral limb for the same reason as mentioned for the above-knee amputation. Bathroom scales are used to record the applied weight on the prosthesis. The amputee steps on the scale, looking at the weight indicator, and continues using the scale until a sense for the desired weight develops. Each session with the parallel bars begins and finishes with the use of the scale. Amputees should not be pressured to walk beyond their tolerance.

The first rigid dressing is usually changed after 10 to 15 days. If wound healing is uneventful, another rigid dressing with a pylon attachment is applied. Ambulation with increased weight bearing is continued to 20 to 30 pounds, and the length of time for rehabilitation increases. If feasible, crutch walking is started with a three-point step-through gait pattern; general conditioning exercises are continued.

The second rigid dressing is removed after another 10 to 15 days. At this point, if the residual limb is healing well, the prosthetist starts fabricating an intermediate prosthesis. A below-knee cast with a cuff for suspension is used to protect the residual limb (Fig. 19–13). The cast fits over an elastic sock. Range of motion and strengthening exercises are begun with the muscle groups that support and stabilize the knee joint. When the intermediate prosthesis arrives, a dynamic alignment is made (Fig. 19–14). The length of the

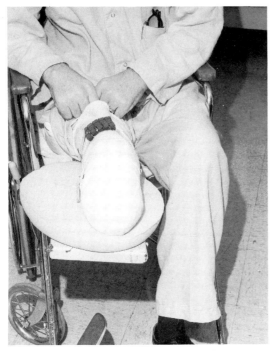

FIGURE 19–13. After removal of the rigid dressing and postoperative prosthesis, a plaster-of-Paris cap is used to protect the below-knee stump from injury. Together with an elastic sock, it controls edema and helps mature and season the residual limb. (*From* Grimm Z: Physical management and rehabilitation of the lower extremity amputee. *In* Rutherford, RB (ed): Vascular Surgery, 2nd Ed. Philadelphia, WB Saunders Co, 1984, p 1525.)

residual limb is checked, as are the length of the step, the width of the walking base, and the range of motion at the knee joint.

Ambulation begins with the amputee balancing in the parallel bars mediolaterally and anteroposteriorly and stepping in place to allow the knee to flex immediately at the heel contact (Fig. 19–15). As the amputee gets the feel of the prosthesis, the cadence and step length are increased to approximate the normal gait pattern (Fig. 19–16). The new intermediate prosthesis is removed every 10 to 15 minutes, and the residual limb is examined for areas of excessive pressure. If there is discoloration, abrasions, or pain, the prosthetist is called. The amputee continues using the three-point gait pattern, increasing weight bearing to tolerance. The intermediate prosthesis is used until the muscles of the residual limb atrophy and mature. As its girth decreases, the residual limb is fitted with socks to compensate for socket fit. All basic techniques of gait are learned while the am-

putee uses an intermediate prosthesis. The transition from intermediate to definitive prosthesis presents no problem. Basically the same component parts are used, and the only difference could be in the type of suspension or foot prescribed.

Residual Limb Care

Care of the residual limb can lead to the success or failure of prosthetic use. Specific factors that can contribute to residual limb problems are body weight changes, inflammation caused by infection, contact dermatitis, and stasis dermatitis. These should be brought to the attention of the physician for treatment or correction.

A poorly fitting prosthesis can contribute to residual limb problems as well as to faulty gait patterns. Choking is a local constriction of the residual limb by the prosthesis at any level above the distal end and has a tourniquetlike effect on returning circulation. Poor counterpressure of the prosthetic socket on the distal end of the residual limb can cause blowout of superficial vessels, with small hemorrhages in the skin and skin breakdown, and a lack of support for the muscle pump

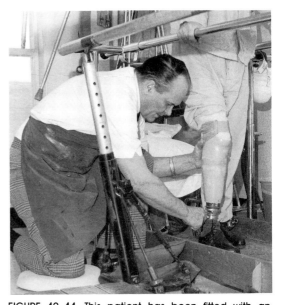

FIGURE 19–14. This patient has been fitted with an intermediate prosthesis after progressing from his last rigid dressing and pylon attachment. The prosthetist is now checking and adjusting the alignment. (*From* Grimm Z: Physical management and rehabilitation of the lower extremity amputee. *In* Rutherford RB (ed): Vascular Surgery, 2nd Ed. Philadelphia, WB Saunders Co, 1984, p 1525.)

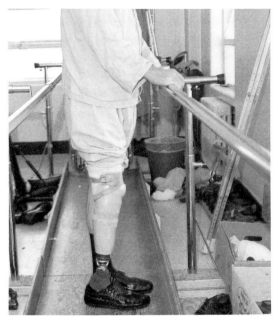

FIGURE 19–15. A patient practices medial-lateral locomotion on an intermediate below-knee prosthesis. Most of the intermediate below-knee prostheses are of the PTB type, with cuff suspension and a SACH foot. (*From* Grimm Z: Physical management and rehabilitation of the lower extremity amputee. *In* Rutherford RB (ed): Vascular Surgery, 2nd Ed. Philadelphia, WB Saunders Co, 1984, p 1525.)

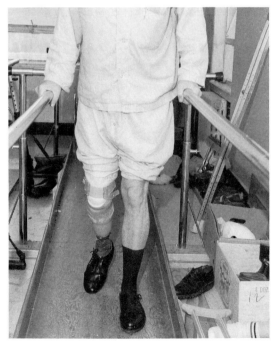

FIGURE 19–16. A below-knee amputee increases his cadence and stride length to approximate his normal gait pattern. (*From* Grimm Z: Physical management and rehabilitation of the lower extremity amputee. *In* Rutherford RB (ed): Vascular Surgery, 2nd Ed. Philadelphia, WB Saunders Co, 1984, p 1525.)

(normally, contraction and relaxation of the muscles milk the veins, assisting in venous circulation). With an immediate postsurgical prosthesis, good counterpressure causes intermittent pressure on the residual limb during ambulation. This pressure, when transmitted to the veins and lymphatic vessels, assists circulation and contains edema. The maintenance of good counterpressure contributes significantly to wound healing; poor counterpressure can cause residual limb breakdown.

The residual limb should be washed daily, preferably at night, and the socket of the prosthesis should also be washed to prevent buildup of body salts. A soft liner should also be kept clean to preserve the leather. Washing at night ensures that the residual limb will be dry in the morning and ready for the prosthetic leg. A liquid antiseptic solution or cake soap containing hexachlorophene should probably be used. The skin should be rinsed and dried thoroughly. The residual limb socks, if used, should be changed daily and washed with a mild wool soap. The wool socks should not be forcibly wrung out but should be laid flat and the excess water blotted out with a towel. They must be completely dry before being worn.

In many cases, residual limb bandaging can be discontinued as soon as the amputee becomes proficient in the use of the prosthesis. A well-fitted prosthesis in many instances helps prevent swelling. If residual limb bandaging is required, the methods described earlier should be used.

SUMMARY

All lower extremity amputees will not be able to use a prosthesis with the same proficiency (Fig. 19–17). The degree of success that an adult amputee will achieve depends on prior athletic abilities and a sense of rhythm. The loss of a foot causes a disruption in proprioception. The foot is a highly complex unit controlled by an elaborate signaling system that includes muscles and tendons. The efficiency of the foot is dependent on the sum of its afferent sensations and the stimuli relating to weight bearing and ground contact; it is intimately bound up in the proprioception of the entire extremity and in coordination of the proximal joints and muscles through its connection with the central nervous system and spinal cord reflexes.

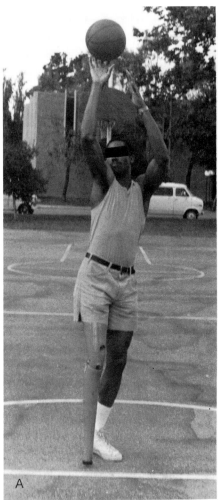

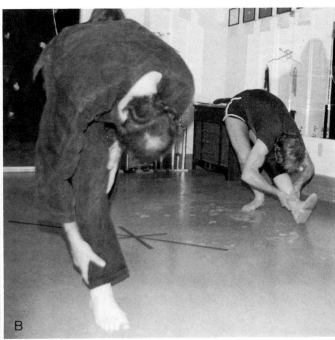

FIGURE 19–17. *A*, A right above-knee amputee shooting baskets. He is using a suction socket, safety knee joint, and pegged foot. By using the peg, he experiences greater pressure feedback and increased stability. *B*, A judo instructor with a below-knee amputation demonstrates flexibility. The prosthesis that he is using is a PTB type with a suction socket and latex rubber sleeve for secondary suspension.

Working with the lower extremity amputee in an acute treatment facility requires an understanding of basic priorities. These priorities are wound healing, prevention of nonspecific disabling complications (e.g., contractures, decubitus ulcers), and evaluation for and prescription of a prosthesis (Fig. 19–18). However, in the functional restoration of the lower extremity amputee, one of the most important aims is the development of motor skills. The mechanics of gait and the pathomechanics of prosthetic function are prerequisites that determine the amputee's full potential for prosthetic use (Fig. 19–19).

The bilateral above-knee amputee is limited in mobility because of the severity of the handicap. In addition to gross proprioceptive disturbances, the energy cost of prosthetic ambulation is great. It is suggested that a lifestyle be adapted to limit the amount of walking to reasonable distances. Such amputees should be offered an opportunity to receive driver education with adaptive hand controls (Fig. 19–20).

All patients who require an amputation of a lower extremity face serious psychological problems. Patients should be prepared to undergo a course of treatment that is directed toward returning them to a realistic level of function within their capabilities (Fig. 19–21). Patients undergoing amputation for vascular conditions may even learn to function at a higher level of productivity than before the amputation.

All amputations should be performed with a surgical technique that will allow the amputee to be fitted with a prosthesis. An unanchored muscle at the distal end of the resid-

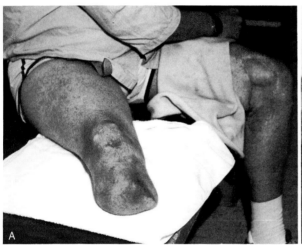
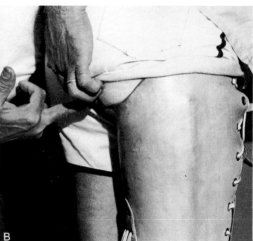
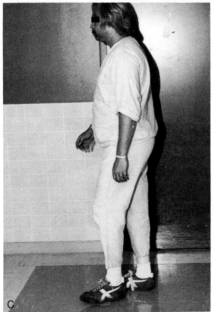

FIGURE 19–18. *A,* A patient with constant residual limb breakdowns is prescribed a prosthesis that will help eliminate intermittent periods when he cannot wear a leg. *B,* This prosthesis is a modified below-knee PTB type with a thigh corset that is reinforced with plastic to form a quadrilateral gluteal-ischial weight-bearing surface, polycentric side joints, a slip socket for the residual limb, and a SACH foot. The therapist is checking the distribution of the vertical load on the ischium, thigh corset, and patellar shelf. *C,* The same patient ambulating with this leg. The transition from the PTS to this leg caused no apparent gait deviations, and the patient felt comfortable. The residual limb problems appear to have been eliminated.

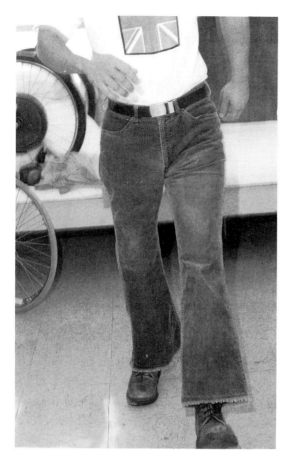

FIGURE 19–19. A right below-knee and left above-knee amputee who walks without the aid of crutches or a cane.

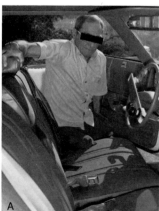

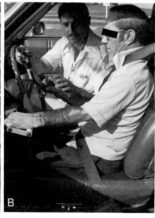

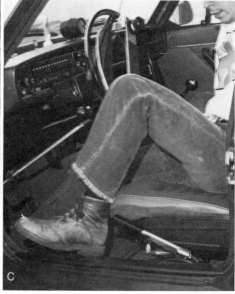

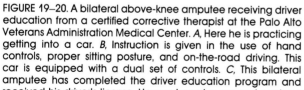

FIGURE 19–20. A bilateral above-knee amputee receiving driver education from a certified corrective therapist at the Palo Alto Veterans Administration Medical Center. *A,* Here he is practicing getting into a car. *B,* Instruction is given in the use of hand controls, proper sitting posture, and on-the-road driving. This car is equipped with a dual set of controls. *C,* This bilateral amputee has completed the driver education program and received his driver's license. He purchased a car and equipped it with hand controls. He is ambulatory and wears his prosthesis all day. (Fig. 19–20*C* from Grimm Z: Physical management and rehabilitation of the lower extremity amputee. *In* Rutherford RB (ed): Vascular Surgery, 2nd Ed. Philadelphia, WB Saunders Co, 1984, p 1526.)

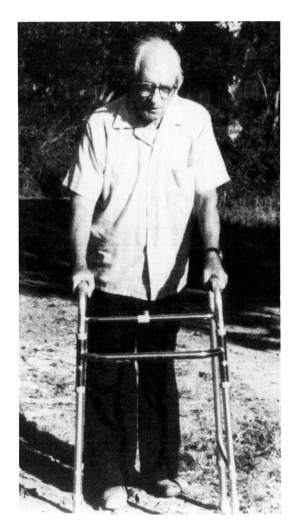

FIGURE 19–21. This right below-knee amputee also has a right hemiparesis. Had he not been given an opportunity to participate in a dynamic functional restoration program, it is doubtful that he would be ambulating.

ual limb destroys muscle pump action and causes uncontrollable edema. Patients' initial levels of functioning are not fair indicators of their potential functioning. Many geriatric amputees are ambulating with the aid of prosthetic legs. Even crutch-supported prosthetic ambulation is preferable to wheelchair-dependent locomotion.

The physical management of amputees should be designed to enable them to achieve the highest level of function compatible with their physical potential. This management also includes the prevention of complications that would inhibit or retard the development of neuromuscular skills.

20

The Amputation Team

James M. Malone, M.D.

To achieve maximal patient rehabilitation after major lower extremity amputation, a modern amputation program must fulfill seven objectives:

1. The use of routine and extended lower extremity arterial reconstructive surgical procedures in order to achieve limb salvage when appropriate

2. The use of quantitative techniques for preoperative amputation level selection

3. The performance of the most distal amputation that will heal

4. The commitment to rehabilitation with a prosthesis

5. The use of early postoperative rehabilitation techniques so that the hospital stay is as short as possible without sacrificing overall rehabilitation

6. The use of cost-effective procedures, techniques, and treatments

7. The coordination of medical and prosthetic care (the team approach)

The first six objectives are discussed in other chapters in the book, and the interested reader is referred to those chapters. This chapter will confine itself to a discussion of the seventh objective, the team approach to rehabilitation after lower extremity amputation.

It is exceedingly difficult to achieve consistently reliable rehabilitation results in the absence of a formal, centralized, dedicated rehabilitation team that includes active participation by all members. Just as some surgical procedures, such as organ transplantation, are confined to regional centers because of their cost and the necessity of skilled personnel, under the best circumstances, amputation rehabilitation should be a centralized resource in a community or among communities in order to achieve the best postoperative results.

Previous studies have clearly suggested that the establishment of centers for amputation rehabilitation has improved wound healing and the rehabilitation rate while decreasing surgical morbidity and the time needed for rehabilitation after lower extremity amputation.[1-3, 5, 9-11, 13] In a previous review of the therapeutic and economic impacts of an amputation program, Malone and associates demonstrated significant economic savings within the 172-hospital Veterans Administration (VA) system if amputation surgery was centralized on a regional basis with appropriate resources.[9] The article concluded that the establishment of modern amputation programs was well justified, on the basis of not only cost but also reduced morbidity and mortality and optimal prosthetic rehabilitation. Similar data were reported by Parhad and colleagues, who reviewed an accelerated postamputation rehabilitation program of 140 lower extremity amputees at the Lakeside VA Hospital in Chicago; they documented a 90-day reduction in hospital stay for patients requiring amputation and rehabilitation and a 50% reduction in hospital stay for patients requiring only preprosthetic and prosthetic training.[12]

TEAM MEMBERS

An overview of the team approach is diagrammatically represented in Figure 20–1. Notice that in the author's view of the amputation team, the patient is the center of the circle of resources and the other members of the team interface with the patient through or with an amputation program coordinator. The exact occupation of the amputation coordinator is not important. This individual could be a physical therapist, an occupational therapist, a nurse, or a lay person. That person, however, is the key in maintaining coordination among other members of the team of health care providers and is especially important in long-term patient follow-up. It has been the author's experience that one break in "the rehabilitation circle" results in at least a 50% failure in amputee rehabilitation.[10] That single factor, a break in the rehabilitation circle, may explain why the average rate of rehabilitation after lower extremity amputation is only 60% or less.[9, 10]

The four primary members of the health care team—the surgeon, the prosthetist, the therapist, and the patient—are equally important in the rehabilitation process. The role of the surgeon is that of team director and provider of health care. The enthusiasm and interest of the surgeon will be directly reflected in all the other members of the health care team. In the absence of an interested surgeon, many rehabilitation failures can be expected. In the presence of an interested surgeon, many complex and difficult rehabilitation successes will be apparent.

The prosthetist is the second coequal member of the health care team but, from a practical standpoint, will be important to the patient long after the surgeon is no longer directly involved. Most rehabilitated amputees identify with the prosthetist, not the surgeon, since most of their long-term problems involve their artificial limbs and not their surgical wounds. The prosthetist has

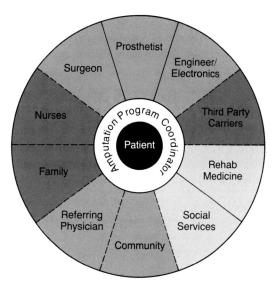

FIGURE 20–1. The circle of resources required for successful rehabilitation after lower extremity amputation. In the author's experience, one break in the circle results in at least a 50% failure of patient rehabilitation.

the long-term responsibility of making sure that the patient is referred to the medical team when medical treatment is required for problems with the residual or contralateral limb.

The best surgery and the use of the best artificial limbs are doomed to failure without the third coequal member of the health care team, the therapist. The therapist is in the unique position of being able to make or break all the efforts of the surgeon and prosthetist. The rehabilitation process runs smoothly only if attention is paid to small details. It is important that the therapist be given a great latitude in patient management during rehabilitation. A skilled therapist should be able to make minor adjustments to the artificial limbs, recognize residual limb and wound problems, and direct the patient back to the physician or prosthetist when appropriate. The therapist will also be important to the patient at various times during long-term follow-up when, for example, the patient receives a new limb and requires some short-term re-education in the techniques of ambulation or daily activities. Elevation of the therapist to coequal status on the health care team relieves the prosthetist of time spent in gait training and minor limb adjustments, and it relieves the physician of a portion of the day-to-day follow-up patient care routine.

The patient is the fourth coequal member of the rehabilitation team. The best team in the world with the best facilities in the world cannot rehabilitate a nonmotivated patient. It is of the utmost importance that the patient be taught to take primary control of the rehabilitation process. Patients need to be actively taught to take charge of their medical, rehabilitative, and prosthetic care. In addition, patients need instruction in the care of their nonamputated contralateral legs since, for example, diabetic patients are at high risk for their loss.[7, 10] Failure of the patients to take an active role in their rehabilitation will ultimately doom the rehabilitation process to failure. This coequal health care team concept significantly improves the patient's overall care, since there are not one but four individuals specifically interested in the medical, prosthetic, and rehabilitative well-being of the patient.

GOALS

Within the rehabilitation circle, there are five primary areas of concern in achieving successful amputation rehabilitation:

1. Coordination of patient care,
2. Education of the patient and family,
3. Access to appropriate community resources,
4. Discharge planning,
5. Centralized long-term follow-up.

The coordination of health care and mobilization of appropriate resources are, in reality, under the direct control and supervision of the surgeon. The surgeon has the responsibility for total patient care and for deciding the overall direction of the surgery and postoperative rehabilitation therapy. However, once postoperative rehabilitation is completed, long-term rehabilitation coordination is a task for which surgeons are poorly trained and in which they rapidly lose interest. In the author's opinion, that task is best directed by the surgeon but executed by the amputation program coordinator.

The education of the patient and family should begin before amputation surgery. It should include discussions about not only surgical morbidity and mortality but also the possibilities of reconstructive arterial surgery

versus primary amputation; the expected physical impairments; the modifications that might be required to the home or auto; the requirements, benefits, and problems with artificial limbs; and the role of other family members in the rehabilitation process. The surgeon is not ideally suited for this task; it needs, in essence, to be performed by several members of the team, including the nurses taking care of the patient, the therapists who will be concerned with rehabilitation, the prosthetist who will fabricate the artificial limb, and, if possible, other amputees. Ideally, before surgery, the prospective amputee should meet an amputee of a similar age and with amputation at the same level. It is important to have potential amputees visit the therapy department and speak with the therapist who will be taking care of them. It is equally important for potential amputees to visit the prosthetic facility, if possible, that will be fabricating their limb and to speak with the prosthetist who will be working with them. This education process is perhaps best organized and orchestrated by the program coordinator, who is actively consulting with the primary health care providers—the surgeon, the prosthetist, and the members of the rehabilitation medicine department—rather than by any of the other individual members of the rehabilitation team. The educational process should also include teaching about long-term medical complications such as wound problems, residual limb breakdown, and, especially in diabetics, the risks of contralateral limb loss and the medical care and treatments that may help avoid those problems.[6, 13]

In an era of economic cost restraint, available community resources, both financial and otherwise, need to be utilized carefully to maximize productivity and minimize cost in rehabilitation. Important among these resources are lay amputee outreach groups, nursing home health care services, in-home skilled and unskilled nursing or therapy care, and homemaker and meal services. This area is clearly the responsibility of the program coordinator and is a job not well performed by the surgeon, therapist, or prosthetist. The amputee's family and referring physician may be very helpful both in deciding the need for these resources and in overseeing the early care after hospital discharge.

Discharge planning should begin before the amputation. It should include a careful analysis of the patient's home environment and expected level of activity after surgery. It needs to include an understanding of the available social and financial resources of the patient. The goal of the discharge planning process is to make the transition from patient to amputee to functional member of society as easy as possible. Discharge planning should include some type of referral to a group of amputees or a counseling group that includes amputee members.[4, 6] This process is best organized by the surgeon in conjunction with the therapist and prosthetist, but the process is best executed by the program coordinator.

Finally, one might argue that centralized follow-up is important only if the team is interested in evaluating treatment protocols or prosthetic components. However, long-term follow-up is mandatory if reliable information on rehabilitation and postoperative complications are to be obtained and integrated into changes and improvements in patient treatment protocols. Careful follow-up is important to long-term medical care, especially as it relates to the risk of contralateral limb loss, residual limb and wound problems, and the prescription and fitting of subsequent prosthetic limbs. Organization of long-term care, obviously, falls under the direction of the physician or surgeon.

ALTERNATIVES

In spite of this prolonged discussion on the benefits and successes of center-directed amputation teams, one should not conclude that successful amputee rehabilitation can be achieved only in dedicated amputation centers. In reality, all that is required are an interested prosthetist, therapist, and surgeon and a motivated patient. Those four individuals working together can achieve successful rehabilitation most of the time in most community hospitals without all the associated personnel and features of "dedicated centers." There are four commandments for successful rehabilitation after amputation:

1. Amputation surgery is a reconstructive procedure;
2. Amputation surgery is not a failure;
3. Rehabilitation of the patient can be defined as the full integration of the patient back into the family and society;
4. Hard-working, motivated individuals

concerned with a particular patient can make the difference between success and failure.

SUMMARY

There is much information on morbidity, mortality, and rehabilitation that suggests that amputee rehabilitation can best be accomplished in dedicated centers.[1–3, 5, 9–11, 13] The data from these centers clearly document decreases in surgical morbidity and mortality, hospital costs, and length of hospital stay and improvements in overall rehabilitation. However, it is also equally clear that interested, motivated members of the health care team can achieve a high degree of successful patient rehabilitation outside of the confines of recognized centers of excellence in amputee care. The overriding factor is that the amputation surgeon owes the patient the debit of rehabilitation after lower extremity amputation.

REFERENCES

1. Burgess E: Amputations. Surg Clin North Am 63:749, 1983.
2. Goldberg RT: New trends in the rehabilitation of lower extremity amputees. Rehabil Lit 45:6, 1984.
3. Hamilton A: Rehabilitation of the leg amputee in the community. Practitioner 225:1487, 1981.
4. Howard DL: Group therapy for amputees in a ward setting. Milit Med 148:678, 1983.
5. Kaplow M, Muruff F, Fish W, et al: The dysvascular amputee: Multidisciplinary management. Can J Surg 26:368, 1983.
6. Lipp MR, Malone ST: Group rehabilitation of vascular surgery patients. Arch Phys Med Rehabil 57:180, 1976.
7. Malone JM: The value of a diabetic education program in reducing contralateral amputation. Presented at the Second Pacific RIM Prosthetic Conference, Maui, Hawaii, April 1986.
8. Malone JM, Goldstone J: Lower extremity amputation. *In* Moore WS (ed): A Comprehensive Review of Vascular Surgery. Orlando, Grune & Stratton, 1983, pp 909–976.
9. Malone JM, Moore WS, Goldstone J, Malone SJ: Therapeutic and economic impact of a modern amputation program. Ann Surg 189:798, 1979.
10. Malone JM, Moore WS, Leal JM, Childers SJ: Rehabilitation for lower extremity amputation. Arch Surg 116:93, 1981.
11. Oh SH: Rehabilitating the geriatric amputee: What the primary MD should know. Geriatrics 37:91, 1982.
12. Parhad A, Gervais B, Wu Y: Beyond the rigid dressing: Pre-prosthetic ambulation for the below-knee amputee. Am Correct Ther J 37:66, 1983.
13. Smith AG: Common problems of lower extremity amputees. Orthop Clin VA 13:569, 1982.

21

Energy Expenditure of Amputee Gait

Robert L. Waters, M.D.
Jacquelin Perry, M.D.
Richard Chambers, M.D.

Normal walking requires continuous muscle activity: in the swing phase, the flexors advance the limb and lift the foot to clear the floor; in the stance phase, the extensors restrain the influence of momentum and gravity. It has been demonstrated that during normal walking, movement of the limbs is patterned so that the least mechanical and physiological energy is expended.[1]

Lower extremity amputation with or without prosthetic replacement imposes energy penalties for ambulation. Without a prosthesis, less energy-efficient upper extremity muscles are used with upper extremity aids for ambulation. With a prosthesis, the remaining muscles of the residual limb must substitute for the lost muscles in addition to performing their customary functions and must also carry and control the additional mass of the prosthesis. Finally, the gait patterns may deviate from the maximally efficient normal pattern because of the inherent limitation of the prosthetic design. Lower

extremity amputation deprives the patient of muscles in the missing limb that are normally active during walking. Although the prosthesis provides a means of vertical support, the extent to which the gait approaches normal depends on the ability of the residual limb to control the prosthesis. Additionally, the patient purposefully deviates from the normal gait pattern to compensate for the inherent limitations of prosthetic gait.

This chapter reviews the physiological energy expenditure of amputee gait and how it is influenced by the amputation level, the reason for the amputation, the length of the residual limb, the use of upper extremity walking aids, and associated medical problems. This information provides clinically useful predictors of the patient's capacity for functional mobility. The basic concepts of exercise physiology and the energetics of normal walking are reviewed to provide a basic framework for understanding the penalty of ambulation for the amputee.

250

PRINCIPLES OF AEROBIC AND ANAEROBIC PHYSIOLOGY

The rationale for energy expenditure measurement in gait disability is that ambulation requires muscle action and physiological response to provide a continuous source of fuel to the muscle. The immediate source of energy for muscle contraction is adenosine triphosphate (ATP). As only a small amount of ATP is stored in the muscle, prolonged exercise requires continuous ATP replenishment via aerobic or anaerobic biochemical pathways.

The use of oxygen consumption as a measure of energy expenditure rests on the fact that during sustained exercise, most ATP is regenerated by oxidative phosphorylation, the metabolic process by which ATP is synthesized by the mitochondria. Since these energy-producing reactions involve oxidative phosphorylation, they are termed aerobic. After several minutes of working at a constant submaximal load, the rate of oxygen consumption is sufficient to meet the aerobic demands of the muscles and the heart, respiratory rates reach approximately constant levels, and the person is said to be in a steady state. Measurement of the rate of oxygen consumption at this time reflects the metabolic power requirement for the activity.

The principal fuels for aerobic metabolism are carbohydrates and fats. In aerobic oxidation, these substrates are oxidized through a series of enzymatic reactions, leading to the production of ATP. A second chain of oxidative reactions that does not require oxygen is also available for the production of ATP. They are thus called anaerobic reactions. In anaerobic metabolism (the glycolytic pathway), glucose is converted to pyruvate and then to lactic acid.

There is an interplay between aerobic and anaerobic metabolism that depends on the intensity and duration of the exercise. The anaerobic pathway provides muscles with an immediate means of regenerating ATP at the start of exercise, before the aerobic pathway can supply ATP. During mild or moderate exercise below the anaerobic threshold (usually less than 50% of the maximal aerobic capacity, for untrained individuals), the oxygen supply to the tissue and the capacity of the aerobic pathway is usually sufficient to satisfy the energy requirements.

During more strenuous exercise, both anaerobic and aerobic oxidation processes occur throughout the exercise period. However, the amount of energy that can be produced by anaerobic means is limited. Nineteen times more energy is produced by the aerobic oxidation of carbohydrates than by anaerobic oxidation. Exercise capability is also limited by the acidosis resulting from the accumulation of lactic acid.

If exercise is performed at a constant moderate rate below the level at which the anaerobic pathway is required to sustain ATP production (the anaerobic threshold), an activity may be sustained for many hours with no easily defined point of exhaustion. When exercise is performed at levels increasingly above the anaerobic threshold, however, the endurance time progressively shortens, and fatigue ensues earlier.

Exercise Capacity

The maximal aerobic capacity ($\dot{V}max_{O_2}$) is the single best indicator of physical fitness.[2] Generally, an individual is able to reach $\dot{V}max_{O_2}$ within 2 or 3 minutes of beginning severe exercise. Any disorder of the respiratory, cardiovascular, muscular, or metabolic systems that restricts the supply of oxygen to the cells decreases the $\dot{V}max_{O_2}$. A physical conditioning program can increase the aerobic capacity by several processes: improving cardiac output, increasing the capacity of the cells to extract oxygen from the blood, increasing the level of hemoglobin, and increasing the muscular mass (hypertrophy). The $\dot{V}max_{O_2}$ is decreased by bed rest, illness, or inactivity.

The oxygen pulse is calculated by dividing the rate of oxygen consumption by the heart rate and is a useful indicator of cardiovascular exercise efficiency. The oxygen pulse may be increased by different mechanisms. A physical training program can increase it by enlarging the cardiac stroke volume so that exercise at a given rate of oxygen uptake is performed at a lower heart rate. A training program that causes muscle hypertrophy increases the oxygen pulse by improving the muscle's capacity to extract oxygen from the blood so that a smaller amount of blood can be circulated to the muscle to achieve the same oxygen supply. The oxygen pulse may be lowered by different mechanisms. Inactiv-

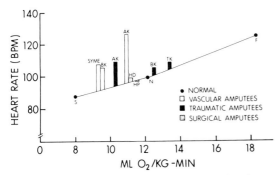

FIGURE 21–1. The relationship between the rate of oxygen consumption and heart rate during slow (S) to fast (F) walking in normal walkers and unilateral amputees. Key to amputation levels: HP = hemipelvectomy, HD = hip disarticulation, AK = above-knee, TK = through-knee, BK = below-knee.

ity or bed rest lowers the maximal exercise capacity and will decrease the oxygen pulse. Arteriosclerotic heart disease, which is commonly present in the older person with amputation for vascular disease, decreases cardiac efficiency and the maximal exercise capacity and decreases the oxygen pulse, since higher heart rates are required to circulate the same amount of blood. Diabetes, commonly present in those persons with amputations for vascular disease, decreases capillary permeability because of basement membrane thickening so that a greater volume of blood must be circulated through the muscle to extract an adequate oxygen supply, thus lowering the oxygen pulse.

In normal subjects and amputees, there is a linear relationship between the rate of oxygen consumption and the heart rate when a specific type of exercise is performed at different submaximal workloads (Fig. 21–1). This relationship also depends on the type of exercise. Less oxygen is consumed per heartbeat for arm exercise (cranking) than for leg exercise (bicycling or walking). Consequently, the $\dot{V}max_{O_2}$ and the oxygen pulse are lower for upper limb exercise than for leg exercise. This fact is particularly relevant to the amputee who requires crutches.

Energy Consumption Measurement

The standard energy expenditure measurement is the rate of oxygen uptake, $\dot{V}o_2$. The rate of oxygen consumption is divided by the body weight of the subject to permit comparisons and is expressed as the milliliters of oxygen consumed per kilogram of body weight per minute (ml O_2/kg-min). The rate of oxygen consumption is the "power" requirement.

There is a second method of expressing oxygen consumption related to the distance of walking. The energy cost, E_w, equals the volume of oxygen consumed in milliliters per kilogram of body weight per meter walked (ml O_2/kg-m). Oxygen cost is calculated by dividing the rate of oxygen consumption by the walking speed. This parameter is the biochemical "work" unit for walking. Either a reduction in velocity or an increase in the rate of oxygen consumption leads to an increased oxygen cost.

There is a considerable body of literature on the energy expenditure of amputee gait.[3–20] However, a comparison of the results of the different studies is difficult for the following reasons. First, young amputees, who usually have undergone traumatic amputation, are not consistently distinguished from older amputees, who usually have undergone amputation for vascular disease. As will be discussed, there are significant differences between these two amputee groups with respect to gait performance. Second, there is often no distinction made between amputees who use crutches or a walker and those who do not. Those amputees who exert their upper extremities using walking aids generally have a higher rate of energy expenditure and a higher heart rate. Third, the adequacy of prosthetic fit and duration of use is not always specified. It is a common clinical experience that those amputees who do not have an adequately fitted prosthesis or who have worn their prostheses only for a brief time will not walk as effectively as more experienced patients with well-fitted prostheses. Fourth, different testing methodologies make it difficult to compare the results of different studies. Some investigators have measured energy expenditure with the subject walking on a treadmill or at a regulated velocity or both. Although velocity-regulated testing enables oxygen uptake to be measured at a specific speed, the data do not indicate the energy expenditure at the patient's customary speed.

The modified Douglas bag method allows subjects to walk at their comfortable walking speeds (CWSs) on a level surface during

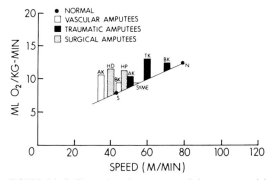

FIGURE 21–2. The rate of oxygen uptake vs speed in normal walkers and unilateral amputees. Key to amputation levels: HP = hemipelvectomy, HD = hip disarticulation, AK = above-knee, TK = through-knee, BK = below-knee.

customary walking conditions. A lightweight air collection system is harnessed to the subject's shoulders, enabling the collection of expired air (Fig. 21–2). The heart rate, respiratory rate, and cadence are all monitored, and the readings are transmitted via a portable radio telemetry system.

The data presented in this chapter are from the authors' studies and others in which energy expenditure was measured at the amputee's CWS and in which the patient's age, the etiology and level of the amputation, the duration of prosthetic use, and the presence or absence of upper extremity walking aids were clearly defined.

Normal Walking

The energy expenditure of normal walking is the baseline against which the penalty imposed by the amputee's gait disability is compared. For adult men and women, the average CWS is 80 m/min, the average rate of energy expenditure is 12.0 ml O_2/kg-min, the average heart rate is 99 beats per minute (beats/min), and the average energy cost per unit of distance traveled is 0.15 ml O_2/kg-m. The minimum value of energy cost occurs at approximately the CWS and increases or decreases with higher or lower velocities.

The relationship between speed and the rate of energy expenditure for normal walking is depicted in Figure 21–2. The rate of oxygen uptake increases with speed. Since the CWS of an amputee is slower than that of a normal individual, the normal energy-speed relationship enables the amputee's rate of energy expenditure to be compared with

the value for a normal subject walking at the same speed as the patient.

The maximal aerobic capacity, $\dot{V}max_{O_2}$, depends on age and is lower in older subjects.[2] The rate of energy expenditure for walking is approximately the same for adults, irrespective of age. Consequently, an older individual has a smaller aerobic reserve and requires a higher percentage of the available maximal aerobic capacity to walk (approximately 32% in those in their third decade versus 45% in those in their seventh decade).

The rate of energy expenditure for normal walking at the CWS in all age groups is below the anaerobic threshold (approximately 50% of the $\dot{V}max_{O_2}$); as a result, normal individuals can sustain exercise for prolonged periods without exhaustion. This accounts for the perception that normal walking requires minimal effort. The fact that older adults have a lower aerobic reserve indicates they are less able to tolerate any added physical penalty. In this regard, the older person who underwent amputation for vascular disease is less able to tolerate the added demand of a gait disability than the younger person whose amputation was congenital or traumatic.

Data Interpretation

Much of the literature on amputee gait focuses primarily on high values of the oxygen cost of amputee walking, which is obtained by dividing the rate of oxygen consumption by the walking speed.[20] Primary consideration of oxygen cost alone may obscure the importance of the two independent parameters used in its calculation: walking speed and rate of oxygen consumption. Speed is the fundamental measure of gait performance. The rate of oxygen consumption (and the heart rate) is the basic measure of physical effort.

The following example illustrates the importance of understanding the difference in the parameters of the rate of oxygen consumption and the oxygen cost. If a vascular below-knee amputee walks slowly at 45 m/min and consumes oxygen at a rate of 9.4 ml O_2/kg-min (halfway between the effort required for normal standing [4.5 ml O_2/kg-min] and that required for normal walking [12.0 ml O_2/kg-min]), the oxygen cost equals

$$\frac{9.4 \text{ ml } O_2/\text{kg-min}}{45 \text{ m/min}} \text{ or } 0.22 \text{ ml } O_2/\text{kg-m}$$

This oxygen cost is 40% higher than during normal walking (0.15 ml O_2/kg-m). It is important to recognize that although the gait is inefficient and costly in terms of oxygen consumption per unit distance, the rate of oxygen consumption is substantially less than that for normal walking, and the patient will not experience physical stress, exertion, or fatigue during customary walking activities. In this case, the patient's mobility is restricted only by the slow speed.

PROSTHETIC AMBULATION

Unilateral

To compare the relative performance of walking with different amputation levels, the authors measured the energy expenditure and gait characteristics of 77 persons with Syme's, below-knee, through-knee, and above-knee amputations.[3, 18] Subjects were divided into two groups: older patients (averaging 60 years of age) whose amputations were performed secondary to vascular disease and younger patients (averaging 30 years of age) whose amputations were performed secondary to trauma. All of the subjects had worn their prostheses at least 6 months and did not use walking aids (with the exception of some patients in the vascular above-knee group who required canes or crutches). Above-knee amputees used a total-contact quadrilateral socket, below-knee amputees used a patellar tendon-bearing (PTB) socket, and Syme's and through-knee amputees used end-bearing sockets.

Speed

Walking speed for all groups of amputees was less than normal and progressively declined at each higher amputation level. In the traumatic group, below-knee amputees averaged 71 m/min, through-knee amputees 61 m/min, and above-knee amputees 52 m/min (Table 21–1). James reported the same average CWS in a group of 34 healthy young above-knee amputees.[10]

Nowroozi and Salvanelli tested 18 patients after hip disarticulation (HD) or hemipelvectomy (HP) for tumor. These amputees were young, were healthy at the time of testing, had not received radiation or chemotherapy for at least 6 months before testing, had no evidence of tumor recurrence, had worn their protheses for at least 6 months, and did not use crutches. In these respects, these amputees were similar to those whom the authors had examined but who underwent traumatic amputation. The average walking speeds for the HD and HP patients were 47 m/min and 40 m/min, respectively. When these two groups are combined, a progressive decline in speed is consistently noted at each higher level, ranging from the below-knee to the HP levels (Fig. 21–3).[17]

When amputees whose conditions were secondary to vascular disease were compared with those whose conditions were secondary to trauma, walking speed was slower in the former than in the latter, when matched for

Table 21–1. ENERGY CONSUMPTION OF UNILATERAL AMPUTEES

Indication and Amputation Level	n	Velocity (m/min)	Heart Rate (beats/min)	Rate of Oxygen Uptake (ml O_2/kg-min)	Oxygen Cost (ml O_2/kg-m)	Oxygen Pulse* (ml O_2/kg-beat)
Normal		80	99	12.1	0.15	0.122
Vascular[3]						
Above-knee	13	36	126	10.8	0.28	0.086
Below-knee	13	45	105	9.4	0.20	0.090
Syme's	15	54	108	9.2	0.17	0.085
Surgical[17]						
Hemipelvectomy	10	40	97	11.5	0.29	0.119
Hip disarticulation	8	47	99	11.1	0.24	0.112
Traumatic[3]						
Above-knee	15	52	111	10.3	0.20	0.093
Through-knee	7	61	109	13.4	0.23	0.123
Below-knee	14	71	106	12.4	0.16	0.117

*Calculated by dividing the average rate of oxygen uptake by the average heart rate for the total group.

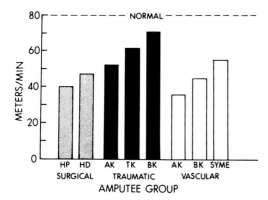

FIGURE 21–3. Walking speed in surgical, traumatic, and vascular amputees. Key to amputation levels: HP = hemipelvectomy, HD = hip disarticulation, AK = above-knee, TK = through-knee, BK = below-knee.

amputation level (Fig. 21–4). For below-knee amputees, the velocity averaged 37% slower for those whose surgery was for vascular disease (45 m/min versus 71 m/min). Gonzales and associates also found a similar average CWS in persons who underwent below-knee amputation for vascular disease.[7] For above-knee amputees, the velocity was 31% slower in those with surgery secondary to vascular disease (36 m/min versus 52 m/min).

Of particular importance was the finding that in persons with amputations for vascular disease, the walking speed for those with Syme's amputations was faster than that for those with below-knee amputations (54 m/min versus 45 m/min). The authors conclude that walking speed in Syme's, below-knee, through-knee, above-knee, HD, and HP amputees is directly dependent on the level of amputation.

Rate of Oxygen Consumption

While walking at their CWS, persons with through-knee and below-knee traumatic amputations showed an average rate of oxygen consumption that was slightly greater than normal (see Table 21–1). The average rate of oxygen consumption in Nowroozi and Salvanelli's subjects with surgical amputations at the HD and HP levels and in the authors' subjects with amputations for vascular disease was lower than normal (see Fig. 21–4).[17]

Although amputees walking at their CWS do not have a rate of oxygen uptake that is significantly greater than that of normal individuals at their CWS, the walking speed of the two groups is different. This difference in walking speeds must be considered when

comparing the rate of oxygen uptake in an amputee with the value for normal walking. The energy-speed relation of normal walking enables one to determine the normal rate of oxygen consumption at the patient's reduced speed and to calculate the added power requirement resulting from the amputation (see Fig. 21–2). The velocity-adjusted values for the percentage rate of oxygen consumption increase due to physical impairment were as follows

1. Traumatic amputation: above-knee, 24%; through-knee, 58%; below-knee, 41%.
2. Surgical amputation: HP, 46%; HD, 37%.
3. Vascular amputation: above-knee, 38%; below-knee, 16%; Syme's, 10%.

In separate studies of persons with above- or below-knee traumatic amputations, James and Molen found that the added power requirement was elevated during treadmill walking throughout the customary range of slow and fast speeds employed by the amputee.[6, 10]

Heart Rate

The average heart rates of persons with unilateral amputation at different levels for trauma, surgical amputation, or vascular disease were approximately the same or slightly higher than the average heart rate for normal subjects (100 beats/min), with the single exception of persons with above-knee amputation, who averaged 126 beats/min (Fig. 21–5). The authors attribute the higher heart rate in this group to the fact that eight of these 13 patients used crutches or canes. The high heart rate and energy cost of walking occurred in dysvascular above-knee ampu-

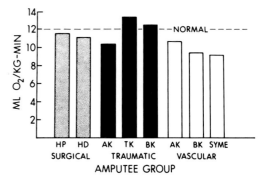

FIGURE 21–4. The rate of oxygen consumption in surgical, traumatic, and vascular unilateral amputees. Key to amputation levels: HP = hemipelvectomy, HD = hip disarticulation, AK = above-knee, TK = through-knee, BK = below-knee.

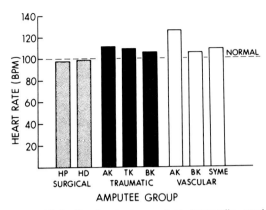

FIGURE 21–5. Heart rate in surgical, traumatic, and vascular unilateral amputees. Key to amputation levels: HP = hemipelvectomy, HD = hip disarticulation, AK = above-knee, TK = through-knee, BK = below-knee.

tees who used a prosthesis despite the fact that the patients in this group were the most rigorously selected subjects in this study. In the authors' hospital, nearly all dysvascular Syme's and below-knee amputees are fitted with a prosthesis, and fewer than one half of the ones included in the study were able to walk 5 minutes and achieve a steady-state condition, a criterion for subject selection. Even the selected above-knee patients did not use a prosthesis for all walking activities. Upper limb assistance (crutches or a cane) was required in more than one half, further increasing energy cost. It must be concluded that, whenever possible, all efforts must be made to protect dysvascular limbs early so that above the knee does not become the amputation site of choice. If the amputation can be kept below the knee, ambulation with a prosthesis becomes practical in the elderly dysvascular patient.

Heart rate is the subjective experience most often associated with physical exertion. Since the heart rate was the same as or slightly higher than normal in all amputees, except those persons with above-knee amputations for vascular disease who did not use walking aids, it can be concluded that the amputee with a well-fitted prosthesis experiences approximately the same or a slightly higher exertion as the normal individual when walking.

Energy Cost

The values for oxygen cost per meter walked parallel the data on velocity. The energy cost increases at each higher amputation level. For persons who underwent am-

putation for vascular disease, the oxygen cost averaged 0.17 ml O_2/kg-m, 0.20 ml O_2/kg-m, and 0.28 ml O_2/kg-m at the Syme's, below-knee, and above-knee levels, respectively. For persons who underwent traumatic amputation, energy cost averaged 0.16 ml O_2/kg-m, 0.23 ml O_2/kg-m, and 0.20 ml O_2/kg-m at the below-knee, through-knee, and above-knee levels. For persons who underwent traumatic amputation, energy cost averaged 0.24 ml O_2/kg-m and 0.29 ml O_2/kg-m at the HD and HP levels (Fig. 21–6). Thus, energy cost tended to vary depending on both the level and cause of amputation.

Cardiovascular Efficiency

The amputee's physical fitness can be assessed by examining the relationship between $\dot{V}O_2$ and heart rate. With the single exception of those persons with through-knee traumatic amputations, most amputee groups at their CWS had a value for the average rate of oxygen uptake that was the same as or lower than that of normal subjects (see Table 21–1). On the other hand, the average heart rate for most groups was slightly higher than normal (see Table 21–1). The heart rate is graphed versus the rate of oxygen consumption in Figure 21–1, enabling the assessment of cardiovascular efficiency. Those persons with above-knee traumatic amputations and all three groups of persons with amputations for vascular disease (above-knee, below-knee, and Syme's amputees) had heart rates elevated above normal at a given rate of oxygen consumption. In a study of 38 healthy above-knee amputees investigated during one-

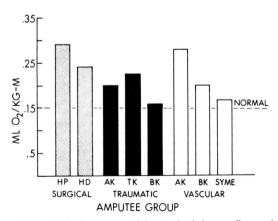

FIGURE 21–6. Oxygen cost in surgical, traumatic, and vascular unilateral amputees. Key to amputation levels: HP = hemipelvectomy, HD = hip disarticulation, AK = above-knee, TK = through-knee, BK = below-knee.

legged and two-legged exercise, James reported similar results. He concluded that the above-knee amputee has a less active lifestyle, resulting in a lower level of physical conditioning.[10] However, since the relationship between the heart rate and the rate of oxygen consumption in Nowroozi and Salvanelli's HD and HP patients (see Fig. 21–6) is normal,[17] the authors conclude that a particular amputation level does not necessarily lead to deconditioning.

In all groups of persons with amputation for vascular disease, an abnormal heart rate to rate of oxygen uptake relationship was observed (see Fig. 21–1). This cardiovascular exercise inefficiency may be quantitated by calculating the oxygen pulse for each group. All three groups of subjects with amputations for vascular disease had oxygen pulses significantly lower than those of the subjects with traumatic amputations (except above-knee amputees), the subjects with surgical amputations, and normal walkers (see Table 21–1).

There are several factors that could account for these findings. First, the older person with an amputation for vascular disease may have a less active lifestyle than the younger patient, accounting for the decreased efficiency. Second, the older person with an amputation for vascular disease is more likely to have arteriosclerotic heart disease or other medical diseases that lower cardiac efficiency. Third, secondary myopathy can occur from peripheral vascular disease or from diabetes, which causes thickening of the capillary basement membrane, decreasing capillary permeability and the ability of the muscle to extract oxygen from the blood. Consequently, more blood must be circulated through the muscle in order to provide an adequate oxygen supply; this accounts for an increase in the oxygen pulse. Finally, more than one half of the persons with above-knee amputation for vascular disease required upper extremity aids, and as previously discussed, the arm work is associated with heart rates comparatively higher than those of leg work.

Residual Limb Length

Gonzales and associates evaluated nine patients with below-knee amputations of unknown etiology to determine the influence of residual limb length.[7] The limbs ranged from 14 to 19 cm in length. Patients wore PTB

prostheses, except for one who had a conventional hard socket. All had used their prostheses at least 6 months and were divided into a group with short residual limbs (three patients) and another group with long residual limbs (six patients). There was no correlation with walking speed. The average rate of energy expenditure was higher in patients with short residual limbs. Nevertheless, the number of subjects was too small to perform statistical analyses.

A similar study was performed at Rancho Los Amigos Medical Center in two groups of amputees: 17 had traumatic amputations, and ten had amputations for vascular disease.[23] The residual limbs ranged from 9 to 24 cm in length, and the minimal length of prosthetic use was 9 months. Fourteen had PTB sockets, six had PTB prostheses with supracondylar suspension, and seven had PTB prostheses with metal-hinged joints and a thigh lacer. No significant differences in walking speed, rate of energy expenditure, and energy cost were observed that related to residual limb length or to the type of suspension used in either diagnostic group. Knee flexion and extension torques were also measured, and there were no significant correlations in either group with residual limb length. It can be concluded that within the residual limb lengths measured, no significant energy differences were demonstrated. Of particular clinical importance is the finding that a residual limb that extends below the knee as little as 9 cm will result in performance superior to that of residual limbs from through-knee or above-knee amputation. Satisfactory prosthetic fit is more easily achieved with longer residual limbs, provided soft tissue coverage is maintained.

Among above-knee amputees, James found a poor correlation between residual limb length and torque, except in adduction.[24] He attributed the stronger correlation in adduction to the fact that adductor muscles insert along the entire length of the femur and are therefore most affected by differences in residual limb length. The authors are aware of no studies relating speed and energy expenditure to residual limb length in above-knee amputees.

Bilateral

Relatively few studies have been performed on bilateral amputees. Table 21–2

Table 21–2. ENERGY CONSUMPTION OF BILATERAL AMPUTEES

Indication and Amputation Level	n	Velocity (m/min)	Heart Rate (beats/min)	Rate of Oxygen Uptake (ml O_2/kg-min)	Oxygen Cost (ml O_2/kg-m)
Traumatic					
Below-knee[22]	3	67	112	13.6	0.20
Above-knee[22]	1	54	104	17.6	0.33
Vascular					
Syme's[22]	3	62	99	12.8	0.21
Below-knee[22]	6	40	113	11.6	0.31
Below-knee[16]	6	40	116	7.8	0.23
Unknown (stubbies)					
Through-knee[15]	1	46	86	9.9	0.22

summarizes data on patients with bilateral traumatic amputations or vascular disease, who were tested in the authors' laboratory. DuBow and colleagues have also tested six persons with bilateral below-knee amputations for vascular disease, three of whom required a cane.[16]

Interpretation of the data on persons with bilateral traumatic amputations must be done with caution, since only a few subjects have been studied. The authors tested three bilateral below-knee amputees who did not require upper extremity assistance. One patient with bilateral above-knee amputations was tested and required crutches. The mean rate of oxygen uptake and the mean heart rate were higher than those of unilateral amputees. The velocities of the bilateral amputees were approximately the same as those of the unilateral amputees, when matched for amputation level. These very limited data suggest that the person with bilateral traumatic below-knee amputations expends a greater physiological effort than the person with a unilateral below-knee amputation. The use of crutches in the bilateral above-knee amputee prevents direct comparison with the unilateral amputees who did not use crutches.

Despite the existence of a large population of dysvascular patients requiring bilateral amputations above the knee, the authors were unable to find any patients with bilateral above-knee amputations or combined above- and below-knee amputations who were able to walk for 5 minutes. The authors were able to find 12 patients with unilateral amputations at the Syme's or below-knee level who subsequently underwent an amputation on the opposite leg and were able to walk with bilateral prostheses for 5 minutes. Those patients who were able to walk with bilateral prostheses were a highly select group; therefore, these data are not reflective of the typical vascular patients in the authors' clinics, who are unable to walk or sustain ambulation for 5 minutes. None of the patients with bilateral Syme's amputations required upper extremity aids. Of the six patients with bilateral below-knee amputations, three required canes, and two required crutches. Analysis of the data on these individuals suggests that the bilateral amputees required more energy expenditure than the unilateral amputees with the same amputation level (see Table 21–2). However, it is not possible to determine to what extent the use of upper extremity aids also accounted for this increase. Of special clinical note is the fact that the bilateral Syme's amputees walked faster and more efficiently than the bilateral below-knee amputees. Also, their heart rates were lower, probably because they did not require walking aids.

Finally, of special interest, Wainapel and coworkers measured energy expenditure in a 21-year-old bilateral through-knee amputee who walked on stubbie prostheses with a walker.[15] This person walked faster at a slightly greater rate of oxygen consumption than with conventional above-knee prostheses and crutches. Although walking on stubbies is cosmetically unacceptable for most patients (except for gait training or limited walking in the home), the data from this single patient illustrate that it can result in a functional gait.

Crutches

Crutch walking without a prosthesis in unilateral amputees may be a primary or secondary means of ambulation when an ade-

TABLE 21–3. CRUTCH WALKING WITHOUT PROSTHESES

Indication and Amputation Level	Velocity (m/min)	Heart Rate (beats/min)	Rate of Oxygen Uptake (ml O$_2$/kg-min)
Vascular[3]			
Above-knee	48	130	12.0
Below-knee	39	124	11.7
Syme's	39	129	10.2
Traumatic[3]			
Above-knee	65	129	12.7
Below-knee	71	135	17.9

quate prosthesis is unavailable or inadequate. Also, in the authors' experience, most persons with above-knee amputation for vascular disease are not able to walk with a prosthesis for all or a portion of their activities and require crutches or a walker.

The energy cost of walking with swing-through crutch-assisted gait and no prosthesis is physiologically stressful for both persons with amputation for vascular disease and those with traumatic amputation. Markedly elevated heart rates were noted in both groups. The mean heart rates average 130 beats/min (Table 21–3). These values approximate the level obtained in normal recreational jogging, indicating the strenuous effort associated with the upper extremity exercise of crutch use. The high heart rate is due to the decreased maximal aerobic capacity associated with arm exercise as compared with leg exercise. As a result of the high heart rate indicating strenuous physical exertion, most amputees are able to walk without a prosthesis using crutches for only short intervals, usually inside the home. Such patients usually prefer to use a wheelchair when required to travel farther distances outside the home.

As compared with walking with a prosthesis but without upper extremity aids, crutch walking without a prosthesis requires higher heart rates in all patient groups tested. The authors conclude that a well-fitted prosthesis that results in a satisfactory gait without the use of walking aids significantly reduces physiological stress. Finally, since crutch walking without a prosthesis requires more physiological exertion than walking with a prosthesis, crutch walking without a prosthesis should not be considered a satisfactory final prosthetic prescription.

Wheelchair

For the older patient with bilateral amputations for vascular disease who is unable to walk with prostheses, the wheelchair is the most common method of transportation. Many persons with unilateral above-knee amputation for vascular disease use a wheelchair. Data on the energy cost of wheelchair propulsion in amputees who customarily used a wheelchair are presented in Table 21–4.[22] All patients were bilateral amputees. Those persons with traumatic amputation wheeled faster than those with amputation for vascular disease. The rate of energy expenditure and the heart rate approximated the values for normal walking. Because the speed was slower than that of normal walking, the oxygen cost was greater.

Wheelchair ambulation is a restricted type of mobility, and performance is best on hard, level surfaces. Uneven terrain or soft surfaces, such as carpet, increase rolling friction; therefore, the amputee must reduce the speed to avoid an increased physiological effort.[25] Wheelchair mobility is also limited by curbs, stairs, and other architectural bar-

TABLE 21–4. WHEELCHAIR PROPULSION IN BILATERAL AMPUTEES

Indication	n	Velocity (m/min)	Heart Rate (beats/min)	Rate of Oxygen uptake (ml O$_2$/kg-min)	Oxygen Cost (ml O$_2$/kg-m)
Vascular[22]	10	50	108	10.7	0.22
Traumatic[22]	5	62	101	12.3	0.20

riers. Hills or inclines increase the required physiological effort. For these reasons, the typical unilateral amputee prefers walking with a prosthesis to wheeling. The unilateral amputee who does not use a prosthesis usually ambulates with crutches or a walker for short distances inside the home. When ambulation for longer distances outside the home is required, the wheelchair is usually preferred to avoid fatigue caused by the severe exertion of prolonged crutch walking.

During wheelchair propulsion, the heart rate was higher in persons with amputation for vascular disease than in those with traumatic amputation (108 beats/min versus 101 beats/min); nevertheless, the rate of oxygen uptake was lower (10.7 ml O_2/kg-min versus 12.3 ml O_2/kg-min). Hence, the amount of oxygen per beat was higher in those persons with traumatic amputation (0.121 ml O_2/kg-beat versus 0.099 ml O_2/kg-beat), indicating greater cardiovascular exercise efficiency. In the previous section on unilateral amputees walking with a prosthesis, decreased efficiency was noted in those patients with amputation for vascular disease and, similarly, may be attributed to a more sedentary lifestyle, older age, associated medical illness, and vascular or diabetic myopathy.

Walker

The older person with a unilateral amputation for vascular disease at the above-knee level or higher and who does not wear a prosthesis is often unable to use crutches and may require a walker. Like crutch ambulation, use of a walker also requires considerable upper extremity exertion, since it is still necessary for the amputee to lift the entire body weight for each step. Because of the slow speed, the person who requires a walker is even more restricted than the one who uses crutches and will rely on a wheelchair for most activities outside the home.

REFERENCES

1. Saunders JB, De CM, Inman VT, Eberhart HD: Major determinants in normal and pathological gait. J Bone Joint Surg 35A:543, 1953.
2. Astrand PO, Rodahl K: Textbook of Work Physiology, 2nd Ed. New York, McGraw-Hill, 1977, p 321.
3. Waters RL, Perry J, Antonelli D, Hislop HJ: Energy cost of walking of amputees: Influence of level of amputation. J Bone Joint Surg (Am)58:42, 1976.
4. Ganguli S, Datta SR, Chatterjee BB, et al: Performance evaluation of amputee-prosthesis system in below-knee amputees. Ergonomics 16:797, 1973.
5. Eberhart HD, Elftman H, Inman VT: Locomotor mechanism of amputee. In Klopsteg PR, Wilson PD (eds): Human Limbs and Their Substitutes. New York, McGraw-Hill, 1954, pp 472–480.
6. Molen NH: Energy-speed relation of below-knee amputees walking on a motor-driven treadmill. Int Z Angew Physiol 31:173, 1973.
7. Gonzales EG, Corcoran PJ, Reyes RL: Energy expenditure in below-knee amputees: Correlation with stump length. Arch Phys Med Rehabil 55:111, 1974.
8. Ganguli S, Bose KS, Datta SR, et al: Ergonomics evaluation of above-knee amputee-prosthesis combinations. Ergonomics 17:199, 1974.
9. Traugh GH, Corcoran PJ, Reyes RL: Energy expenditure of ambulation in patients with above-knee amputations. Arch Phys Med Rehabil 56:67, 1975.
10. James U: Oxygen uptake and heart rate during prosthetic walking in healthy male unilateral above-knee amputees. Scand J Rehabil Med 5:71, 1973.
11. Pagliarulo MA, Waters R, Hislop HJ: Energy cost of walking of below-knee amputees having no vascular disease. Phys Ther 59:538, 1979.
12. Ganguli S, Datta SR, Chatterjee BB, Roy BN: Metabolic cost of walking at different speeds with patellar tendon-bearing prosthesis. J Appl Physiol 36:440, 1974.
13. Huang CT, Jackson JR, Moore NB, et al: Amputation: Energy cost of ambulation. Arch Phys Med Rehabil 60:18, 1979.
14. Erdman WJ II, Hettinger TH, Saez F: Comparative work stress for above-knee amputees using artificial legs or crutches. Am J Phys Med 39:225, 1960.
15. Wainapel SF, March H, Steve L: Stubby prostheses: An alternative to conventional prosthetic devices. Arch Phys Med Rehabil 66:264, 1985.
16. DuBow LL, Witt PL, Kadaba MP, et al: Oxygen consumption of elderly persons with bilateral below knee amputations: Ambulation vs wheelchair propulsion. Arch Phys Med Rehabil 64:255, 1983.
17. Nowroozi F, Salvanelli ML: Energy expenditure in hip disarticulation and hemipelvectomy amputees. Arch Phys Med Rehabil 64:300, 1983.
18. Waters RL, Hislop HJ, Perry J, Antonelli D: Energetics: Application to the study and management of locomotor disabilities. Orthop Clin North Am 9:351, 1978.
19. Waters RL, Hislop HJ, Perry J, et al: Comparative cost of walking in young and old adults. J Orthop Res 1:73, 1983.
20. Fisher SV, Gullickson G: Energy cost of ambulation in health and disability: A literature review. Arch Phys Med Rehabil 59:124, 1978.
21. James U, Oberg K: Prosthetic gait pattern in unilateral above-knee amputees. Scand J Rehabil Med 5:35, 1973.
22. Waters RL: Unreported data, 1979.
23. Hunt AR: Unreported data, 1983.
24. James U: Maximal isometric muscle strength in healthy active male unilateral above-knee amputees with special regard to the hip joint. Scand J Rehabil Med 5:55, 1973.

22

Biomechanics of Ambulation

J. H. Bowker, M.D.
M. Kazim, M.B., B.S., F.R.C.S.(C)

This chapter will provide a concise explanation of what the surgeon who performs lower limb amputations needs to know about normal gait. In the past, knowledge of gait has been considered essential to the research prosthetists, engineers, and kinesiologists who design prostheses; to the prosthetists who make and fit them; and to the therapists who train amputees in their use. Relatively little emphasis has been placed on making the amputation surgeon—the single person most responsible for the individual patient's functional outcome—"gait wise." An appreciation of the significance of residual limb length and of the preservation of joints and end–weight-bearing capabilities comes with the study of normal gait patterns. This in turn should lead to a striving for more perfectly executed, more distal, and hence more useful amputations.

The unique walking pattern of each individual represents his or her solution to the problem of how to get from one place to another with minimal energy expenditure, adequate stability, and acceptable appearance.[1] During this century, the many elements of human gait have been delineated and then systematically studied in a variety of sophisticated ways, each of which has shed light on the subject from a particular viewpoint.[15] In the analysis of these findings from various methods and their subsequent synthesis lies the key to understanding normal gait. The proven methods of gait investigation will be examined and incorporated in a description of normal gait. Finally, a discussion of amputation levels will explain why many amputees have such awkard, energy-wasting gaits.

STUDIES OF NORMAL HUMAN GAIT

Photographic Methods

The motion of limb segments—the pelvis, thigh, leg, and foot—relative to each other were first evaluated by a study of multiple still photographs.[11] With the advent of movie cameras, individual movie frames and slow motion films were used to delineate the phases of gait further. In a significant advance, strips of reflective tape are fixed to the pelvis, thigh, leg, and foot, and stroboscopic photographs are taken at the rate of 20 per second as the subject walks in a darkened room.[9] Viewed from the side, the marked limb segments resemble articulated

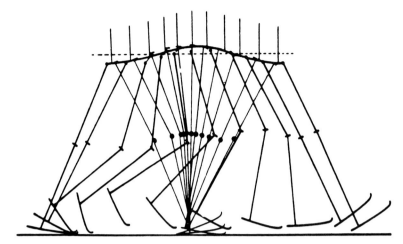

FIGURE 22–1. Action of the limb during stance and swing phases, derived from interrupted light photography (20 frames per sec). Note the sinusoidal path of the body's center of gravity, with its low point at heel strike and high point at midstance. (*From Perry J: Anatomy and biomechanics of the hindfoot. Clin Orthop 177:9, 1983.*)

sticks moving through space, allowing the viewer to focus on one limb or limb segment at a time (Fig. 22–1).

Analysis of Muscle Function

It must be kept in mind, however, that the articulated segments of the lower limb can function during gait only as levers that are acted on by muscles crossing the hip, knee, and ankle joints. Generally speaking, muscles accelerate, decelerate, or stabilize the limb segments. Thus, they may act while shortening, lengthening, or remaining the same length. If a muscle contracts concentrically, as in the shortening of the tibialis anterior when the toes clear the floor during swing phase, the work performed can be readily calculated. Other muscles act primarily as shock absorbers by undergoing a progressive but resisted increase in length, termed an eccentric contraction. For example, the hamstrings are performing significant work during controlled hip flexion (deceleration of the thigh) in terminal swing just before heel strike. Acting as joint stabilizers, however, muscles undergo no change in length while still performing significant biological work. This isometric contraction is illustrated by the triceps surae (gastrosoleus) as it maintains a relatively fixed relationship between the leg and foot during terminal stance, allowing the forefoot to act as a propulsive rocker.[17]

To comprehend normal gait more fully, it is essential to know exactly when and how each muscle group functions in the cycle. Information on muscle activity during gait has been provided by electromyography (EMG) in which, for greatest accuracy, wire electrodes are placed directly in each muscle. A multiple-channel recorder allows simultaneous monitoring of several muscles. For the exact temporal correlation of the firing of a given muscle with the location in the gait cycle, the EMG signal can be synchronized with foot-switch signals, which indicate heel strike and toe-off (preswing).[6] Another method synchronizes EMG signals with the videotaped image of the walker; this is especially useful because of the instant replay feature. For the most part, muscle function during gait will require short bursts of activity and longer periods of relaxation during each complete cycle (Fig. 22–2).

Center of Gravity and Gait Efficiency

The relative motions of the jointed limb segments, controlled by their muscles, determine the efficiency of gait in terms of the forward progression of the body mass, which is represented by the center of gravity (CG). The CG of the body is that point at which its mass would be perfectly balanced in any position. In the human, the center of gravity lies just anterior to the second sacral vertebra, within the true pelvis. Viewed from the front, this is just above the symphysis pubis; from the side, just above the tip of the greater trochanter (Fig. 22–3). To study the path of the CG, one may mark its projections on the body surface with a pinpoint light source and walking in a darkened room, photograph the subject, with an open-shuttered still camera. From the side, the lighted CG describes a sine wave rising and falling a total of only 5 cm (2 inches) (Fig. 22–1). From above, the CG during gait is also seen to move 5 cm from side to side as the weight is transferred from one foot to the other. The resultant path of the CG is thus a horizontal spiral confined within a 5 cm tube. These very modest shifts are an expression of the efficiency of human gait, which is accomplished by the coordination of pelvic, knee, and ankle motion, including the transverse rotation of the pelvis and lower limb.[15] The latter motion consists of internal rotation of the pelvis and lower limb from heel strike until foot-flat (loading response), after which there is progressive external rotation until toe-off (preswing), when internal rotation begins again (Fig. 22–4).

Ground Reaction Forces

Other important considerations in the study of the gait cycle are the reactions between the lower limbs and the ground. The factors involved are gravity and friction. Without these, ground contact would be un-

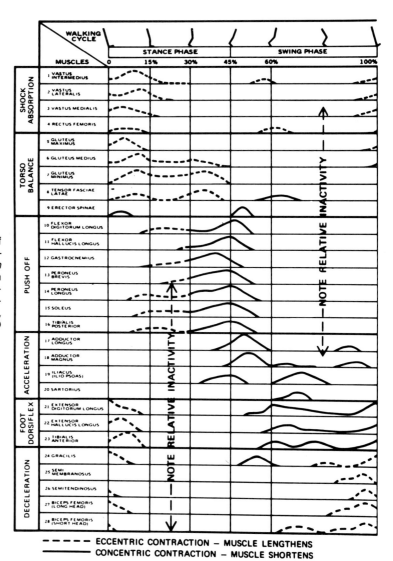

FIGURE 22–2. Electromyograph of the lower limb during walking. (*Reproduced by permission from* Bowker JH, Hall CB: Normal human gait. *In* American Academy of Orthopaedic Surgeons: Atlas of Orthotics. St Louis, The CV Mosby Co, 1975. *Courtesy of* Dr Charles O Bechtol, Los Angeles, CA.)

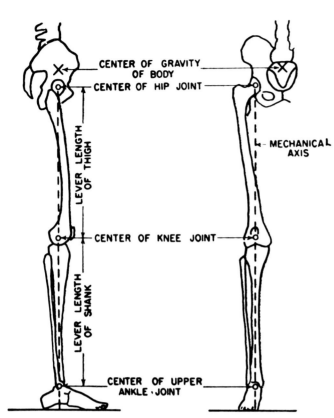

FIGURE 22–3. Lateral and anterior views of the skeletal pelvis and lower limb. Note the position of the body's center of gravity and the joint centers of the hip, knee, and ankle. (*From* Anderson MH, Bechtol CO, Sollars RE: Clinical Prosthetics for Physicians and Therapists, 1959. *Courtesy of* Charles C Thomas, Publisher, Springfield, Illinois.)

dependable, and adequate functional stabilization of the limbs for acceleration and deceleration would be absent.

The primary determinants of balance and, therefore, of the demands upon the lower limb muscles during walking, are the position of the trunk and its CG at each instant. The approximate location of the trunk's CG is anterior to the tenth thoracic vertebra. If the body is viewed from the side at any instant in the stance phase and if the location of the trunk's CG is known, a line can be drawn

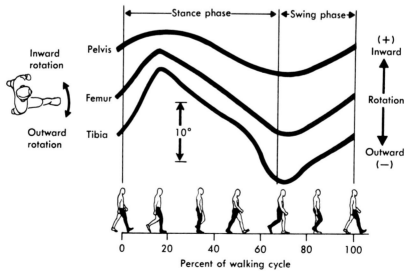

FIGURE 22–4. Transverse rotation of the pelvis, femur, and tibia during a gait cycle. Internal rotation reverses to external rotation during loading response and back again to internal rotation during preswing. (*Reproduced by permission from* Mann RA: Biomechanics of the foot. *In* American Academy of Orthopaedic Surgeons: Atlas of Orthotics, 2nd Ed. St Louis, The CV Mosby Co, 1985.)

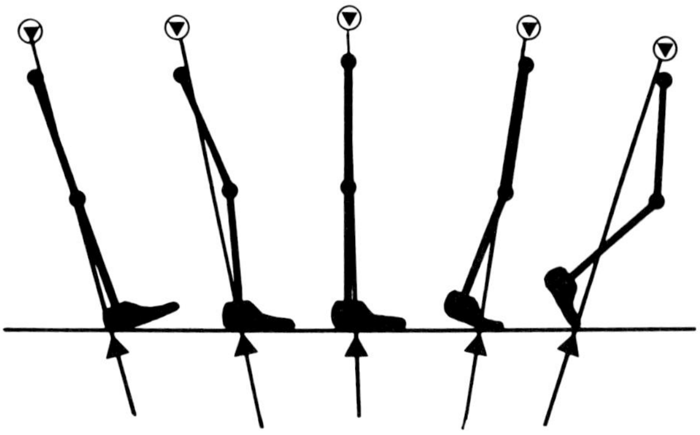

HEEL STRIKE   LOADING RESPONSE   MID-STANCE   TERMINAL STANCE   PRE-SWING

FIGURE 22–5. Changes in the direction of the ground force reaction vector during stance phase. (*Modified by permission from* Fernie GF: Biomechanics of gait and prosthetic alignment. *In* Kostuik JP (ed): Amputation Surgery and Rehabilitation: The Toronto Experience. New York, Churchill Livingstone, 1981.)

from the point of contact of the stance foot to the CG of the moving trunk. This line is known as the ground force reaction vector or, conversely, as the body weight vector if the latter is considered the primary vector. Depending on the position of the limb segments at that instant, this line will pass either in front of or behind the ankle, knee, and hip joints' centers (of rotation) (Fig. 22–5). It is then easy to deduce the specific muscle actions needed to provide stability or to control the motion of the limb segments in that position. For example, at heel strike, the vector is applied at the heel, passes behind the ankle joint's center and in front of the knee's and hip's centers. Muscle contraction is thus required of the ankle dorsiflexors to prevent immediate foot-slap.

Because of the varying angles at which the stance limb contacts and leaves the ground, the forces associated with ground contact are complex. In addition to vertical loading, they include fore and aft shear, medial and lateral shear, and internal and external torque. These can all be measured by a calibrated force plate set in a walkway (Fig. 22–6).

Energy Measurement

Finally, the study of energy consumption during normal walking has formed an important baseline against which to measure the performance of amputees using a prosthesis, crutches alone, or a wheelchair. Fortunately, these findings can be easily related to the wide range of ages found among amputees.

There are two types of energy supply: aerobic and anaerobic. Briefly, the aerobic

pathway entails the oxidation of substrates to carbon dioxide and water via enzymatic action and yields adenosine triphosphate (ATP) for muscle contraction. The production of ATP by the anaerobic pathway, in contrast, does not require oxygen, as the glycolytic pathway is used for the conversion of glucose, via pyruvate, to lactate. This has two drawbacks: the energy produced is 19 times less than in the aerobic pathway,[4] and the body can tolerate only a limited accumulation of the end product, lactic acid. The aerobic pathway is, therefore, used for prolonged energy supply, via oxygen delivered to the tissues, whereas short bursts of energy can be supplied via the anaerobic pathway.

Energy consumption during walking can be expressed as oxygen consumed either in

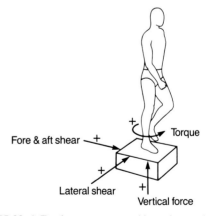

FIGURE 22–6. The forces measured by a force plate set in a walkway. (*From* Eberhart HD, Inman VT, Bresler B: The principal elements in human locomotion. *In* Klopsteg PE, Wilson PD (eds): Human Limbs and Their Substitutes. New York, McGraw-Hill Book Co, 1954. *Reprinted with the permission of* the National Academy of Sciences, Washington, DC.)

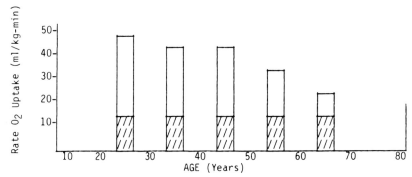

FIGURE 22–7. Maximal aerobic capacity related to age. Note that the overall aerobic reserve decreases with age. Hatched areas show the proportional increase in the rate of energy expenditure required in walking as age increases. (*Reproduced by permission from* Waters RL, Lunsford BR: Energy expenditure of normal and pathologic gait: Application to orthotic prescription. *In* American Academy of Orthopaedic Surgeons: Atlas of Orthotics, 2nd Ed. St Louis, The CV Mosby Co, 1985.)

walking at a certain speed (ml O_2/kg-min) or, better, in covering a given distance (ml O_2/kg-m). It should also be noted that there is actually an optimal walking speed for each person if maximum efficiency is to be realized. This is known as the comfortable walking speed (CWS).[5] Although going slower than one's CWS will decrease step length and energy expenditure per unit of time, the cost per unit of distance increases.[14] The maximal aerobic capacity ($\dot{V}max_{O_2}$) is the best indicator of *physical fitness*, accurately reflecting the oxygen supply to the tissues.[19] Any disorder that restricts the supply of oxygen to the tissues will result in a decrease in the $\dot{V}max_{O_2}$, which can be measured experimen-

tally. This is seen in disorders of the respiratory, cardiovascular, and metabolic systems. Independent of these disorders, the $\dot{V}max_{O_2}$ also decreases with advancing age (Fig. 22–7).

There are various ways of determining the energy cost of walking. All require the subject's achievement of a steady state of metabolic demand, followed by collection of samples of expired air and determination of their oxygen and carbon dioxide content with spirometers and mass spectrometers (Fig. 22–8).[2] One method of study involves the use of a treadmill to simulate walking across a floor. Although a normal gait pattern is easily achieved by normal individuals using this

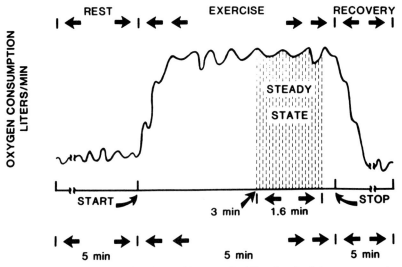

FIGURE 22–8. Oxygen consumption curve showing achievement of the steady state necessary for energy studies. (*From* DuBow LL, Witt PL, Kadaba MP, et al: Oxygen consumption of elderly persons with bilateral below knee amputations: Ambulation vs wheelchair propulsion. Arch Phys Med Rehabil 64:255, 1983. *Reprinted with the permission of* the Archives of Physical Medicine and Rehabilitation.)

method, it is almost never attained by any amputee. For this reason, the treadmill method for amputees has since been discarded in favor of one using a level track.

More recently, mobile gas-analysis modules have been developed that allow the subject to walk at the CWS, as well as at speeds above and below it, with simultaneous sampling of respiratory gases. In this way, the subject is minimally encumbered by the test equipment. The results obtained from these machines can be expressed in several valuable parameters from which the energy cost can be deduced:

1. Distance walked (m)
2. Comfortable walking speed (m/min)
3. Oxygen utilized per minute (ml O_2/min)
4. Oxygen utilized per meter walked (ml O_2/m)
5. Maximum aerobic capacity ($\dot{V}max_{O_2}$)

If the third and fourth values are expressed per kilogram of the patient's body weight, comparisons can be readily made from person to person to study energy expenditure during ambulation.[3]

THE GAIT CYCLE

The normal gait cycle has, by convention, been defined as the period between successive heel strikes of one limb.

Stance Phase

The stance phase of gait comprises 60% of the gait cycle and has five subdivisions—heel strike, loading response, midstance, terminal stance, and preswing (Fig. 22–9).[13] At *heel strike*, the limb meets the floor, with the hip flexed 30°, the knee fully extended, and the ankle in the neutral (90°) position. The foot contacts the floor at a 25° angle. As previously mentioned, the ground force reaction vector passes behind the ankle's center and in front of the hip's and knee's centers (see Fig. 22–5). The ankle dorsiflexors contract to prevent instant foot-slap. Heel strike also marks the beginning of a period of double-limb support that lasts until the opposite limb begins its swing phase (Fig. 22–10). The CG is at its lowest point in the sine wave during double stance (see Fig. 22–1).

Loading response is the time period when the body weight is accepted by the ground in a stable manner, chiefly by a combination of ankle plantar flexion, knee flexion, and subtalar and midtarsal eversion. The ground force reaction vector moves backward until it passes behind the knee's center and close to the hip's center, resulting in the following responses (see Fig. 22–5). After the initial contact of the point of the heel, the body weight is applied through the ankle joint, forcing the foot rapidly into plantar flexion because of the heel lever arm, which extends from the point of the heel to the ankle joint's center. This motion is resisted strongly by the eccentric contraction of the ankle and toe dorsiflexors, allowing controlled descent of the forefoot (Fig. 22–11). The compliance of the plantar surface of the foot to the walking surface is improved by eversion of the subtalar joint. This unlocks the midtarsal joints, allowing dorsiflexion for shock absorption. The limb is forced into internal rotation by this action, improving the alignment of the ankle joint with the plane of progression.

As the ankle and toe dorsiflexors contract to dampen ankle plantar flexion, they also pull the tibia forward, resulting in 15° of knee flexion. The quadriceps undergoes eccentric contraction to dampen and control this motion. Restraint of hip flexion to ap-

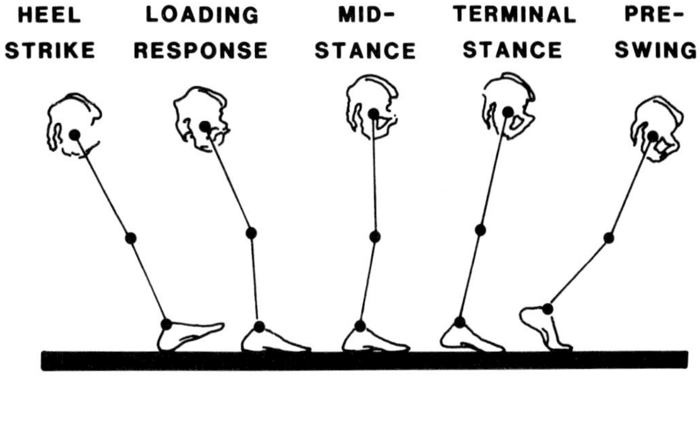

| HEEL STRIKE | LOADING RESPONSE | MID-STANCE | TERMINAL STANCE | PRE-SWING |

FIGURE 22–9. The five subdivisions of the stance phase.

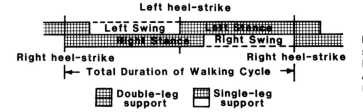

FIGURE 22–10. Phases of the gait cycle, showing periods of single- and double-limb support. (*From* Murray MP, Drought AB, Kory RC: Walking patterns in normal men. J Bone Joint Surg 46:335, 1964.)

proximately 15° is accomplished by the eccentric contraction of the gluteus maximus. Note that knee and ankle motion have a reciprocal relationship that tends to maintain a relatively constant limb length, hence allowing less vertical displacement of the CG. That is, when the foot plantar flexes, thereby increasing limb length, the knee flexes to reduce it; when the foot dorsiflexes, decreasing limb length, the knee extends. Force plate studies show that vertical force increases steadily from heel strike to foot-flat, even exceeding body weight momentarily as the descending mass of the CG loads the new stance foot. Shear recordings demonstrate a forward peak just after heel strike. Initial medial shear on heel contact quickly shifts to lateral shear.

Midstance is characterized by the advance of the body and stance limb over the fixed foot and by the initiation of the swing phase by the opposite lower limb, resulting in a period of single-limb support (Fig. 22–10). During midstance, the ground force reaction vector gradually moves forward along the length of the foot, passing anterior to the knee's center at the midpoint of midstance (see Fig. 22–5). From an initial position of slight plantar flexion, the ankle gradually dorsiflexes to a maximum of 10°, creating an ankle rocker that allows the tibia and, thus, the superincumbent body weight to move forward toward the forefoot. This forward rotation of the tibia on the fixed foot is stopped chiefly by the eccentric contraction of the soleus. By thus restraining the tibia, the femur is free to advance by knee extension, as a result of body momentum produced by the opposite or swing leg. As the knee reaches full extension, the quadriceps relaxes, and knee stability is obtained passively by the strong posterior knee ligaments. With the onset of single stance, the pelvis drops on the swing limb side. This is corrected by contraction of the gluteus medius of the stance limb. During midstance, the vertical loading may actually drop below body weight as the CG passes through its highest point in the sine wave (see Fig. 22–1). Aft

shear occurs as the foot pushes back with reacceptance of body weight.

Terminal stance is initiated by heel rise and ankle dorsiflexion allowing the CG to fall forward of its area of support in the forefoot. This forward fall gives the propulsive force for walking. The resulting ground force reaction vector now passes upward from the forefoot and anterior to the knee's center (see Fig. 22–5). Ankle motion reverses to 5° of plantar flexion and is strongly maintained there by the triceps surae throughout terminal stance. The knee fully extends passively secondary to the forward momentum of the CG, while hip hyperextension beyond 10° is restrained by the iliacus. As weight is transferred to the forefoot, the 30° external slant to the metatarsal head support area (in relation to the long axis of the foot) induces

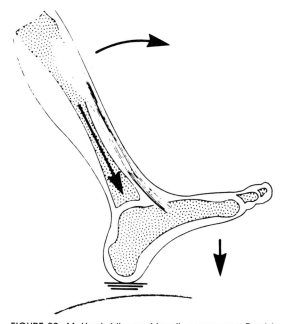

FIGURE 22–11. Heel strike and loading response. Rapid plantar flexion due to the heel lever arm is decelerated by the pretibial muscles, which also pull the tibia forward. (*Reproduced by permission from* Perry J: Normal and pathologic gait. *In* American Academy of Orthopaedic Surgeons: Atlas of Orthotics, 2nd Ed. St Louis, The CV Mosby Co, 1985.)

locking of the subtalar, midtarsal, and midfoot joints; this transforms the previously supple foot into a rigid lever, hence a more efficient rocker. The subtalar joint is maintained in this locked position medially by the tibialis posterior and laterally by the peroneales. The metatarsophalangeal joints dorsiflex, and the toes then contribute to the base of support. Aft shear occurs again as the stance foot thrusts to the rear. Lateral shear forces increase as the CG shifts to the opposite side in preparation for the transfer of body weight to the opposite foot.

Preswing of the stance limb is simultaneous with heel strike of the opposite limb, initiating a second period of double-limb support (see Fig. 22–10). The ground force reaction vector passes from the metatarsal heads anterior to the ankle's center and behind the knee's and hip's centers (see Fig. 22–5). The forward shift of body weight passively flexes the knee to 45° with no quadriceps response because the body weight has been transferred to the new, opposite stance limb. The hip actively flexes to prepare the limb for the swing phase.

Swing Phase

During the swing phase, which comprises 40% of the gait cycle, the foot is lifted from the ground, and the limb is advanced and made ready for acceptance of weight bearing. The swing phase is subdivided into initial swing, midswing, and terminal swing (Fig. 22–12).[13] During *initial swing*, the hip rapidly flexes to 20° because of the concentric contraction of the iliacus, thus advancing the limb. The momentum created produces forward propulsion of the body on the opposite stance limb and, with an assist from the short head of the biceps femoris, gives the 60° of knee flexion needed to allow toe clearance (see Fig. 22–2). During *midswing*, limb advancement continues as the hip and knee each flex 30° and the tibia becomes vertical. Concentric contraction of the ankle dorsiflexors allows the foot to clear the floor in the neutral position. During *terminal swing*, limb advancement ends as it is prepared for stance. Hip flexion is maintained at 30° while the hamstrings decelerate the thigh, leg, and foot with an eccentric contraction; this allows the quadriceps to fully extend the knee and prevents hyperextension. The ankle continues to be held in a neutral position. In summary, during swing phase, the limb is advanced, toe clearance is accomplished, step length is established, and the swing limb is prepared for weight acceptance.

APPLICATION OF GAIT STUDIES TO THE AMPUTEE

The proper integration of the factors previously described will, in the intact human, result in a smooth, energy-efficient gait as reflected not only in minimal displacement of the CG but also in minimal oxygen consumption.

The spiral described by the CG during the gait cycle is determined by the integrated limb and pelvic motions.[15] These in turn depend on the presence of intact, muscle-powered limb segments. Loss or modification of any of these components changes the spiral path of the CG, more so with higher levels or bilaterality of amputation. To compensate for an increased energy requirement, amputees will find progressively slower CWSs to minimize energy use per unit of time with progressively higher levels of amputation

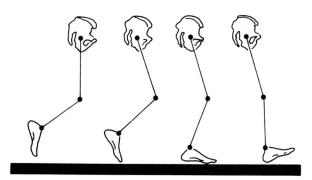

FIGURE 22–12. The three subdivisions of the swing phase.

INITIAL SWING   **MIDSWING**   **TERMINAL SWING**

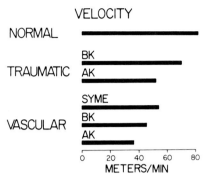

FIGURE 22–13. Normal gait velocity compared with the average gait velocities for persons with different levels of amputation. (*Reproduced by permission from* Perry J, Waters RL: Physiological variances in lower limb amputees. *In* American Academy of Orthopaedic Surgeons: Atlas of Limb Prosthetics. St Louis, The CV Mosby Co, 1981.

(Fig. 22–13). Even within the category of below-knee amputation, energy expenditure during ambulation increases with progressively shorter residual limb length (Fig. 22–14).[5] There are limitations, moreover, to the possibility of functional ambulation for amputees. There is a point at which no matter how slowly the amputee walks, the anaerobic pathway for energy production must be used. Irrespective of the walking speed, this incurs a great expense. The switch from the aerobic to the anaerobic pathway occurs as the oxygen requirement for ambulation becomes more than 50% of the amputee's $\dot{V}max_{O_2}$.[19] This is normally seen in amputation levels

through the knee and higher. For example, the energy cost per unit of distance (ml O_2/kg-m) is 65% above normal for the above-knee amputee.[5] In a study of younger tumor patients, the energy cost was increased 82% with hip disarticulation and 125% with hemipelvectomy.[12]

For bilateral amputees, energy expended during ambulation rises in a more dramatic fashion. A bilateral below-knee amputee requires 41% more energy to walk than does the normal individual; whereas a unilateral below-knee amputee requires only a 25% increase (see Fig. 22–14). A bilateral above-knee amputee, on the other hand, requires 280% more energy to walk than does the normal individual, and a unilateral above-knee amputee requires only a 65% increase.[7] As previously noted, it may not be possible for the amputee to meet these high levels of energy demand.

The question of mobility aids, such as a walker, crutches, and a wheelchair, must also be addressed. It has been found that a unilateral above-knee amputee expends slightly less energy walking with axillary crutches than with an above-knee prosthesis, irrespective of whether the prosthetic knee is locked (Fig. 22–15).[16, 18] Indeed, if the amputee cannot meet the demands of ambulation, wheelchair mobilization—at an energy cost only slightly above normal—may be the answer.[18] This is especially so for older patients with hemipelvectomy, hip disarticulation, or bilateral above-knee or below-knee amputations.[2]

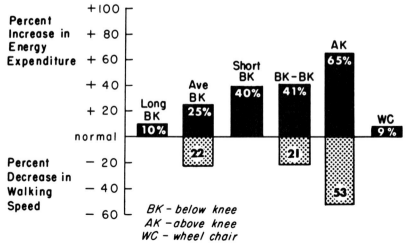

FIGURE 22–14. Energy cost and walking speed for different lengths of below-knee amputation compared with those for above-knee amputation and wheelchair use. (*From* Gonzalez EG, Corcoran PJ, Reyes RL: Energy expenditure in below-knee amputees: Correlation with stump length. Arch Phys Med Rehab 55:111, 1974.)

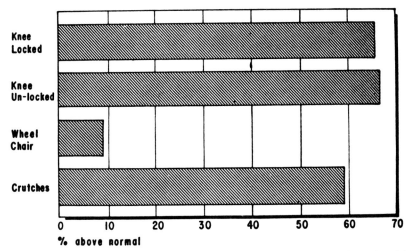

FIGURE 22-15. Comparative energy studies of above-knee amputees using a prosthesis, a wheelchair, or crutches alone. Note that there is no advantage, energy-wise, in using an above-knee prosthesis. (*From* Traugh GH, Corcoran PJ, Reyes RL: Energy expenditure of ambulation in patients with above-knee amputations. Arch Phys Med Rehab 56:67, 1975.)

Relation of Amputation Level to Functional Loss

The toe break in the prosthetic foot at the metatarsophalangeal joint level substitutes for toe dorsiflexion but not for metatarsophalangeal stabilization, subtalar and tarsal motions, and tibial rotation. Controlled descent of the foot after heel strike, a function of the foot dorsiflexors, is provided in the commonly used SACH (solid ankle, cushion heel) foot by compression of its cushion heel and not by an ankle joint. The solid ankle provides a smooth terminal stance by simulating the ankle-joint–stabilizing action of the triceps surae. Subtalar and ankle motions can be simulated by more complex designs, but these add further weight to the prosthesis, a consideration in elderly amputees. Nevertheless, in the case of above-knee amputees, regardless of age, the more rapid forefoot descent inherent in a single-axis foot may, by its increased safety, be worth the extra weight. Younger, athletic individuals may benefit, without significant energy penalty, from a variety of newer energy-storing/releasing foot designs now available.

Syme's amputees enjoy a significant proprioceptive advantage through their end–weight-bearing capability as compared with below-knee amputees, who must bear weight through the proximal tibia, which does not provide proprioceptive feedback on foot placement during normal gait. The strength of the long Syme's lever arm is also an ad-

vantage over the shorter below-knee residual limbs, as is reflected in energy studies.[20]

If the knee joint is removed in the amputation, a marked rise in disability occurs. In through-knee (knee disarticulation) and above-knee amputations, one additional actively controlled joint and proprioceptive source is lost. Prosthetic substitution is even more complex and additional gait motions are lost or modified, resulting in further deviation of the CG from the optimal gait spiral. Control of the prosthetic knee is accomplished by active hip flexion and extension along with the momentum of the below-knee portion of the prosthesis. Various refinements can be added, but each increases the weight and complexity of the prosthesis. For example, hydraulic knee control allows a wider range of walking speeds with a virtually normal duration of stance and swing phases;[10] however, it is suitable chiefly for younger persons with traumatic amputations, with their greater vigor, agility, and tolerance of design complexity. Ankle-knee synchronization is also lost in these amputations but is not substituted for prosthetically. In through-knee, as in Syme's, amputations, proprioception through end–weight-bearing is preserved.[8] In contrast, the above-knee amputee with the standard quadrilateral socket must rely on proprioceptive feedback from the ischial tuberosity, again not a source of feedback in normal gait. Of course, the longer the above-knee residual limb, the more skin area is available for feedback and the greater is the lever arm strength, given a residual limb with proper myodesis.

Moving to an even higher amputation level sacrifices yet another joint. If a hip disarticulation or hemipelvectomy was necessary or if the femoral remnant distal to the hip joint is too short for standard above-knee prosthetic fitting, further substitution is required in the form of a hip disarticulation or hemipelvectomy prosthesis. Active hip control is replaced by the appropriate pelvic and lumbar spine movements, that is, the loss of hip flexion and extension now entails an increased hiking and rotation of the pelvis, with even further straying of the CG from a smooth sinusoidal path. In summary, even though the appropriate prosthesis for higher levels may weigh less than 50% of the limb's ablated portion, its components allow minimal active control by the wearer and provide little vital feedback in terms of proprioception and sensation required for coordination of the prosthesis.

Other Factors Affecting Amputee Gait

In addition to the level of amputation and bilaterality, several other factors, already mentioned briefly, bear directly on the individual amputee's ability to become a functional ambulator. Disorders of the central or peripheral vascular systems—for example, congestive heart failure and peripheral vascular occlusive disease—will restrict the flow of oxygen-bearing blood to the tissues. Diabetes mellitus also affects oxygen delivery to the tissues by impairment of the microvascular circulation. Diseases of the respiratory system that restrict the flow or exchange of

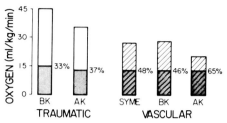

FIGURE 22–16. Aerobic capacity of amputees. The shaded area represents the percentage of the total capacity used for walking. (*Reproduced by permission from* Perry J, Waters RL: Physiological variances in lower limb amputees. *In* American Academy of Orthopaedic Surgeons: Atlas of Limb Prosthetics. St Louis, The CV Mosby Co, 1981.)

gases, such as chronic obstructive pulmonary disease or edema from left-sided cardiac failure, restrict the flow of oxygen at its source. Any of these factors alone can account for diminution of the maximal aerobic capacity. More often than not, in the amputee population, there is a summation effect when more than one factor is involved. This is seen in the common example of the diabetic amputee with peripheral vascular occlusive disease and cardiac and renal decompensation, who is already deconditioned from prolonged bed rest related to the hospital stay. Trauma and tumor amputees, usually younger and in better health, contend with fewer of these factors (Fig. 22–16).

Loss of knee extension (knee flexion contracture) is usually seen in below-knee amputees whose knees did not have the benefit of rigid immobilization during the critical first few postoperative days. Such amputees' increased energy cost is proportional to the severity of the contracture (Fig. 22–17). If their $Vmax_{O_2}$ is borderline, it may be the critical factor preventing functional household ambulation.

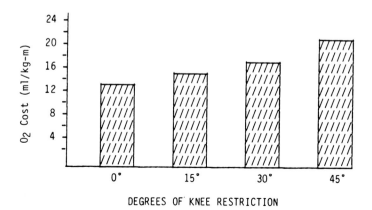

FIGURE 22–17. Increasing energy cost of walking with progressively greater knee flexion contracture. (*Reproduced by permission from* Waters RL, Lunsford BR: Energy expenditure of normal and pathologic gait. Application to orthotic prescription. *In* American Academy of Orthopaedic Surgeons: Atlas of Orthotics, 2nd Ed. St Louis, The CV Mosby Co, 1985.)

SUMMARY

This chapter has tried to provide, as concisely as possible, a biomechanical-physiological rationale applicable to the needs of amputation surgeons and the therapists and prosthetists who assist them in providing the amputee with the best possible mobility options. It remains true, however, that the surgeon's informed decision as to the level of amputation is the single most important factor determining the patient's functional outcome. In short, the preservation of residual limb length, of joints, and of end–weight-bearing capability at the operating table either limits or expands the amputee's subsequent mobility options. Also, since energy expenditure rapidly increases with each higher level of amputation (because of the progressive loss of bone lever length, motors [muscles], articulations, sensory feedback capabilities, and their precisely integrated functions), an effort should be made to determine the lowest possible amputation level that has a reasonable chance to heal, based on methods thoroughly described in Chapters 3 through 9.

There is yet another compelling reason for the surgeon to perform always the most distal amputation feasible. This is the likelihood of vascular failure of the contralateral lower limb if the dysvascular amputee lives long enough. On the basis of the studies of bilateral amputees' functional capabilities presented in this chapter, the opportunity for tissue conservation within the boundary of good surgical judgment should always be taken. The result of this approach in terms of self-care cannot be overestimated. For example, if a Syme's or below-knee amputation was the primary procedure and, later, knee disarticulation or above-knee amputation is unavoidable on the other side, the amputee may still be able to ambulate in the house because the first knee joint was preserved. Last, the amputation surgeon and the team should, ideally, also provide long-term prosthetic follow-up care, as they are the persons most attuned to prevention of amputation of the contralateral limb.

REFERENCES

1. Bowker JH, Hall CB: Normal human gait. *In* American Academy of Orthopaedic Surgeons: Atlas of Orthotics: Biomechanical Principles and Application. St Louis, CV Mosby Co, 1975, pp 133–143.
2. DuBow LL, Witt PL, Kadaba MP, et al: Oxygen consumption of elderly persons with bilateral below knee amputations: Ambulation vs wheelchair propulsion. Arch Phys Med Rehabil 64:255, 1983.
3. Fisher SV, Gullickson G: Energy cost of ambulation in health and disability: A literature review. Arch Phys Med Rehabil 59:124, 1978.
4. Ganong WF: Energy balance, metabolism, and nutrition. *In* Review of Medical Physiology, 12th Ed. Los Altos, Lange Medical Publications, 1985, pp 225–257.
5. Gonzalez EG, Corcoran PJ, Reyes RL: Energy expenditure in below-knee amputees: Correlation with stump length. Arch Phys Med Rehabil 55:111, 1974.
6. Gronley JK, Perry J: Gait analysis techniques. Rancho Los Amigos Hospital Gait Laboratory. Phys Ther 64:1831, 1984.
7. Huang CT, Jackson JR, Moore NB, et al: Amputation: Energy cost of ambulation. Arch Phys Med Rehabil 60:18, 1979.
8. Mensch G: Physiotherapy following through-knee amputation. Prosthet Orthot Int 7:79, 1983.
9. Murray MP, Drought AB, Kory RC: Walking patterns of normal men. J Bone Joint Surg 46A:335, 1964.
10. Murray MP, Mollinger LA, Sepic SB, et al: Gait patterns in above-knee amputee patients: Hydraulic swing control vs constant-friction knee components. Arch Phys Med Rehabil 64:339, 1983.
11. Muybridge E: The Human Figure in Motion. New York, Dover Publications, 1955.
12. Nowroozi F, Salvanelli ML, Gerber LH: Energy expenditure in hip disarticulation and hemipelvectomy amputees. Arch Phys Med Rehabil 64:300, 1983.
13. Perry J: Normal and pathologic gait. *In* American Academy of Orthopaedic Surgeons: Atlas of Orthotics: Biomechanical Principles and Application, 2nd Ed. St Louis, CV Mosby Co, 1985, pp 76–111.
14. Ralston HJ: Energy-speed relation and optimal speed during level walking. Int Z Angew Physiol 17:277, 1958.
15. Saunders JBdeCM, Inman VT, Eberhart HD: The major determinants in normal and pathological gait. J Bone Joint Surg 35A:543, 1953.
16. Sulzle H, Pagliarulo M, Rodgers M, Jordan C: Energetics of amputee gait. Orthop Clin North Am 9:358, 1978.
17. Sutherland DH, Cooper L, Daniel D: The role of the ankle plantar flexors in normal walking. J Bone Joint Surg 62A:354, 1980.
18. Traugh GH, Corcoran PJ, Reyes RL: Energy expenditure of ambulation in patients with above-knee amputations. Arch Phys Med Rehabil 56:67, 1975.
19. Waters RL, Lunsford BR: Energy expenditure of normal and pathologic gait: Application to orthotic prescription. *In* American Academy of Orthopaedic Surgeons: Atlas of Orthotics: Biomechanical Principles and Application, 2nd Ed. St Louis, CV Mosby Co, 1985, pp 151–159.
20. Waters RL, Perry J, Antonelli D, Hislop H: Energy cost of walking amputees: The influence of level of amputation. J Bone Joint Surg 58A:42, 1976.

23

Lower Extremity Prosthetics

Timothy B. Staats, M.A., C.P.

The field of lower limb prosthetics has recently experienced major revolutions in both below-knee and above-knee fitting techniques. The pertinent points of these changes are explained along with classic prosthetic principles. In addition, partial foot, Syme's, hip disarticulation, and hemipelvectomy amputation levels and prosthetic fittings are reviewed.

This chapter examines recent prosthetic developments, such as energy-storing feet, which were developed for very active, athletic, and young individuals. Under pressure from older amputees, prosthetists have begun to experiment with and apply these advanced designs for geriatric patients. In general, the less active patient will benefit from these new prosthetic designs; however, the benefits may not be as dramatic as those in the younger individual. Accordingly, these new advances are presented for the sake of completeness and with the belief that they offer something more to those elderly amputees who do not want to sit still during their golden years.

BELOW-KNEE PROSTHETICS

There are several basic factors that are important in below-knee amputations (BKAs) and that must be considered to produce a

"good" residual limb. First, the tibia and fibula should be 6 to 8 inches in length. Although many texts recommend that the fibula be transected about one half of an inch shorter than the tibia, some progressive surgeons suggest that equal bone length can be biomechanically advantageous. The angle of the transection of both bones should be perpendicular to their shafts, and the cut tibia must be meticulously beveled (45 to 60°) and smoothed. Second, the nerves must be carefully transected under tension and allowed to retract deep into the soft tissue. Third, the muscles and skin must be tailored to avoid redundant tissue. A flabby residual limb is difficult to fit and prone to socket interface problems. Last, poor skin, scarring, skin grafts, and unusual residual limb shapes all create special problems for the prosthetist.

Although problem residual limbs are a prosthetic challenge, they increase the risk of rehabilitation failure. The maturation of the residual limb can be followed up with measurement of the circumference and monitoring of distal edema and suture line appearance. When the residual limb has ceased to atrophy, the prosthetist will recommend that a definitive prosthesis be fitted. This maturation point may be reached as early as 3 weeks after amputation, but usually takes 4 to 6 months or longer, depending on the patient's rate of healing and level of activity.

Before fabricating a permanent prosthesis,

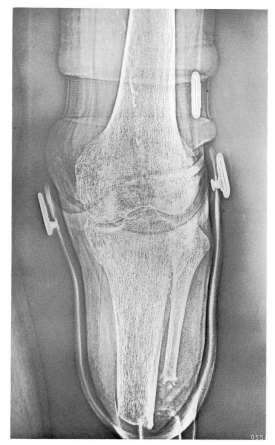

FIGURE 23–1. Xeroradiograph of the residual limb of a BKA, in a prosthesis. Note the bone configuration and spurs.

Measurement and Casting Techniques

Measurements of the residual limb of a BKA normally include anteroposterior and mediolateral dimensions at the level of the mediotibial plateau (MTP) along with a series of circumferential measurements (Fig. 23–2). A plaster impression of the residual limb can be taken in a number of ways; the text describes the diagonal four-stage casting technique.[2] A nylon stocking is applied over the residual limb to act as a compression and shaping barrier between the skin and the plaster. An anterior shell composed of several layers of a rigid plaster splint is molded over the bony anterior compartment, encasing the head of the fibula and the medial flare of the tibia (Fig. 23–3). Vacuum (Fig. 23–4)[3] or controlled pressure[4] may be used to enhance the definition of this first stage of the cast. A second, circular wrap is applied with elastic plaster. This wrap draws the soft posterior tissues forward, compressing them and locking the tibia in position in the cast. This second stage of the cast must be kept well below the popliteal crease of the knee. The third stage, which involves molding the cast

the prosthetist may request X-ray films or xeroradiographs of the amputated limb. These studies provide the prosthetist with information on residual limb maturation, bone configuration, and potential pressure-sensitive areas. Although xeroradiographs expose the patient to more radiation than do X-ray films, their clarity and detail make them preferable for the prosthetist's use.[1] Xeroradiographs can also be used to study the socket fit of the residual limb. Figure 23–1 illustrates the benefits the prosthetist derives from this technique. Notice that the distal tibia has a sharp edge and that the fibula has been cut about 2 inches shorter than the tibia. It looks as if the fibula was bitten off by a beaver rather than removed by modern surgical techniques. The loss of fibula length will limit the mediolateral prosthetic socket stability available to this patient, and the sharp tibia edge will most likely cause pressure tenderness or skin problems.

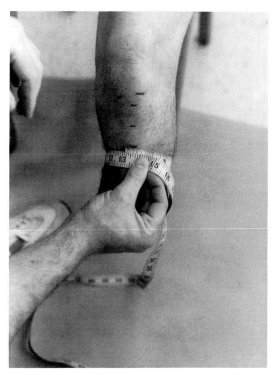

FIGURE 23–2. Circumferential measurement of the residual limb of a BKA.

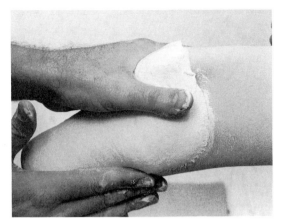

FIGURE 23–3. Anterior stage of the diagonal four-stage procedure for casting the residual limb of a BKA.

brim, forms the posterior trim line of the cast and the hamstring tendon reliefs (Fig. 23–5).

An optional fourth stage may be used to create supracondylar suspension: a plaster splint is carefully molded over the femoral condyles and compressed firmly. The completed cast is carefully removed from the patient and mounted in a gimbal-ring casting stand so that alignment lines can be plumbed on the cast. Alginate dental impression material is applied to the inner surface of the cast in a thick slurry, and the cast is quickly placed back on the patient, who then bears weight into it to create an intimate pressure fit (Fig. 23–6).[5] The cast is removed and immediately filled with plaster of Paris. A mandrel or pipe is placed in the plaster to provide a mount for modifying the cast. The

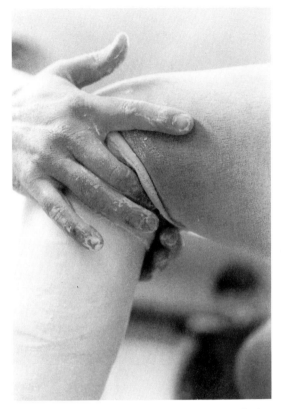

FIGURE 23–5. Hamstring reliefs are created by flexing the knee in the third stage of casting the residual limb of a BKA.

outer wrap cast is removed from the plaster master model, and modification procedures are performed to improve and enhance the fit of the socket (Fig. 23–7).

There are two main philosophies of model modification: total-surface–bearing (TSB) technique[6] and patellar tendon-bearing (PTB) technique.[7] The TSB technique represents a significant advance in the time-honored below-knee PTB modification and fitting technique. In the PTB prosthesis, socket forces are distributed so that more weight is borne by tissues that are thought to be pressure tolerant, and forces are relieved over tissues that are pressure sensitive. In the TSB prosthesis, weight is distributed more or less equally over the entire residual limb surface. No one spot bears more weight than do other areas. The TSB below-knee prosthesis is precision fit, whereas the PTB below-knee prosthesis is designed to be worn with thick residual limb socks. It is beyond the scope of this chapter to thoroughly discuss the detailed differences between the two phi-

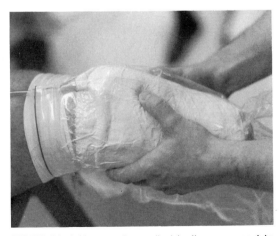

FIGURE 23–4. Vacuum is applied to the wrap cast to compress and define anatomical structures.

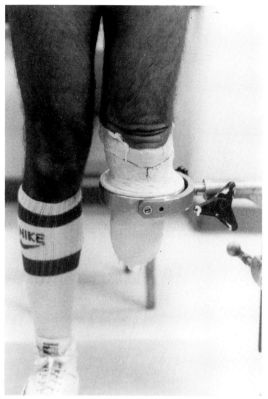

FIGURE 23–6. As the patient stands in a gimbal mount to pressure-fit the cast, alginate is injected into the plaster wrap.

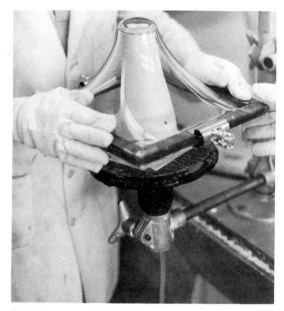

FIGURE 23–8. Molten transparent plastic is thermoformed over the master model.

losophies; however, the author presently teaches TSB techniques and discusses the PTB techniques only for historical purposes.

When modification of the master model is complete, a check socket, used to perfect the fit, is fabricated over the model. The master model is mounted on a vacuum table, and heat-softened transparent plastic is drawn over it. When the plastic has cooled, the transparent socket is removed from the model, trimmed, and polished. Figure 23–8 shows a below-knee socket being formed with a plastic called Surlyn. The prosthetist can visualize and correct socket fit problems with excellent accuracy by further modifying the master model as indicated by fitting problems detected with one or more transparent check sockets (Fig. 23–9).

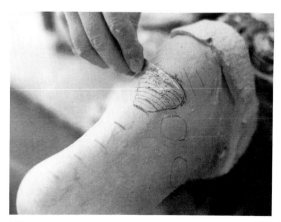

FIGURE 23–7. The master model is altered to match the patient's actual measurements.

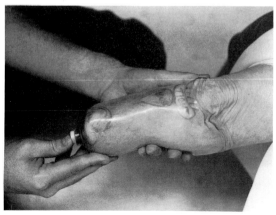

FIGURE 23–9. The prosthetist checks the fit of a flexible transparent test socket on a patient.

Alignment Systems

A variety of adjustable pylon systems are available to align the socket over the prosthetic foot. Generally, these pylons permit angular or slide adjustments, or both, at the junction between the socket and the pylon tube or at the foot and pylon tube interface, or at both. The prosthesis shown in Figure 23–10 illustrates the Otto Bock pylon system,[8] which has angular adjustments at the foot-pylon and socket-pylon interfaces. This type of assembly is known as a nonvertical pylon system. The Otto Bock alignment system is particularly well suited to being left permanently in the prosthesis and enclosed in a cosmetically shaped soft foam cover. For the alignment procedure, the patient is instructed to walk (usually between parallel bars for safety) and is closely observed. The gait pattern may be videotaped (Fig. 23–11) in front and side views so that gait deviations, if any exist, may be analyzed. Slow motion is helpful in the video gait analysis to determine if the prosthetic foot is reacting correctly and if the fit and alignment of the prosthesis are satisfactory. When alignment problems are recognized, adjustments can be made at the pylon-socket or pylon-foot junctions. With the Otto Bock system, only angular adjust-

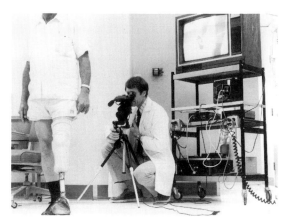

FIGURE 23–11. Video examination of the patient's gait pattern assists in prosthesis alignment.

ments can be made. To effect a lateral adjustment, an angular adjustment must be made at both the foot-pylon and the distal socket-pylon areas to maintain the foot flat on the floor during midstance.

Socket Fabrication

The permanent below-knee prosthesis can be fabricated in a number of ways that include the following features: (1) sockets and liners, (2) suspension systems, (3) endoskeletal and exoskeletal systems, and (4) feet.

The below-knee socket and liner are fabricated over the modified master plaster model, which has been perfected through check sockets and pressure fittings. Once socket fit has been achieved, there are probably 30 different combinations of the four variations listed that can be used in construction of the prosthesis. Laminate materials that can be used as liners include foamed polyethylene, silicone, pelite, leather/Kemblo, and latex, or no liner at all may be used, as in the case of a hard-socket prosthesis. Normally, when a hard-socket prosthesis is made, a foam distal end pad is used to protect the distal limb tissues. Socket liners are generally chosen for their durability and their appropriateness for a particular patient's needs, such as skin condition or sensitivity, climatical environment, or level of activity.

Below-knee suspension systems (the methods of maintaining the prostheses on the patient) include the cuff suspension, shown in Figure 23–12. In that type of suspension system, perhaps the most popular for a be-

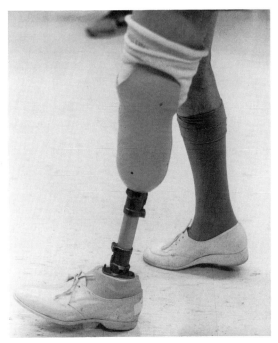

FIGURE 23–10. An adjustable pylon-socket-foot system is used for dynamic prosthesis alignment.

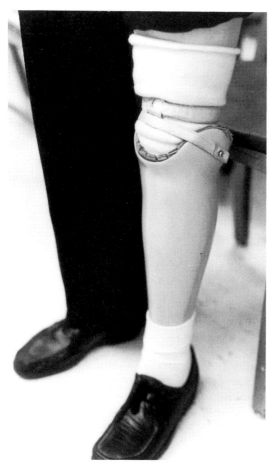

FIGURE 23–12. PTB prosthesis with a Washington cuff suspension system.

cure the socket in position. Latex or Neoprene sleeves (Fig. 23–14) are also very popular suspension systems because they afford a greater degree of movement and comfort. Occasionally, there are problems with sleeve suspension systems, including skin chafing, allergic skin reactions or rashes, and, in some cases, undesirable odors.

The knee side joint and the thigh lacer, or conventional, suspension is used less frequently now than it was 20 years ago. Such a design offers mediolateral stability and transfer of weight distribution to the leather lacer, but important disadvantages of the system include its bulk and the added weight of the lacer and joints. The least bulky and most cosmetic suspension system is suction suspension, in which the intimate fit of the socket creates its own suspension, which is augmented by the patient's natural muscular contractions (Fig. 23–15).

low-knee prosthesis, a cuff of Dacron tape, leather, or a combination of the two is applied across the proximal patella. The cuff both suspends the prosthesis and maintains the knee in flexion, thereby opening the knee joint space and permitting better weight-bearing characteristics between the residual limb and the socket. The knee is held in flexion by the cuff opening; the knee joint space allows it to better contact the socket surfaces.

Another popular suspension system, the supracondylar, is designed so that the socket shape cups over the femoral condyles, thereby suspending the prosthesis. This design is called a PTS or KBM socket design.[9] Figure 23–13 shows one variation of this, called the removable medial wall (RMW) prosthesis.[10] The medial proximal portion of the RMW socket is removed before and replaced after the prosthesis is donned, to se-

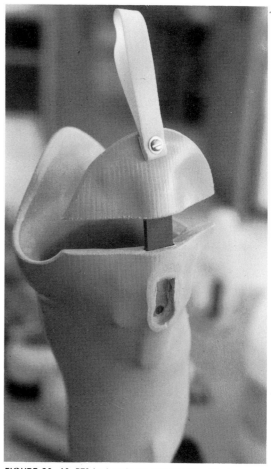

FIGURE 23–13. PTS below-knee prosthesis with a removable medial wall.

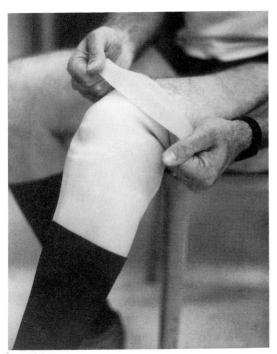

FIGURE 23–14. A patient dons a below-knee prosthesis with a latex sleeve suspension.

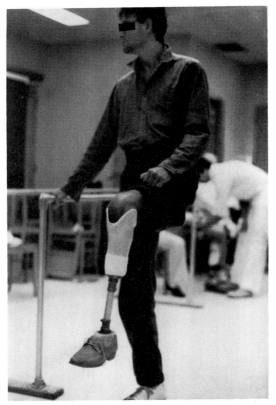

FIGURE 23–15. UCLA below-knee prosthesis with suction suspension. Note the absence of straps, cuffs, or sleeves.

Structural integrity of the prosthesis (attachment of the socket to the foot) can be provided either endoskeletally or ectoskeletally, depending on the patient's preference, level of activity, and weight and durability considerations. In exoskeletal (or hard-finish) limbs, the alignment coupling (socket-pylon-foot system) is removed from the aligned prosthesis and is replaced with rigid urethane foam, balsa wood, or some other lightweight material. The material between the socket and foot is shaped to the measurements of the sound leg, and a lamination of rigid resin and nylon is applied over the outside surface of the prosthesis. When a limb is to be finished using endoskeletal procedures, the inner pylon-foot-socket system is left in place. This inner skeleton can be the actual metal pylon system that was used to align the prosthesis, or the alignment pylon system may be removed from the prosthesis and replaced with a strong and lightweight laminated structure. The final shape of an endoskeletal prosthesis is created with a soft foam cover that is carved to the proper shape or is made by casting the sound leg of the patient and reversing the mold to make a "mirror image."[11] The cosmetic mirror image shell is wrapped around the endoskeletal system, and flexible urethane foam is injected into the cavity between it and the pylon system. When the foam has cured, the outer shell is removed, leaving a soft-finish prosthesis with a cosmetic shape identical to the sound leg. Most men prefer the more durable finish of the exoskeletal prosthesis over the soft foam of the endoskeletal limb. However, most women prefer the cosmetics of the "mirror image" technique. Further cosmetic finishing[12] may be provided through the use of prosthetic skin coverings. Prosthetic skin may be colored to match the patient's skin with air-brushed or hand-applied paints and dyes that are compatible with the skin material.

Recent experiments with computer-aided design and computer-aided manufacturing (CADCAM) have explored the feasibility of applying this technique to below-knee prosthestic sockets.[13] Figure 23–16 shows a graphics display of a prosthesis model that can be modified on the monitor screen (rather than with check sockets and plaster model modifications). When the graphic model modification is complete, the digital measurements are sent to a computer-driven milling machine, which carves a limb model from a block of urethane foam or wax. This

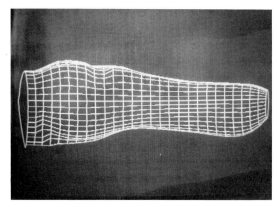

FIGURE 23–16. Graphic display of the computer-aided below-knee socket design technique.

limb model can then be used for fabrication of the permanent prosthesis as previously described. Although the technical feasibility of such systems has been convincingly demonstrated, the economic feasibility has yet to be proved. At present, the limited capability and expense of the computer-directed milling equipment may not permit such CAD-CAM systems to be practical other than in very large centers or for education or research activity.

ABOVE-KNEE PROSTHETICS

The above-knee amputee is much more difficult to fit properly than the below-knee amputee. In addition, the loss of knee function increases the difficulty of making a prosthesis that is safe for ambulation. Above-knee amputations (AKAs), although not ideal from the standpoint of prosthetic design, are nevertheless not unusual and represent the range of problems under discussion. Figure 23–17 illustrates the long residual limb of an AKA in a patient with obvious obesity. The top circumference measurement of this residual limb was almost 30 inches. The very short residual limb (four and one-half inches) of an AKA is shown in Figure 23–18; such very flaccid residual limb tissues are not at all unusual in very short AKAs. The problems of scar tissue from multiple surgical procedures are illustrated in Figure 23–19; skin breakdown, ulceration, osteomyelitis, and numerous surgical revisions have made consistent prosthetic fits difficult for the patient.

As discussed in the prior section on below-knee prosthetics, the use of xeroradiography is very important to the prosthetist for the

discovery and analysis of bony anomalies. Figure 23–20 demonstrates one of the most spectacular bone spurs, or osteophytes, the author has encountered in an above-knee amputee. Most prosthetists would refuse to even attempt a prosthetic fitting with such a bone spur, if they knew it was present; however, not all prosthetists require X-ray films or xeroradiographs of their patients and therefore do not have the opportunity to

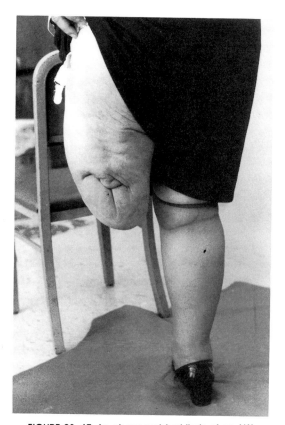

FIGURE 23–17. An obese residual limb of an AKA.

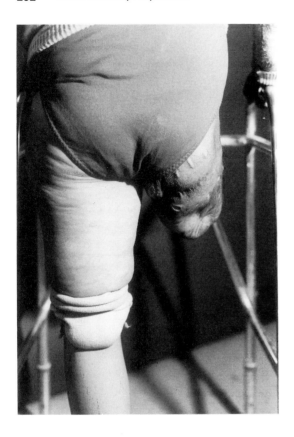

FIGURE 23–18. A short residual limb of an AKA, with heavy scarring.

visualize these sorts of problems before prosthetic fitting. Old femoral shaft fractures may or may not cause fitting problems (Fig. 23–21). In the example shown, the fracture is well healed; it will not present a fitting problem because most of the bony deformation is out of harm's way in the socket and good proximal femur shaft bone is present and can be used to stabilize the residual limb in the socket.

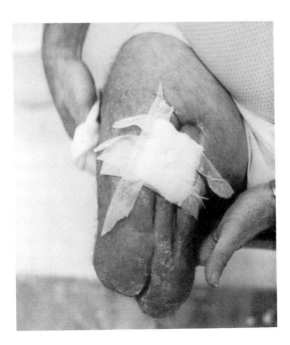

FIGURE 23–19. A residual limb of an AKA, with many surgical scars and drainage from osteomyelitis.

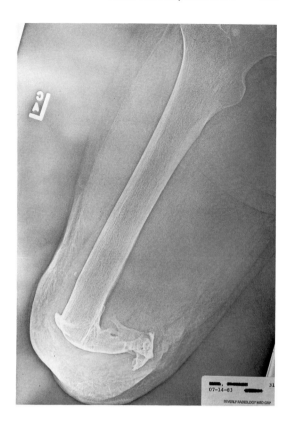

FIGURE 23–20. A xeroradiograph of a residual limb of an AKA, with a giant bone spur.

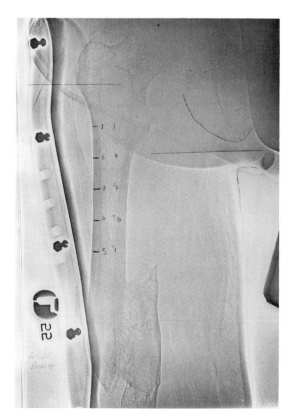

FIGURE 23–21. A residual limb of an AKA, with an old femoral fracture. (*Courtesy of* John Sabolich, Oklahoma City, Oklahoma.)

Measurement and Casting Techniques

As part of the initial process for fitting an above-knee amputee, a series of measurements are taken of the residual limb. The anteroposterior (AP) measurement, the dimension between the ischial tuberosity and the adductor longus tendon (Fig. 23–22), is important for the construction of an above-knee prosthesis with a quadrilateral socket. Generally, the AP measurement on the normal adult will range from about two and one-half to four and one-half inches. The caliper measurement is always checked with a scale. The inner dimension is called the *net* AP, whereas the measurement that actually loads the ischium on the posterior wall of the quadrilateral socket is called the *gross* AP. Accurate circumferential measurements of the residual limb are also extremely important. Consistency of technique is the most important concept in above-knee circumferential measurement. The normal method is to place the tape around the limb at 2 inch intervals, beginning at the ischial level and

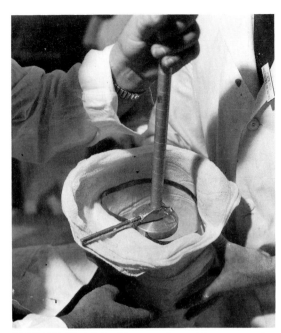

FIGURE 23–23. A Schmid gauge is used to measure the inner cast circumference.

moving down the residual limb. The tape is drawn snug, and the patient is requested to contract the muscles of the residual limb. The tape is allowed to expand to the limit of this contraction, and the measurement is recorded. This skintight measurement is later used in the modification of the master model of the residual limb.

After completion of the circumferential measurements, an elastic plaster bandage is carefully applied to the residual limb in such a way that the tissues do not appreciably elongate. The plaster is wrapped well above the groin and covers the greater trochanter of the femur and the gluteal fold. The patient is then quickly placed in a casting machine, which will deform the proximal portion of the cast into a near quadrilateral socket shape. This deformation may also be done by hand. After the cast hardens, it is carefully removed, and a Schmid gauge is used to evaluate the inner circumferential dimensions (Fig. 23–23). These dimensions are compared with prior AP and circumferential measurements.

The checked wrap cast (Fig. 23–23) may be trimmed and premodified by the application of a plaster slush to help form the shape of a finished socket.[14] This modified cast is reapplied to the patient (Fig. 23–24) with weight bearing while the cast is mounted or

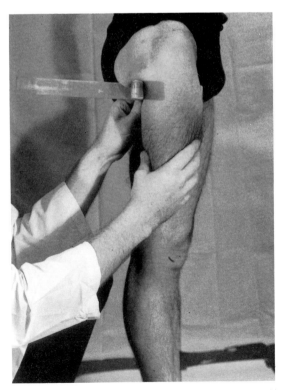

FIGURE 23–22. Taking the anteroposterior measurement of the residual limb of an above-knee amputee.

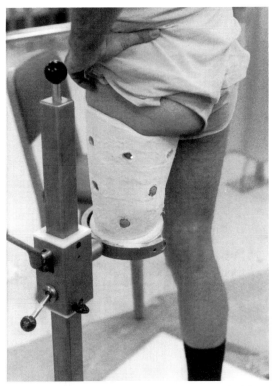

FIGURE 23–24. An above-knee amputee is fitted in a corrected or modified wrap cast by weight bearing.

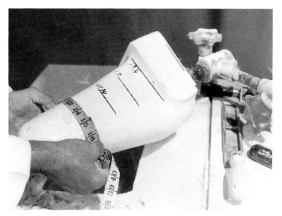

FIGURE 23–25. The master plaster model is modified to the patient's measurements and contour criteria.

suction socket, the tension value measurements are extremely important. When the master model has been completely modified, it is carefully smoothed in preparation for the fabrication of either a transparent check socket or a definitive laminated socket.

There are several techniques for fabricating above-knee transparent plastic check sockets. One method is to use a preformed plastic cone, which is heated and drawn over the model with a vacuum source. Sockets may also be made with flat sheets of heat-softened plastic. For large casts or unusual shapes, pulling the plastic sheet over the plaster model to form a transparent socket may require the precise teamwork of two or three skilled individuals. The socket is then trimmed and removed from the plaster cast.

balanced on a gimbal-ring casting stand. Holes have been cut in the cast so that tissue tension and total skin contact can be assessed by the prosthetist. When the premodification fitting check is completed, the cast is removed from the patient and filled with plaster. The resultant cast model is then modified following the procedure described by Bray[15]—a series of about 30 steps, each related to information gathered during the previous measurement and evaluation procedure.

The final stage of model modification is to match the circumference measurements of the plaster cast to those of the residual limb (Fig. 23–25). The final socket circumference measurements will be somewhat smaller than the residual limb values. This reduction of circumferences is called the tension value. Tension value tables[16] are used to modify the model cast. If a residual limb sock will be used with a pelvic joint and waist belt for prosthesis suspension, tension value measurements are not critical to socket fit. The patient's ability to walk, gait, and general rehabilitation success will also reflect this less critical fitting procedure. However, for the creation of a suction socket or flexible brim

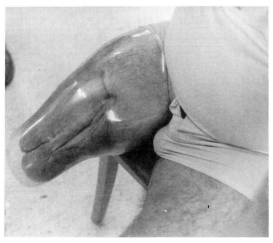

FIGURE 23–26. A transparent test socket is fitted to an above-knee amputee. Note the lack of total contact when the patient is sitting. Total contact should be achieved when the patient is standing.

The plaster cast is saved so that if changes in the socket are required to perfect the fit, a new cast need not be made. The transparent check socket is now fitted to the patient; corrections, if required, are noted, and the plaster model is modified appropriately. In Figure 23–26, the check socket does not make total contact; however, the patient is seated. When this patient stands, with full weight bearing, the socket void should be filled with tissue; however, if after several trials total contact is not achieved, it may be necessary to correct the cast and make a new check socket.

Alignment Systems and Socket Fabrication

Transparent sockets may be bench-aligned and used in dynamic fittings and walking trials. Bench alignment is a basic starting alignment of the socket in relation to the knee bolt axis and the foot. It represents a starting relationship only and will most likely be altered during dynamic (walking) alignment of the prosthesis. The prosthesis is held in an alignment fixture to establish these stationary relationships accurately. When the socket is fitted to the patient (Fig. 23–27), the following factors become extremely important:

1. Is the prosthesis the correct length when the socket is correctly fit?
2. Is the knee stable and safe?
3. Is the knee bolt axis aligned so that it swings-through without deviation on the line of progression?
4. Is the foot positioned correctly under the socket, and does it support the patient to create a natural gait?

Usually, all walking trials should be done with safety rails or parallel bars. If gait deviations are spotted during a dynamic alignment session, the alignment must be changed to eliminate them. Some components have built-in alignment features. In the Otto Boch alignment system shown in Figure 23–28, adjustments are made with Allen wrenches. Screws in the alignment coupling oppose a pyramid-like projection, and angular adjustments are made by adjusting two Allen screws simultaneously. Rotation and linear adjustments are also possible, although linear adjustments must be accomplished through opposing angular adjustments.

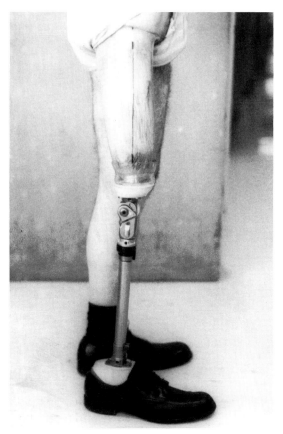

FIGURE 23–27. Dynamic alignment of the prosthesis using a transparent test socket and modular endoskeletal components.

Alternative alignment units include the Berkeley above-knee adjustable leg and the Staros-Gardner Veterans Administration Prosthetic Center (VAPC) coupling. The Berkeley was one of the first units developed;

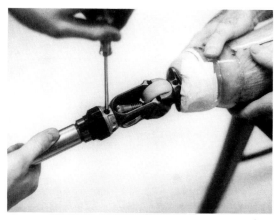

FIGURE 23–28. The built-in alignment feature of the Otto Bock knee-pylon system is clearly shown in this photo.

it is easy to use and offers angular, linear, and length adjustment. However, a basic disadvantage of this unit is that it does not allow for alignment of the prosthesis with the knee mechanism that will be incorporated into the finished prosthetic limb. If the geometry and action of the definitive knee mechanism are different than those of the alignment unit, as it often is, the final alignment with the Berkeley system may have to be readjusted when the knee mechanism is fitted into the prosthetic limb. The VAPC coupling does not have this disadvantage. Normally, a new above-knee amputee will be given basic instructions and initial gait training by the prosthetist. After satisfactory alignment parameters for the new limb have been achieved, the prosthetist may arrange long-term gait training with a physical therapist if needed. Amputees who have consistently worn a lower limb prosthesis will rarely need physical therapy training when a new limb is fabricated.

There are probably over 50 knee mechanisms that can be used in the definitive above-knee prosthesis. It is beyond the scope of this chapter to discuss all of them. The prescribing physician should consult the prosthetist when selecting an appropriate knee design to suit a particular patient's needs. Knee mechanisms fall into two general categories: exoskeletal (crustacean) and endoskeletal (skeletonlike). Within each of these major categories are the following subcategories: constant friction, hydraulic and pneumatic, locking, and polycentric systems.

A Hydracadence[17] hydraulic knee mechanism with a VAPC adjustable coupling is shown during dynamic alignment (Fig. 23–29). This particular knee unit permits hydraulic swing-phase cadence response, controlled ankle motion, and heel height adjustment. It was one of the first modular knee mechanisms in which the hydraulic cartridge could be changed very quickly. A more modern modular hydraulic knee unit,[18] which has a compact design that allows it to be used in patients with very slender limbs, is shown in Figure 23–30. With the built-in alignment system of the Otto Bock hydraulic modular knee, changes and quick replacement are possible even after the unit has been delivered in a definitive prosthesis.

The finished quadrilateral above-knee socket has a classic shape (Fig. 23–31). All edges are smoothed and rounded, and the

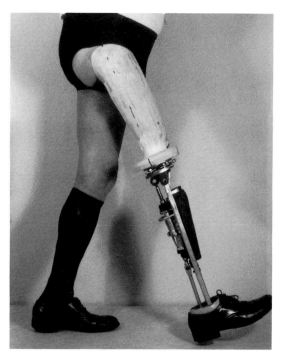

FIGURE 23–29. Dynamic alignment of an above-knee prosthesis with a Hydracadence hydraulic knee and a VAPC adjustable alignment system.

inner socket surface is highly polished. The outer finish of the prosthesis is either a durable hard finish or a cosmetic soft foam cover that, while not durable, is pleasing to

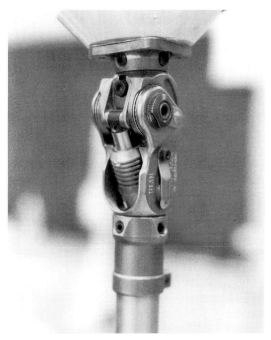

FIGURE 23–30. The Otto Bock hydraulic modular knee.

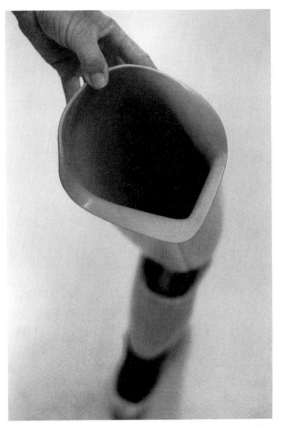

FIGURE 23–31. The standard quadrilateral socket brim of a finished above-knee prosthesis.

Very obese above-knee amputees may be comfortably fit with standard quadrilateral sockets. However, donning a prosthesis in the conventional manner, using either a pull sock or an Ace bandage, can be extremely difficult or virtually impossible. With very fleshy patients, it is possible to use a "wet fit" procedure in which the residual limb is lubricated with lotion or cream, permitting easy entry into the prosthesis without the use of a pull sock. It will take several minutes for all tissues to arrange themselves in correct location in the socket, but very satisfactory fitting results can be obtained using this technique.

The development of the contoured adducted trochanteric-controlled alignment method (CAT-CAM) above-knee socket [20] in 1985 was the first significant departure from quadrilateral socket shape theory in about 30 years. The CAT-CAM is a socket design variation in which the mediolateral dimension is compressed and the ischial tuberosity slides inside the medial socket wall; this is unlike the quadrilateral design, in which the anteroposterior dimension is compressed and the ischial tuberosity rests on the socket brim (Fig. 23–34). The socket is unusual in that it

feel and very lightweight compared with exoskeletal finishes. Wearers of suction-socket above-knee prostheses don them using either a length of tubular cotton stockinette or an elastic Ace bandage (Fig. 23–32). By loosely winding the elastic wrap around the residual limb and feeding the loose end through the air valve hole in the middle of the prosthesis' bottom, the residual limb may be gently pulled into the socket. The patient must develop the skill to don the limb in the correct toe-in or toe-out position, as it is possible to pull the leg on incorrectly, as much as 5° out of rotational alignment.

A new above-knee socket fabrication technique used with the quadrilateral design is called the Swedish flexible socket[19] or the Icelandic-New York (ISNY) socket (Fig. 23–33). The socket consists of a very thin transparent flexible socket supported by a heavily reinforced medial wall strut. Patients have reported improved comfort, but prosthetists are reporting durability problems with the inner sockets.

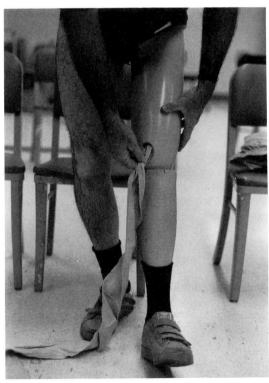

FIGURE 23–32. An above-knee amputee dons his prosthesis.

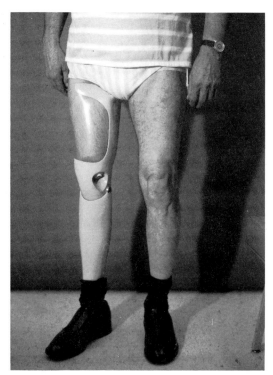

FIGURE 23–33. An above-knee amputee wears the ISNY flexible socket combined with a quadrilateral brim.

is totally flexible and made of thermoplastic materials, such as low-density polyethylene or Surlyn or of flexible resin laminate. Improved suspension and gait have been reported with this technique, but fabrication and fitting are more difficult than with the standard quadrilateral design.

There are rare above-knee prosthetic situations that call for unusual solutions. The patient in Figure 23–35 has a completely flail

and paralyzed residual limb as a result of childhood polio. The waist belt performs the dual function of creating a cosmetic buttocks shape build-up while providing artificial muscle control through elastic straps. An anterior "adductor" elastic strap holds the leg under the patient during swing phase. A "hamstring" elastic strap prevents excess hip flexion at the end of swing phase. This patient has been able to control his prosthesis without the aid of canes or crutches.

Many bilateral above-knee amputees find that "stubbie" prostheses are useful as a steppingstone to wearing full-length prostheses (Fig. 23–36). The stubbies are also practical for many activities of normal daily living. The decision to fit stubbies may relate to the question of whether the patient is really capable of handling artificial limbs. If the amputee cannot be made comfortable in stubbies, it would appear to negate the possibility of using full-length prostheses successfully. If the patient can demonstrate balance and agility in stubbies, it may be an indication not only that normal length prosthetic legs will work but that the patient is motivated to strive for success. The shape of the "feet" on stubbies can be developed to the patient's needs. In the case of the patient in Figure 23–36 blocks of rock-hard maple with hiking boot soles were used. Some patients will use

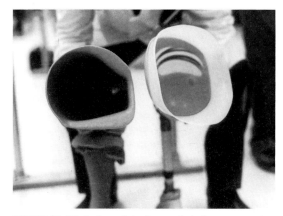

FIGURE 23–34. A down-into-the-socket view comparing the quadrilateral (left) with the CAT-CAM (right) socket design.

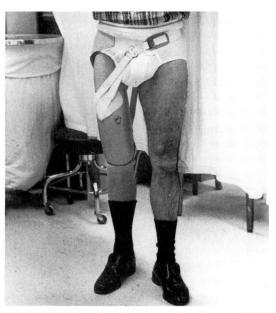

FIGURE 23–35. An above-knee amputee whose residual limb is paralyzed as a result of childhood polio uses elastic webbing for artificial muscle control of his prosthesis.

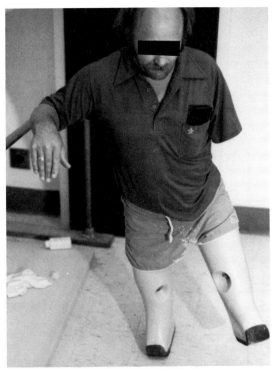

FIGURE 23–36. A bilateral above-knee amputee wearing stubbie prostheses.

solid ankle, cushion heel (SACH) feet mounted in reverse on the bottom of the sockets. The flexible toes of the SACH feet give the patient some sensation of pushoff.

The final cosmetic finish of an above-knee prosthesis depends on whether it is endo-skeletal or exoskeletal; the finishes are similar to those discussed for the below-knee systems.

PROSTHETIC FEET

Prosthetic feet designs are as varied as socket liner materials. Popular styles include the SACH foot, the SAFE (stationary ankle, flexible endoskeleton) foot,[21] the Seattle foot,[22] and the Flex-foot.[23] The SACH foot is the most widely used design. It is inexpensive, durable, and offers a reasonably good gait when properly fitted. The foot is constructed around an inner keel made of hard wood and rubber belting. The outer shape is high-density flexible urethane foam, and the heel is also urethane foam, the density depending on the weight of the patient. Variations of the SACH foot include either an internal or external keel and models with or without molded toes.

The SAFE foot was designed to emulate the windlass action of the plantar fascia of the normal foot. It incorporates a keel made of flexible urethane elastomer with a none-lastic Dacron strap that connects the heel and toe sections. As the amputee rolls over the toe during plantar flexion, the strap stiffens, much like the plantar fascia in a normal foot. The combination of "restive plantar flexion" and heel and foot flexibility has made the SAFE foot very popular with many wearers, particularly those whose activities require that they walk on uneven surfaces.

The concept of energy storage in prosthetic feet has recently been incorporated into several new prosthetic foot designs. The Seattle foot (Fig. 23–37) uses a keel design (much like a leaf spring) of high-strength, nondeformable Delrin plastic. The foot stores energy during foot roll over (the plantar flexion phase of walking) then returns the stored energy in the form of a "push" that propels the wearer forward at toe-off. Early versions of the Seattle foot featured a composite carbon-graphite keel. Although very lightweight, the original keel was prone to breakage. The present design has been field tested on 500 patients and is now commercially available. The Flex-foot (Fig. 23–38) is the most advanced design available in energy storage prosthetic foot systems. Fabricated of carbon-graphite and fiberglass, the Flex-foot is individually designed and tailored to the weight and activity level of each particular patient. The foot consists of two components, a toe/shaft and a heel. Both components compress when weight is ap-

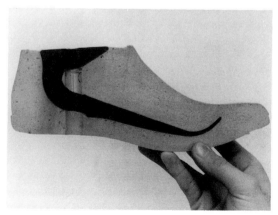

FIGURE 23–37. Longitudinal cut-away view of the Seattle foot.

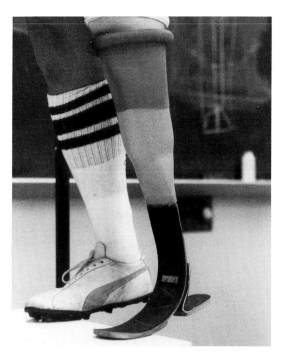

FIGURE 23–38. A below-knee Flex-foot prosthesis without a cosmetic cover is shown in stance phase.

plied, and the stored energy is released as the body weight rolls over the individual foot structures. The Flex-foot is cosmetically finished with foam blocks that are modified to create a normal limb shape.

UNCOMMON AMPUTATION LEVELS

Partial Foot Amputation

Partial foot amputations (including Chopart's and Lisfranc's amputations) present difficult challenges for the prosthetist. If the remaining bones do not migrate after amputation, the prosthetist has a reasonable chance of making the patient comfortable. The primary problem is the construction of a prosthesis that will both be cosmetic and fit inside a shoe. Fabrication of such a prosthesis is very time consuming, and failure is very common, especially when the foot bones migrate or go into fixed plantar flexion (contracture). One prosthetic solution is a slipper-style prosthesis made of latex rubber and polyethylene foam (Plastozote) and covered with horsehide leather.[24] Such a prosthesis

will last about a year with normal use. A more advanced type of prosthetic limb is shown in Figure 23–39; the prosthesis was fabricated with a complicated mold-making process developed by Chuck Childs, CPO; it is called the STEP prosthesis.[25] The prosthesis is injection molded from a tough polyurethane elastomer reinforced with nylon and Dacron belting. The final result is a prosthesis that blends well with the shape of the patient's residual foot and is difficult to detect if cosmetic hose are worn over it.

Syme's Amputation

The Syme's amputation is fairly uncommon, particularly among those patients whose amputations were due to the complications of vascular insufficiency or diabetes mellitus. However, Syme's amputees make excellent candidates for prosthetic rehabilitation if they are capable of full weight bearing and if the distal fat pad is secure and not prone to migration. Probably the worst candidates for a Syme's amputation are those persons who place undue emphasis on their physical appearance—irrespective of the reason for the amputation—because neither the amputated limb nor the Syme's prosthesis is very cosmetic.

The long length of the residual limb forces the prosthetist to carve into the prosthetic foot to achieve equal leg length. The combination of a bulbous distal limb end, long limb length, and the narrow midshaft of the leg requires very accurate casting and many cast modifications to fabricate a good-fitting prosthetic limb. A two-stage wrap cast is used,

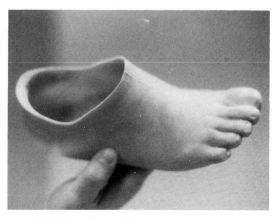

FIGURE 23–39. The STEP partial foot prosthesis.

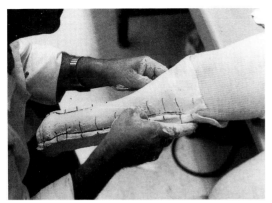

FIGURE 23-40. The posterior stage of the two-stage casting procedure for a Syme's amputation.

and the anterior and posterior stages are keyed together along alignment lines (Fig. 23-40). The prosthesis is dynamically aligned without an alignment coupling system between the prosthesis and the foot; this is because of the lack of space between the distal end of the limb and the prosthetic foot. The patient shown in Figure 23-41 is wearing a Syme's prosthesis with a medial window.

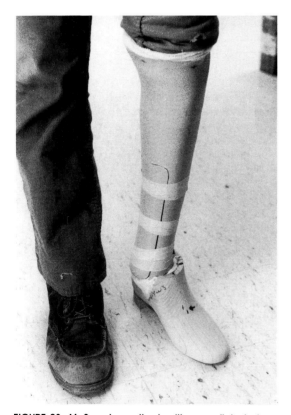

FIGURE 23-41. Syme's prosthesis with a medial window is shown in the fitting stage. Notice that the socket is sunk into a carved-out foot.

The opening is necessary so that the bulbous distal end of the limb can pass into the socket without getting stuck in the narrow ankle area of the prosthesis. Other techniques for solving this problem of fitting and fabrication involve special liners or expandable wall sockets. The final prosthetic limb is aligned by approximation, and the amputee walks and is evaluated. If the alignment is incorrect, the foot and socket are separated and carefully reconnected in a more optimal relationship. When the correct alignment is achieved, the entire limb is laminated with a final coat of plastic in order to reinforce and cosmetically finish the prosthesis. The medial window cutout is usually secured with straps, Velcro fasteners, or buckles.

Hip Disarticulation

The hip disarticulation amputation is perhaps even more uncommon than the Syme's amputation. This amputation is most often performed for cancer or trauma and rarely for vascular disease. The prosthesis (Fig. 23-42) is made in stages similar to those used for other lower limb prostheses. A plaster

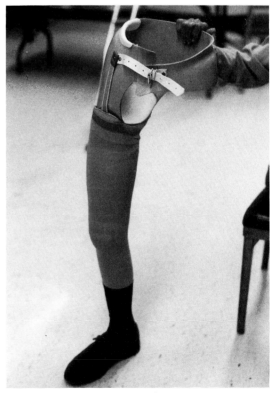

FIGURE 23-42. A modular hip disarticulation prosthesis.

cast is taken from the amputated limb, modified, and laminated as previously described. The prosthetic limb is then fabricated over the laminated socket; it is usually composed of an endoskeletal system with a foam cover in order to minimize weight. The socket is made flexible across the back portion by laminating the proper areas with flexible plastic resins. Total firm skin contact with the residual limb is important.

Patients who receive hip disarticulation prostheses are divided into two categories: those who wear their limbs and those who don't. Patients who are successful prosthetic limb-wearers can again be divided into three subcategories: those really rare individuals who walk unaided, the more common group who wear their prostheses but walk with two crutches, and those who wear their prostheses only while sitting or only on special occasions. What distinguishes hip disarticulation patients from all other lower limb amputees is that they have to be very motivated if they are going to learn to walk. Most persons with amputations at this level will not ambulate, but they often do not want to be seen in public without their prosthetic limb. Unfortunately, it is difficult to make an attractive hip disarticulation prosthesis. Prosthetic skins have been developed, but they usually cannot tolerate the excessive stretching required at the hip joint in the ambulatory patient. Therefore, its use for hip disarticulation is confined to those patients who walk only some of the time or who want the prosthetic limb for only cosmetic reasons.

Hemipelvectomy

The hemipelvectomy prosthesis is similar in construction to the hip disarticulation prosthesis. Since the amputee has no pelvis on the amputated side, it is very difficult to achieve true socket stability. Body weight is supported in the socket in the areas of residual limb tissue, and also under the rib cage. These prostheses tend to be heavy (10 to 20 pounds), despite the use of lightweight materials in their construction. Ambulation with this level of amputation is even more uncommon than at the hip disarticulation level.

Multiple Limb Amputation

The prosthetist will occasionally fit very complex multiple limb amputation cases. A quadruple amputee with his prostheses is shown in Figure 23–43. The right-sided lower extremity prosthesis was a Canadian hip disarticulation prosthesis with a stance-phase locking-knee mechanism and a SACH foot; the left limb had a proximal femoral focal deficiency that required a modified above-knee prosthesis with a stance-phase locking-knee mechanism and a SACH foot. In addition, special pelvic straps were required to prevent socket rotation during ambulation. The locking knees permitted the patient to roll into a seated position from a standing one using his upper extremity prosthesis, without fear of having the knees buckle. This patient is a full-time ambulator and enjoys elk hunting with his friends. This is probably a good case to recall whenever the decision is being made to either pursue or give up on the rehabilitation of a particular patient. Patient attitude is all important.

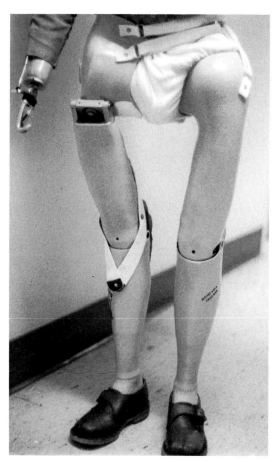

FIGURE 23–43. A multiple amputation patient.

REFERENCES

1. Varnau D, Vinnecour K, Luth M, Cooney D: The enhancement of prosthetic fit through xeroradiography. Orthot Prosthet 39:14, 1985.
2. Staats T: Advances in prosthetic techniques for below knee amputations. Orthopedics 8:249, 1985.
3. Hittenberger D, Carpenter K: A below knee vacuum casting technique. Orthot Prosthet 37:15, 1983.
4. McQuirk A, Morris A: Controlled Pressure Casting Technique Teaching Manual. London, Hanger Co, 1982.
5. Hayes R: A below knee weight bearing pressure formed socket technique. Clin Orthop Prosthet 9:13, 1985.
6. Stokosa J: Prosthetics for lower limb amputees. *In* Haimovici H: Vascular Surgery, 2nd Ed. Norwalk, Connecticut, Appleton-Century-Crofts, 1984.
7. Radcliffe C, Foort J: The Patellar-Tendon–Bearing Below-Knee Prosthesis. University of California, Berkeley Biomechanics Laboratory, 1961.
8. Otto Bock Orthopedic Industries, Minneapolis, Minnesota.
9. Marschall K, Nitschke, R: Principles of the PTS BK prosthesis. Orthop Prosthet Appliance J 21:33, 1967.
10. Fillauer C: The removable medial wall below knee prosthesis. Orthot Prosthet 25:26, 1971.
11. Childs C: The Mirror Image Finishing Technique Teaching Manual. UCLA Prosthetics and Orthotics Education Program, Advanced Below Knee Seminar, Fall 1984.
12. Lundt J, Staats T: The USMC prosthetics skin. Orthot Prosthet 37:59, 1983.
13. Saunder CG: Computer Aided Socket Design Teaching Manual. Vancouver, Medical Engineering Research Unit, Shannessey Hospital, March 1984.
14. Otto Bock Orthopedic Industries: Technical Manual. UCLA Prosthetics and Orthotics Education Program, Advanced Prosthetics Techniques Seminar, 1984.
15. Bray J: Total Contact Plastic Suction Socket Manual, 6th Ed. UCLA Prosthetics and Orthotics Education Program, 1981.
16. Anderson M, Bray J: Prosthetic Principles, Above Knee Amputations. Springfield, Illinois, Charles C Thomas, 1960.
17. Hydracadence Technical Manual. Pasadena, United States Manufacturing Co.
18. Otto Bock Orthopedic Industries: Hydraulic Module Knee Mechanism.
19. Swedish Flexible Socket Technical Manual. Chattanooga, Durr Fillauer Inc.
20. Sabolich J: The CAT CAM above knee socket. Clin Prosthet Orthot 9:15, 1985.
21. Campbell J, Childs C: The SAFE foot. Orthot Prosthet 34:3, 1980.
22. Burgess E, Hittenberger D, Forsgren S: The Seattle foot. Orthot Prosthet 37:25, 1983.
23. Leal J: The Flex-foot prosthesis. UCLA Prosthetics and Orthotics Education Program, Advanced Prosthetics Techniques Seminar, 1984.
24. Sethi PK, Udawat MP, Kasliwal SC, Chandra R: A Vulcanized rubber foot for lower limb amputees. Prosthet Orthot Int 1:125, 1978.
25. Childs C: The STEP prosthesis. UCLA Prosthetics and Orthotics Education Program Teaching Manual, 1983.

24

New Developments in Prosthetics

Jan J. Stokosa, C.P.

There is nothing more difficult to take in hand, more perilous
to conduct, or more uncertain in its success, than to take the
lead in the introduction of a new order of things, because
the innovator has for enemies all those who have done well
under the old conditions, and lukewarm defenders in those
who may do well under the new.
NICCOLÒ MACHIAVELLI (1469–1527)

The best we have to offer the amputee is none too good.
WALTER STOKOSA, C.P. (1919–1971)

A review of the literature reveals that the desire to improve the rehabilitation of amputees has created a surge of research in amputation surgery and prosthetics. There is little question that such efforts have improved almost every area within the prosthetist's domain of amputee rehabilitation. Undoubtedly, many amputees are being increasingly better served. However, there is, and always will be, an opportunity to further improve lower extremity prosthetics.

Effeney and associates[9] and Hoaglund and colleagues[15] conducted a survey and an evaluation of the problems and needs of veterans with traumatic amputations and amputations for vascular disease; they discovered that most members of these groups had residual limb pain. Within the dysvascular group, 75% of the below-knee amputees complained of pain while walking. Within the traumatic amputation group, 58% associated pain with wearing the prosthesis, and 37% noted pain without the prosthesis. Evaluation of the quality of the prosthesis revealed improper socket fit in 59% of below-knee amputees and in 78% of above-knee amputees. Additional noteworthy deficiencies were the high frequency of mechanical skin irritation, skin breakdown, prosthesis misalignment, improper suspension, and foot dysfunction. Most of these deficiencies were found to be due to improper initial socket design and prosthesis construction in general. The investigators concluded that new research in socket design is needed to reduce the incidence of residual limb pain effectively.

Wilson[41] and Rose[33] argue cogently that the government has lost interest in prosthetic research and development and that the Veterans Administration has lost its position as the world's leader in the field of prosthetics. Wilson expands his view by citing that less than one fourth of the reports contained in the Fall 1979 issue of the *Bulletin of Prosthetics Research* (BPR #10-32) relate to prosthetics. Wilson concludes that perhaps the prosthetics profession has grown to assume leadership in research, development, evaluation, and education and states that most manuscripts submitted to *Orthotics and Prosthetics* (the journal of the American Orthotics and Prosthetics Association) are from private practitioners.

New developments are competing with established achievements that have been serving amputees well—some for decades. Many new theories have emerged that promise an improved life for the amputee. Such new thoughts include

1. An amputee should not experience pain as a natural consequence of amputation.

2. The amputee, surgeon, and prosthetist are the primary players on the rehabilitation team—when necessary, other specialists are consulted.

3. It is not possible to determine the details of a prosthesis before the actual fitting and trial by the amputee; therefore, the most efficient, functional socket design or prosthetic foot, ankle, knee, or hip mechanism that will best suit the varied and individual requirements of an amputee cannot be "prescribed" in advance of fitting.

4. Amputees can do things that heretofore were believed to be beyond their abilities.

Each new applied theory, each development, is vying for "paradigm" status.

Paradigms gain their status because they are more successful than their competitors in solving a few problems that the group of practitioners recognizes as acute. Some new paradigms will create a revolution within the community of amputee rehabilitation specialists. The use of this metaphor emphasizes that when an existing paradigm—one that has served both the amputee and the prosthetist well—has ceased to function adequately for the amputee, a crisis situation exists, and a new paradigm is initiated. It will by nature meet with resistance from those within the community who adhere to the older paradigm (hence this chapter's epigraph). Proponents of a new paradigm claim that it can solve the problems that led the old one to crisis.

Some paradigms are clearly well established, whereas others are gallantly competing to attract supporters. This chapter provides the reader with clinically useful information on some new developments in extremity prosthetics.

TREATMENT PROCESS OVERVIEW: A UNIFIED APPROACH*

The proliferation of new developments has touched nearly every aspect of prosthetic fitting; therefore, it may be beneficial to review this entire process. Some procedures are dealt with in detail as they appear in this section; others are expanded in later sections.

The desideratum in lower extremity prosthetic fitting is comfort to the wearer, with maximal mobility, function, and cosmesis. The author agrees with Murdoch[26] that the patient, surgeon, and prosthetist should thoroughly discuss the patient's next 30 years of prosthetic wear and establish a plan accordingly.

The goal of the prosthetist is to aid amputees in re-entering and regaining their

---

*Most discussion in this section concerns the below-knee and above-knee amputation levels, for simplicity. The same general principles apply to patients with amputations at other levels—from partial foot amputation to hemipelvectomy—and those with multiple amputations.

places in society—working, playing, and engaging in a full range of human relationships. Progress in this endeavor is marked by the amputee's placing a diminishing emphasis on the amputation and prosthesis. Ideally, the amputation and prosthesis will move outside the inner circle of the amputee's life concerns. The prosthetist's role in this process, in the broadest terms, is to enhance the amputee's mobility and appearance, with maximal comfort.

Achievement of the prosthetist's goal is ultimately dependent on five factors: (1) the general physical and mental condition of the amputee, (2) the amputee's understanding of the rehabilitation process, (3) the level of amputation, (4) the quality of the surgery and the physiology of the residual limb, and (5) the degree of comfort, mobility, and cosmesis afforded by the prosthetist.

These five factors can be achieved *only* through the cooperation of the *essential* participants: the patient, the surgeon, and the prosthetist. The physiatrist, nurse, physical therapist, rehabilitation counselor, family members, and others may also be productively involved. Although it is generally accepted that the multidisciplinary team approach to rehabilitation yields maximal results,[4, 18, 25] it should be noted that most amputees do not follow a rehabilitation program that includes such a defined team. Consequently, for any particular amputee, the members of the treatment team may vary in their relative importance to that process. The surgeon and the prosthetist usually have the greatest impact on the rehabilitation of the amputee.

An alternative to the full team is the team of three: the amputee, the surgeon, and the prosthetist.[37] With open communication, effective results are possible.

Prosthetists should, from their first contact with an amputee, provide counsel regarding the complex interplay of the genuine physical or technical limitations and the individual amputee's aspirations and will. In light of ever-emerging prosthetic techniques and procedures, the question of "what is possible?" should always be left open. A good mental formula for assessing what is possible for an individual amputee is

(Objective Physical Capability + Available Relevant Technology + Prosthetist's Ability and Willingness to Innovate)
× Amputee's Aspirations and Will =
What Is Possible[38]

It is the prosthetist's fundamental purpose to help the amputee in realizing a whole life and existence in his or her environment; this approach is expressed by maintaining a personal dialogue, showing compassion, sharing personal experiences, cultivating a deep empathy, and adhering to technical excellence. Keeping this philosophy in mind, the prosthetist gains an understanding of the amputee's somatic, psychic, and emotional resources; perceptions; and short-, medium-, and long-range goals; these are translated into a specific, realistic treatment plan.

THE IDEAL RESIDUAL LIMB

From the prosthetist's perspective, the ideal residual limb may be described as pain free, strong, well muscled, and as functional as the original limb as is possible; the residual limb's bone(s) should be as long as possible,[20, 38] with the distal end capable of bearing 100% of the body weight. In the below-knee amputation, the fibula should be stable (ideally as in the Ertl tibiofibular synostosis[12]). The muscles should have distal insertions and be able to contract in their usual antagonistic manner without pain. The skin should be smooth and conforming, with natural tension, a good vascular supply, movable underlying subcutaneous tissue, and a well-healed surgical scar (Fig. 24–1).

Very seldom is a residual limb ideal. Many surgeons consider the distal one third of the tibia unacceptable as an amputation site because of the preponderance of tendinous structures, which they say "predisposes to poor circulation and an unstable, painful stump."[35] Certain pathological conditions may cause surgeons to apply this presumptive thought further. In the author's experience, the surgeon's use of a careful biological approach to amputation renders the best possible condition for the body's healing powers to create a functional, pain-free residual limb for the amputee.

As early as 1939, Ertl[10–12] described an improved surgical technique to maximize residual limb function, biologically and mechanically, by emphasizing terminal tibial loading. Many below-knee amputees were able to bear 100% of their body weight on the end of their residual limb. Ertl's work was subsequently reported in the American

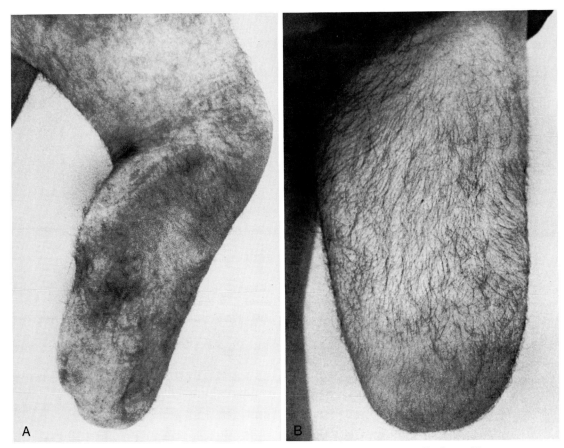

FIGURE 24–1. The ideal residual limb: below the knee *(A)* and above the knee *(B)*.

literature by Loon,[23, 24] who cited research results indicating a superior residual limb both physiologically and mechanically. The author also finds that this technique increases the area of weight-bearing distribution, thereby reducing the pressure per cm². Deffer,[7, 8] prompted by Loon's articles, used Ertl's technique and reported superior results: increased proprioception, diminished residual limb pain, improved control of the prosthesis, and, above all, increased certainty in the amputee's sense of the foot's location—something that comes only with end-bearing amputations. The author has worked with amputation surgeons John Ertl and William Ertl,* who continued to expand their father's technique here in the United States.[11, 12]

Investigations by Katz and associates[16] and

---

*I cannot emphasize enough the indebtedness I feel to these surgeons, for they have made my chosen profession of prosthetic replacement more enjoyable. Prosthetists are just beginning to appreciate the benefits of interested, concerned, and skilled surgeons.

Persson and Liedberg[29] have shown that below-knee amputees can bear from 3 to 79% of their body weight on the end of the residual limb. These investigations were carried out without regard for surgical technique. Good healing may be hindered by physiological circumstance. Often, the amputation is performed under emergency conditions that preclude time-consuming osteomyoplastic procedures. It is under these circumstances that the prosthetist is challenged to mitigate the consequences of a residual limb that is less than ideal.

EXAMINATION AND EVALUATION

A precise understanding of the detailed anatomy of the residual limb is paramount to successful socket design, prosthesis fitting, and amputee rehabilitation. The residual

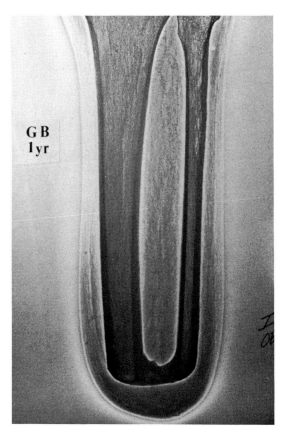

G B
1 yr

FIGURE 24–2. Xeroradiograph of a below-knee residual limb—internal oblique view.

limb is composed of bone and soft tissue (the chief component of which is water). Soft tissues are subject to day-to-day changes in volume. Also present is active or, in some cases, inactive muscle. Muscles may hypertrophy or they may atrophy, depending on their particular physiological make-up, whether they have distal insertions, and, to a large extent, the amputee's physical activity and desire to maintain muscle density. The residual limb's shape is necessarily dynamic and is the greatest challenge confronting the amputee and the prosthetist in establishing and maintaining a comfortable fit.

The application of xeroradiography to the examination of the lower extremity residual limb provides valuable insight into the condition of the underlying bone, muscle, and other soft tissues (Fig. 24–2).[39] In xeroradiography, contours are intensified so that the boundaries between different thicknesses or densities are especially pronounced. This information aids the prosthetist in forming a multidimensional image of the socket design that provides an optimal fit. Xeroradiogra-

phy also assists in assessing particularly difficult fitting problems. By imaging the residual limb within the socket during controlled weight bearing, the relationship between the socket and the residual limb can be better analyzed.

PROSTHETIC FABRICATION

The entire design, fitting, and fabrication process consists of six basic steps:
1. Impression molding
2. Cast reduction modification
3. Test fitting—static and dynamic biomechanical analysis of the socket and the foot, ankle, knee, and hip components and their alignment
4. Fabrication and design theory of the definitive prosthesis
5. Definitive dynamic biomechanical alignment and component testing
6. Final finishing

This process may take from 10 to more than 20 appointments with the prosthetist. The number of appointments depends on the overall case complexity, the number of test socket fittings needed, and the number of different components tested. Each appointment lasts approximately 1 to 2 hours. In addition, technicians may perform as many as 15 laboratory fabrication procedures, taking from 25 to more than 40 hours.

Impression Molding and Cast Reduction Modification

To meet the high demands of new socket design, many investigators have pursued improvements in molding that will reduce the possibility of human error. The impression mold will be a function of the prosthetist's mental image of the desired geometric configuration. The goal is twofold: (1) to place the residual limb under stress in a manner similar to that encountered during weight bearing within the prosthetic socket and (2) to then capture and translate the residual limb's dimensions under these conditions into a mold.

All molding techniques require various degrees of hands-on contour enhancement, depending on the prosthetist's innovation, experience, and goals. No particular technique has achieved universal acceptance. Rather, the skills and experience of each prosthetist must be applied to the needs of each individual amputee. After the molding procedure, a cast is prepared and then modified to create a model consistent with the residual limb's parameters and the prosthetist's mental image of the desired geometric configuration. Seldom is the prosthetist successful in achieving comfort and function on the first fitting. This is due, in part, to the complex contour and cross-sectional changes that occur as the residual limb goes from static to dynamic states and from activity to activity. It is for this reason that transparent plastic test sockets have become a popular diagnostic tool in achieving optimal socket fit and efficient biomechanical alignment.

Transparent Test Socket Fitting—Static and Dynamic Biomechanical Analysis

Murphy discussed the use of plaster "trial sockets" in fitting below-knee amputees in 1954.[27] Although these sockets were not transparent, he reported that rectifications could be made to the trial socket until a satisfactory fit was achieved, thus minimizing expensive and time-consuming changes in the final socket. For the most part, trial sockets were used in the research laboratory and, ironically, were *routinely* used in fitting upper extremity amputees. Also, trial sockets were purported to be used occasionally as an aid to the prosthetist in fitting the difficult case. Most reports in the literature discuss the materials and fabricating methods of the transparent socket, with little emphasis placed on using diagnostic methods to achieve optimal socket design.

For the past 8 years, the author has used the transparent plastic test socket routinely on all amputee patients in the manner described later in the text. The transparent plastic test socket offers the amputee and prosthetist the opportunity to analyze socket fit and biomechanical alignment more accurately. The effects of pressure on the residual limb's skin are observed through the plastic and are empirically evaluated. Deficiencies of socket fit may include isolated areas of high or low pressure. Socket fitting refinements can easily be made in one of two ways: (1)

direct modification to the test socket (e.g., grinding, heating and reshaping, injecting molding material) or (2) rectification of the model and fabrication of another test socket. The degree of refinement required dictates the modification procedure. This process is necessarily iterative, often requiring a number of test sockets, with each new test socket fitting better than the previous one. The complex nature of human anatomy requires this serial approach. The intent is to achieve the best possible fit while the amputee is standing before the fitting proceeds to walking trials (Fig. 24–3). Walking and other activities of daily living introduce greater and more complex pressure and forces.

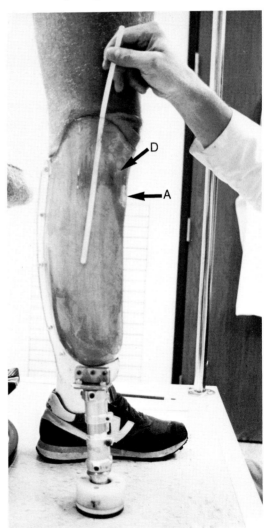

FIGURE 24–3. Test socket fitting—static analysis. Note the air pocket (A). The darker area (D) indicates that there is less skin pressure than in the area below, which appears much lighter.

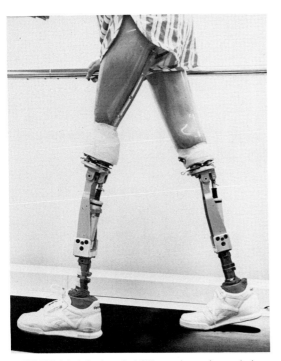

FIGURE 24–4. Test socket fitting—dynamic analysis.

The purpose of dynamic biomechanical analysis is to establish a stable and efficient gait while maintaining comfort. Appropriate components (foot, ankle, knee, and hip) are attached to the test socket and positioned (aligned) under the amputee's center of gravity. It is at this time that the amputee first experiences the capabilities and deficiencies of the residual limb and prosthesis. It is reassuring for the amputee to know that the first experience is not the sole indicator of the future but simply one of many compared in achieving the most comfortable and functional prosthesis for the individual's requirements (Fig. 24–4).

There are more than 20 different prosthetic feet, and an equally large number of prosthetic knees, commercially available. A new procedure that departs from conventional practice and that the author has been using for many years is to provide amputees the opportunity to test a number of different components, initially within the controlled environment of the rehabilitation facility and later in their own environments and daily activities. The author has been surprised many times when an amputee reported greater stability, smoother heel-to-toe mo-

tion, and generally more confidence with one particular prosthetic foot than with the one predicted to be best. It may be valuable to reassess the practice of "prescribing" prosthetic components.

Although the designers of prosthetic feet strive to replace the lost original function, the practical result may vary significantly in function from amputee to amputee. Each component requires a different dynamic biomechanical position, and a number of factors may influence the outcome: the residual limb's length and condition; the amputee's general physical condition (e.g., height, weight, strength, stamina); and the amputee's functional and aesthetic requirements for simple mobility, vocation, and recreation. Some prosthetic feet are lifelike in appearance (see Components).

Therefore, it is best for the amputee to thoroughly test different components, especially in cases of higher level amputations involving combinations of components (foot-ankle-knee-hip). Refined modular systems provide quick and easy repositioning of the prosthetic foot (and knee and hip), which achieves a smoother walking pattern and greater efficiency and reduces energy expenditure (Fig. 24–5). Modular systems also allow the quick and easy exchange of components for functional comparison (Fig. 24–6).

It is important to emphasize that effective communication between the amputee and prosthetist is critical in achieving optimal socket fit and biomechanical alignment. Most amputees can "feel" beyond the ability of the prosthetist to observe. Many times, the observing prosthetist may conclude that optimal socket fit and biomechanical alignment have been achieved only to have the amputee report discomfort in the socket or instability in walking.

The subtlety of socket geometry (explained in greater detail under Modern Socket Design Theory) is not always observable. Likewise, a 2 or 3° inversion or eversion of the prosthetic foot may go undetected by the prosthetist's eye but may be experienced by the amputee as unstable. The amputee's proprioceptive and kinesthetic abilities are affected, in part, by socket design, components, function, biomechanical alignment, efficiency, and weight. In an attempt to refine and quantify prosthetic gait, audiovisual feedback systems have from time to time been used clinically, with unclear results.

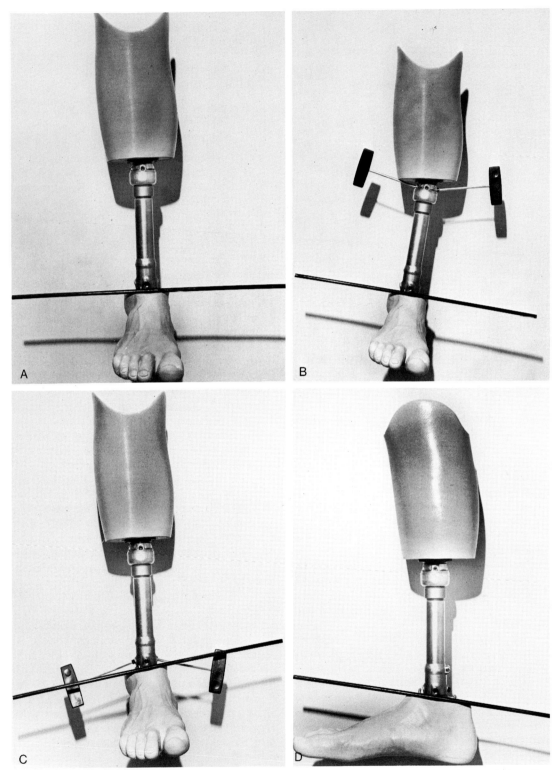

FIGURE 24–5. Below-knee prosthesis showing the angular adjustability of the alignment coupling: neutral position *(A)*, abduction *(B)*, inversion *(C)*, and dorsiflexion *(D)* (an equal amount of plantar flexion is also available).

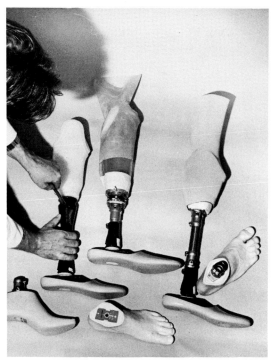

FIGURE 24–6. Modular systems allow quick, easy exchange of components for amputee comparison trials.

Staats[36] reports that videotape replay significantly benefits both the amputee and the prosthetist by providing an opportunity to review general and specific elements of prosthetic design and function and the amputee's performance—without exhausting the amputee.

Boyd[3] investigated the use of videotape with a control group and an experimental group of four above-knee amputees and found that the learning rate and quality of gait were equal in both groups. The author recognizes the benefit of repeated viewings of various gait parameters for determining the cause of a problematic deviation and for investigative purposes but has found limited clinical utility beyond historical recording for comparison.

The best method of assessing prosthetic fit seems to be one of open communication between the amputee and the prosthetist. The amputee describes aberrant sensations and makes suggestions for correction. The prosthetist observes and assesses the biomechanical situation and makes appropriate adjustments. The amputee immediately comments on the degree of comfort and the smoothness of gait.

Definitive Prosthesis Design Theory

The artistic ability of the technician and the cosmetic properties of new materials are clearly evident in the improved aesthetics of prostheses (Fig. 24–7). There are two basic finishing designs in lower extremity prosthetics: exoskeletal and endoskeletal. The exoskeletal design has historically proved very reliable and reasonably cosmetic, but the solid attachment of the components does not allow them to be easily exchanged or aligned. Most endoskeletal designs, on the other hand, are modular, allowing easy and quick exchange of components and alignment alterations. Lightweight, adjustable alignment couplings of titanium or graphite composites add to the advantages of endoskeletal systems. In addition, the appearance of the finished prosthesis seems to be slightly better with the endoskeletal design.

Modern Socket Design Theory

In discussing the relationship between the amputee and the prosthesis, the socket can be said to be the reciprocal correlate of the ideal residual limb. Through its design, the socket provides a way for the residual limb to ascertain information about the forces acting on the prosthesis and body. A socket that produces pain in the residual limb reduces its ability to function, in turn diminishing the overall function of the person. It can be said that the socket is the most important aspect of the prosthesis—much more important than component function or weight.

Prosthetic socket design theory continues to be rather unsophisticated, exhibiting minimal understanding of the body's tolerance of pressure and shear forces. The ideal socket for all levels of lower extremity amputation should

1. Be comfortable to the wearer
2. Support the load of the body during stance phase and the load of the prosthesis during swing phase
3. Allow maximal weight bearing up through the end of the bone (the tibia in below-knee amputation and the femur in above-knee amputation)
4. Maintain the residual limb bone struc-

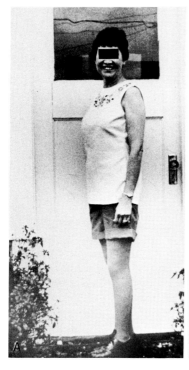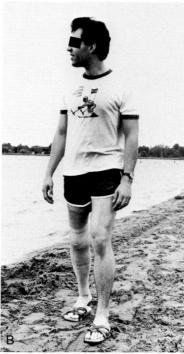

FIGURE 24–7. The excellent cosmetics of endoskeletal prostheses: above the knee *(A)* and below the knee *(B)*.

ture in a position that allows or approaches natural locomotion (the amputee's walking pattern before amputation or one that consumes the least energy)

5. Be intimately connected to the body and respond efficiently to the residual limb's action (maximal efficiency exists when the bone's position in relation to the socket does not change during activity)

6. Be anatomically conforming, using the entire surface area for support and allowing maximal joint motion

7. Maintain the biomechanics of body segments in a posture as near to natural as possible

8. Allow physiological, kinesthetic, and proprioceptive functioning of the residual limb and body that are as natural as possible, working as a whole under all static and dynamic conditions.

Current socket design theory diverges significantly from conventional paradigms that proscribe the transfer of weight-bearing loads to a few specific anatomical areas of the residual limb and dictate that the biomechanical alignment should be altered from its natural configuration to take advantage of the remaining muscles. The old design theories are best exemplified by the patellar tendon-bearing (PTB) socket for below-knee amputees and by the quadrilateral design for above-knee amputees. These previous socket designs, based on conceptual research at the University of California, Los Angeles, were improvements over previous paradigms and provided increased comfort and function, which in turn improved the amputee's quality of life.[1, 31] These sockets were designed so that floor reaction forces and weight-bearing loads were applied to specific areas on the residual limb. Very often, the small radius of the socket created tangentially increased pressures that often resulted in skin and subcutaneous disorders, nonpathogenic terminal edema, and irritating phantom pains. These conditions frequently led to more serious complications that often required involved medical treatment.

Growing numbers of prosthetists are beginning to realize that there is no single geometric configuration that fits all amputees within a particular amputation level—not even most amputees. Each individual's anatomy is unique, and it alone determines the socket shape necessary to achieve optimal comfort and function. Even so, there have been new developments in socket design specific to the level of amputation.

Partial Foot Amputation

Although this level of amputation is perceived by many as the least severe because it removes the least amount of the extremity, prosthetists have looked upon fitting persons with partial foot amputations with dismay. Some feel that a simple shoe filler of any readily available soft material will suffice—often recommending a foot sock be stuffed into the toe section of the shoe. This choice, unfortunately, results in less than acceptable levels of mobility, function, and comfort.

Socket design for amputations of the foot varies with the functional capability of the remaining portion. Maximal function is possible in persons with amputations at the metatarsophalangeal joint that leave at least slightly more than 20% of the metatarsal length. In this situation, the socket can usually be designed with its margins below the tibial and fibular malleoli, allowing a full range of motion and maximal cosmesis. Care is taken to achieve an intimate fit of the socket to the remaining longitudinal and metatarsal arch contours. The posterior aspect of the socket is designed to grasp behind the calcaneus and hold the socket in place.

Generally speaking, the extent of activity and desired functional performance of the amputee dictate socket margin levels. Low designs may not allow high-level function because of the insufficient biomechanical response of the prosthesis and the high pressures generated at the socket margin. A more proximal anterior margin may be necessary to spread pressure over a larger area. This is especially important during activities such as running, jumping, walking long distances, and carrying heavy loads. The amputee can best determine proper socket design and margin level during the dynamic testing phase of the fitting process.

Persons with amputations removing more of the foot usually achieve greatest function with a socket designed so that its anterior margin is at a level just below the inferior point of the patella, immobilizing the ankle joint (Fig. 24–8).

Below-Knee Amputation

The improved surgical techniques that increase the capability of the below-knee residual limb, combined with sockets designed to potentiate these capabilities, have provided greater functional opportunities for the below-knee amputee. The socket's suspension and the overall weight of the prosthesis also

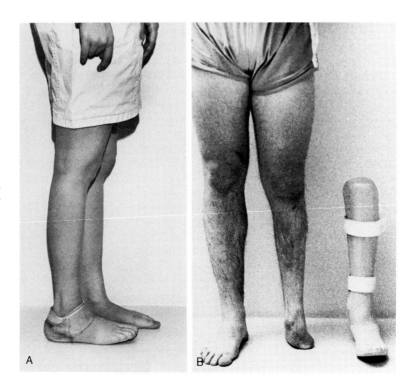

FIGURE 24–8. Partial foot prosthesis: low (A) and high (B) designs.

A   B

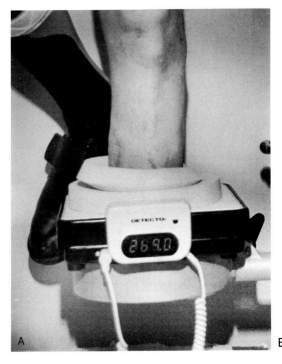

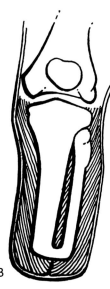

FIGURE 24–9. Superior end weight bearing after Ertl's osteo-myoplastic amputation. *A,* A below-knee amputee weighing 207 pounds is able to bear 269 pounds. *B,* Schematic of osteo-myoplasty.

play important roles in prosthetic function. Most amputees can bear a percentage of their body weight on the terminal aspect of the tibia. Maximal end weight bearing is best achieved when a synostosis exists between the tibia and fibula, with myoplasty (Fig. 24–9).[26]

Newer approaches in socket design emphasize anatomical contouring that incorporates total surface bearing (TSB) and maximizes terminal loading. TSB[38] is a recent term and is often mistaken for the older term total contact. Total contact is the condition brought about when the entire surface of the residual limb is in total contact with the socket but is not necessarily under compression. TSB is the condition brought about when the entire surface of the residual limb is in total contact with the socket while every unit of area is under compression to its appropriate and tolerable level. TSB socket design theory contrasts with that of PTB, which advances the notion that certain pressure-tolerant areas of the residual limb, in contact with the socket, should bear the vast majority of the body weight.

If the amputee is asked to compare the PTB total-contact socket and the TSB socket, the usual response is that in the PTB, weight is supported by a few isolated areas (under the kneecap, behind and on both sides of the knee, and over the termination of the lateral

distal fibula), whereas in the TSB socket, body weight is supported by the entire residual limb surface, including the distal end.

The TSB socket design differs from that of the PTB in a few easily observed ways:

1. The patellar ligament protuberance is greatly reduced and conforms more to the natural profile of the ligament (seeing the relationship between the residual limb and the socket in this perspective provides the opportunity to observe causes of traumatic skin lesions and associated disorders).

2. The posterior surface better resembles the anatomical contour, using muscle expansion whenever possible to aid in prosthetic suspension. (Some amputees are able to wear a TSB socket designed to be held on by muscles expanding against the socket wall (Fig. 24–10).[21] The author has found that the amputee who can voluntarily contract muscles without discomfort is more likely to be successful at such physiological suspension.)

3. The socket margins are generally lower, containing only those structures above the tibial plateau that are necessary for support and stability. (The "Old" rationale for a mid-patellar socket margin [in the PTB socket] was to provide strength to the medial and lateral socket walls. In some cases, the author has found that the lateral socket margin need

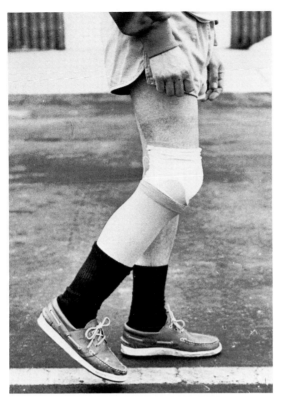

FIGURE 24–10. Partial suspension is derived from muscle expansion within a specially designed socket.

sleeve has been the suspension of choice by 98% of all below-knee amputees treated by the author since 1971.

Knee-Disarticulation

A true knee-disarticulation amputation, which retains the femoral condyles untouched and a patella capable of full end weight bearing, offers the amputee many functional advantages. Intact, fully functioning muscles are able to provide superior planar stability. Full end weight bearing reduces tangential socket tensions on the vertical surfaces of the residual limb's thigh and provides more natural kinesthetic and proprioceptive function.

Socket margins vary depending on the capabilities of the individual's residual limb but are usually at or near the subischial level. Suspension can often be achieved by designing the socket to grasp the superior flares of the femoral condyles, and this design can not be higher than the tibial plateau [Fig. 24–11].)

Suction (negative atmospheric pressure) is the best means of suspending the above-knee prosthesis. Suction is superior in suspending the below-knee prosthesis as well, with either an elastic sleeve (of various materials) or an atmospheric pressure valve (Fig. 24–12).[6, 14] The advantages of suction suspension are the reduction or elimination of friction between the skin and the prosthesis and the reduction of destructive subdermal tissue shear.

Not all amputees are able to use suction suspension with the suction valve alone. Key elements to success are an experienced prosthetist (the socket must be designed to be most intimate); a motivated, reliable, and, above all, patient amputee; a mature residual limb (being at least one year after amputation); a residual limb with an amount of subcutaneous tissue that is greater than average; and a residual limb greater than 5 inches in length.

Most amputees, regardless of age, are able to use the latex sleeve successfully as a means of suction suspension (Fig. 24–13). The latex

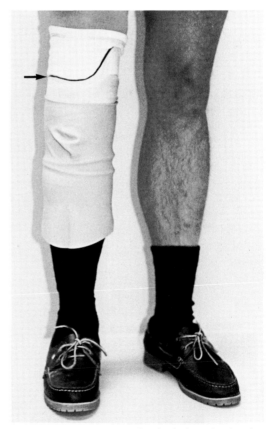

FIGURE 24–11. Socket margins (arrow) are kept as low as possible, while maintaining the prosthesis' biomechanical advantage.

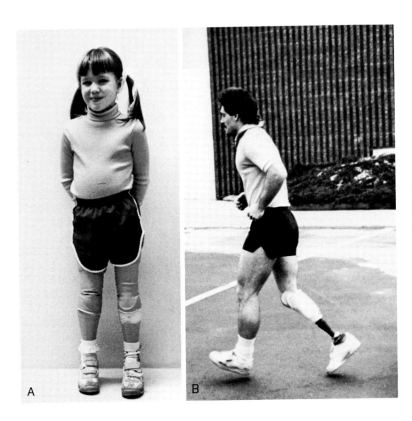

A   B

FIGURE 24–12. Suction suspension of below-knee prostheses with a latex sleeve (A) and with an atmospheric pressure valve (B).

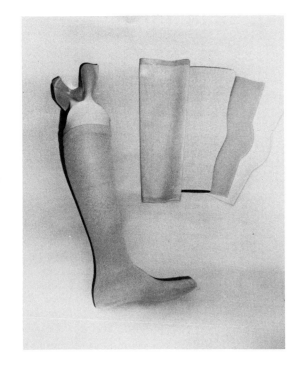

FIGURE 24–13. Various designs of suction suspension sleeves.

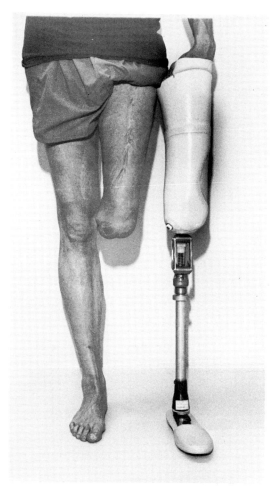

FIGURE 24-14. Knee-disarticulation socket designed with suction as a means of suspension.

also be used in conjuction with suction (Fig. 24-14).

Above-Knee Amputation

The quadrilateral socket design has held paradigm status for about 30 years in the United States. This design theory holds that a geometric socket shape can be established based on anatomical measurements, residual limb musculature (soft, average, or firm), residual limb length, and position of the trochanter.[1] The most obvious characteristic of this design is its rectangular shape—the narrow anteroposterior dimension (the medial, proximal one third) and the broad, flat, horizontal posterior margin, which provides a seatlike shelf for the ischial tuberosity to rest upon. A specific transverse pattern (at the subischial level) that incorporates several

design principles is desired: the medial wall of the socket is parallel with the path of progression; the posterior wall is at a specified angle away from the medial wall to accommodate muscle characteristics; the medial first inch of the anterior wall is at right angles to and higher than the medial wall to hold the ischium on the seat, and then it bulges outward to accommodate the rectus femoris, sartorius, and anterior fibers of the tensor fasciae latae muscles; the lateral socket wall is parallel to and 3 inches higher than the medial wall; and all proximal margins are flared upward and outward.

The weight-bearing and stabilizing mechanism of the quadrilateral socket is based on the concept that the inferior aspect of the ischial tuberosity will be the major contributor in supporting vertical loads and will act as a fulcrum for the lever system (the femur/hip abductors) to stabilize the pelvis. Additional vertical support is gained from hydrostatic pressure developed within the socket. Stability is achieved by designing the lateral wall of the socket to maintain the femur in an adducted position—the notion being that the femur will move only slightly when the gluteus medius and minimus muscles contract, thereby stabilizing the pelvis during the contralateral limb's swing phase.

In practice, however, the author has found that the quadrilateral socket inconsistently achieved comfort and stability for the amputee. During single-limb stance on the prosthetic side, the opposite-side pelvic-stabilizing muscles, which normally pull against a *fixed* femur to control the tilt of the pelvis, often cause abduction of the thigh. The distal aspect of the femur presses against the socket, pushing it away laterally. In turn, the ischial tuberosity tends to move medially, proximally, and, occasionally, anteriorly (caused by contraction of the hamstring muscles). Those forces result in high pressure and shear on the skin and subcutaneous tissues at and below the perineum, ischial tuberosity, and medial one third of the inguinal crease and over the lateral distal femur. Furthermore, the narrow anteroposterior dimension of the medial one third of the socket creates harmful pressure over the femoral vessels, which is exacerbated by high circumferential tension-compression values. Typical circumferential tension (the amount the socket is smaller than the residual limb) from the proximal ischial tuberosity level to the most

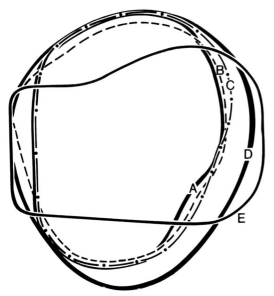

FIGURE 24–15. Schematic cross section (approximately 1 cm below the ischial tuberosity) of the right thigh residual limb and four socket designs: contoured adducted trochanteric-controlled alignment method (CAT-CAM) socket (A); anatomical-biological design (B); natural shape, natural alignment (NSNA) design (C); thigh (D); quadrilateral design (E). The anterior portion of the leg is at the top of the figure.

distal end is 1¼ to one half of an inch, respectively.

These factors result in trauma, including skin ulcerations, soft tissue lesions, nonpathogenic terminal edema, and mediolateral instability of the pelvis and upper body. Complications often progress to a degree requiring medical treatment. Other potential problems include the tendency of the lateral proximal socket margin to gap, noticeably asymmetric walking patterns with a wider than usual base, altered arm swing, gross upper body sway over the prosthetic side, and reduced pelvic rotation. There is some doubt as to whether the quadrilateral socket's failure to accommodate the residual limb is a problem of poor execution or of poor design; many above-knee amputees are well satisfied with their quadrilateral-designed sockets.

A number of new design approaches seem to be successful in reducing the incidence of the previously mentioned problems. These designs, however, may not differ as much as the theories themselves suggest. Common to all is the containment of the ischial tuberosity within the socket margin, a narrow mediolateral socket dimension, a wide anteroposterior dimension, and greater conformity of the

socket to the lateral surface of the residual limb's thigh. In general, these new designs provide greater residual limb stability and more amputee comfort (Fig. 24–15).

Long was the first to describe a socket design with a narrow mediolateral dimension.[22] He called it the natural shape, natural alignment (NSNA) socket, and it contained the ischium within the posteromedial margin. He also stressed the importance of coronal alignment, referring to "Long's line"—a straight line (in the coronal plane) passing through the center of the head of the femur ("located approximately at the center of a narrow socket"), through the center of the distal femur, lateral to the center of the prosthetic knee (with the knee in an appropriate degree of valgus), and through the center of the heel. This line relates to a line clinically known as the weight-bearing line and scientifically termed the mechanical axis of the lower limb (Fig. 24–16).

Other important features of the NSNA design include the medial wall of the socket being parallel to the path of progression and the proximal first inch of the socket being flared outward at 45° (Fig. 24–17). The circumferential tension of the socket ranges from three fourths or one inch at the subischial level to zero at the most distal end. (Compare these measurements with the previously stated numbers for the old quadrilateral socket design.) The mediolateral dimen-

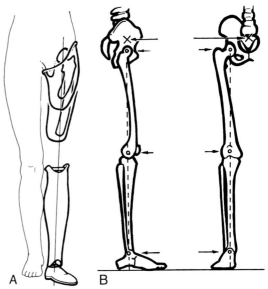

FIGURE 24–16. A, "Long's line." B, The weight-bearing line, or the mechanical axis of the lower limb.

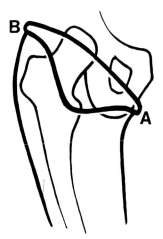

FIGURE 24–17. Schematic of the natural shape, natural alignment (NSNA) socket, posterior view. The proximal first inch of the medial wall (A) is angled 45° outward. The lateral margin (B) is well above the greater trochanter.

sion of the socket at the ischial level is a function of the residual limb's circumference. (A table of subischial residual limb circumferences and the corresponding mediolateral socket dimensions was established from data on 500 sockets designed and fitted by Long.) The transverse pattern of the socket at the ischial level is very similar in shape for all amputees, differing in size only with slight alterations for muscle variance.

Sabolich,[34] calling his work the contoured adducted trochanteric-controlled alignment method (CAT-CAM, and later SCAT-CAM [skeletal CAT-CAM]) was inspired by Long and others. Sabolich described a more contoured surface for ischial tuberosity support along the socket's inferior, posterior, and medial surfaces. He further described three "ischial tuberosity-ramus" types or shapes— alpha, beta, and gamma. The alpha shape is well defined and extends downward almost vertically, thereby being the most ideal to grasp the residual limb within the socket, providing the most stability. The gamma shape possesses a very shallow protuberance and therefore is the most difficult to fit, resulting in much less stability. The beta shape is midway between the alpha and gamma.

Other enhancing features of the CAT-CAM include an intimately contoured, high lateral wall that combines with the subtrochanteric support of the femur and the medial surfaces of the ischial tuberosity and ramus to form a "three-point pressure system to lock the femur into adduction" (Fig. 24–18). The adduction angle of the femur (and the socket) is established for each individual during walking trials through the use of an adjustable alignment coupling. The design assumes that the femur can better accept a percentage of the amputee's weight by being at a hyperadducted angle. The mediolateral dimensions of the socket are determined by the residual limb's measurements. This design results in the socket's mediolateral dimension being much wider at the ischial level. This variation serves to encapsulate as much of the bony anatomy as possible. The mediolateral dimension reduces sharply at the subtrochanteric level, in an attempt to secure the femur firmly in the proper adduction angle, for greater mediolateral stabilization. The lateral wall (viewed from the transverse plane) is V-shaped along its entire length, contributing to femur stabilization in the anteroposterior plane.

Last, Sabolich's design incorporates an inner flexible socket with an outer rigid frame that allows the upper three fourths of the posterior socket wall, the entire proximal 3

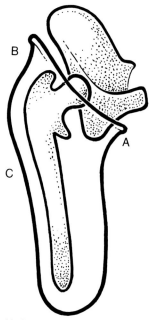

FIGURE 24–18. The contoured adducted trochanteric-controlled alignment method (CAT-CAM) socket design has a "three-point pressure system to lock the femur into adduction: medial, inferior to the ischial tuberosity and the ischiopubic ramus (A); superior to the greater trochanter (B); and along the shaft of the femur (C).

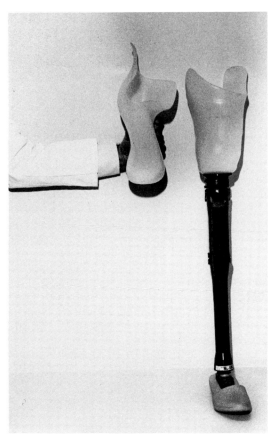

FIGURE 24–19. Demonstration of the flexibility of the contoured adducted trochanteric-controlled alignment method (CAT-CAM) socket.

to 4 inches of the circumference of the socket, and an anterior window to be exposed. It is claimed that such a design allows the socket to change shape dynamically as forces are applied and to deform naturally when the amputee is sitting (Fig. 24–19).

For amputees using sockets with this design, Sabolich recommends that those who previously used quadrilateral sockets undergo intensive physical therapy to strengthen hip abductor muscles and to break lateral trunk-bending habits established while using the quadrilateral socket. In addition, the use of a pelvic joint and waist belt "has been eliminated even in very short amputations."

Redhead[32] reports the development of a total-surface–bearing, self-suspending socket based on the hypothesis that soft tissues behave as an elastic solid with low stiffness, rather than as a fluid, when they are adequately supported. Changes in residual limb shape are limited by the arrangement of the tissue structures bounding the fluid compartments. The residual limb is contained within the socket, and the skin is stretched down to a predetermined tension. Ischial weight bearing is avoided. The retention of the socket is first dependent on the friction of the interface of the socket and the residual limb; this factor enables the socket to be held to the residual limb with a force approaching or equal to the weight of the prosthesis. Suspension can be increased temporarily by voluntarily contracting the residual limb muscles to increase the interface pressure. For loads greater than the weight of the prosthesis, atmospheric pressure holds the socket in place.

About 100 persons using the Redhead socket design over a 15-year period have remained healthy, with no evidence of progressive soft tissue shrinkage or skin breakdown. However, the cornerstone of the Redhead method is a very technical and sophisticated molding procedure. The complexity of this procedure is thought to be the reason that this technique has not been pursued by other prosthetists.

Another approach that the author has been pursuing begins with the premise that each amputee and each residual limb are unique. The prosthetic socket must be designed to use the entire available surface and take advantage of the residual limb's capabilities in achieving body and prosthesis efficiency and amputee comfort. The socket must be shaped to conform to the anatomy intimately, with specific geometric alterations to enhance biomechanical efficiency (Fig. 24–20).

The physical characteristics and capabilities of a particular residual limb will be unlike those of any other (see The Ideal Residual Limb). The individual's anatomy, the pathological condition, and the surgeon's technique all influence the residual limb. If the four major pelvis types are examined, eight variations are evident in the inferior aperture and the subpubic arch (Fig. 24–21). The average bituberous diameter (the distance between the ischial tuberosities) is 85 mm in the adult male and 118 mm in the female. The ischial tuberosity conjoined with the branch of the ischium creates an important angle that varies morphologically and with the degree of pelvic tilt.[13, 40] The angle of inclination of the femur's neck may vary from 150° in infants to 120° in the elderly person, and the angle of torsion of the femur may vary from 8 to 25° across individuals and sexes.[28]

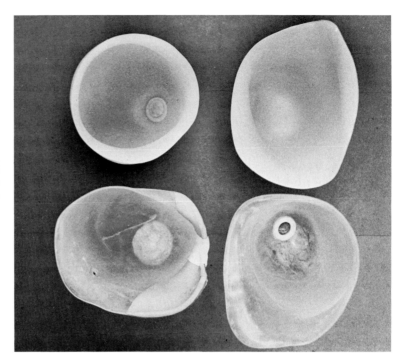

FIGURE 24–20. Two left-sided and two right-sided sockets for above-knee amputation show the viability in shape that is possible.

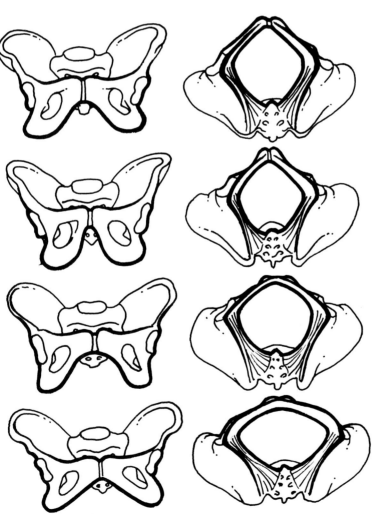

FIGURE 24–21. Variations in pelves' shapes.

The level of amputation also affects socket shape. A longer residual limb more closely resembles the original. When the muscle insertions remain intact, there appears to be less muscular atrophy over time. Muscles naturally expand, assisting in prosthetic suspension and rotation stability; less socket tension is required, and the lateral wall is somewhat concave. As the amputation level moves closer to the hip joint, the muscle bellies are transected, reducing their strength and size, and the residual limb tends to move into abduction and flexion. Rotational instability increases because of the increased amount of soft tissue in relation to bone. Active muscle contraction usually results in proximal distraction and distorted, irregular shapes (in residual limbs without muscle fixation) and pain. In addition, the loss of the muscle pump creates a tendency for nonpathogenic edema to form.

A flexible, biological approach to socket design is necessary to allow for all the variations described; consequently, the end result is not often clearly visualized before prosthetic fitting. In addition to these variations, one must consider how the socket's complex weight-bearing mechanism transmits the ground reaction forces to the pelvis. The hip joint of the intact limb is the focal point of weight bearing during times of standing and walking (see Fig. 24–16*B*). It is also the point of all rotation when the limb moves. At times of single-limb stance, the hip abductor muscles act directly on the hip joint through the weight-bearing line. During single-limb stance on the amputated limb with a socket designed for ischial weight bearing, the hip joint is no longer the focal point of support or rotation, and the normal biomechanics are disrupted. To a lesser degree, the same applies when the inferior portion of the ischial tuberosity shares in weight bearing, i.e., the hip joint on the amputated side no longer bears all the body's weight. At its contact with the socket, the ischial tuberosity becomes an additional point of rotation to the hip joint. The ischial tuberosity and its associated skeletal structures lie below, medial, and behind the hip joint (in coronal and sagittal planes) (Fig. 24–22). This situation creates a mechanical disadvantage for the hip abductors and imposes complex pressures and shear forces on the residual limb. It is the prosthetist's objective to minimize these discrepancies by designing the socket to resolve the floor re-

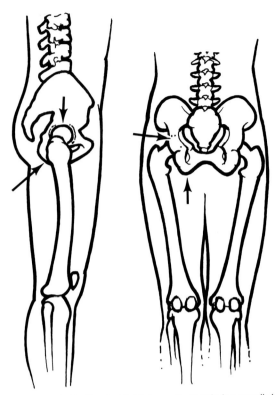

FIGURE 24–22. The ischial tuberosity is inferior, medial, and posterior to the center of the hip joint.

action forces to the body in as normal a manner as possible.

Hip Disarticulation and Hemipelvectomy

Socket designs for persons with hip disarticulation and hemipelvectomy follow the same principles as those for above-knee amputees, but more emphasis is placed on intimately fitting the prosthesis to the anatomical structures and on encapsulating only those structures necessary to effect maximal comfort and stability. A combination of flexible, elastic, and rigid materials is used selectively to enhance comfort (Fig. 24–23).

Overview

The described techniques and practices, when diligently applied by interested, dedicated, and skilled practitioners, can result in a socket that provides an acceptable degree of comfort and function. Consistency in reconstructive amputation surgery would serve to reduce the broad variations seen in resid-

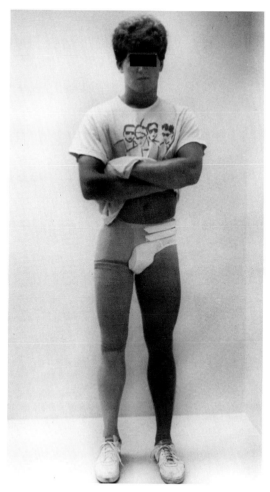

FIGURE 24–23. Total-surface–bearing socket for hip disarticulation.

ual limbs and to make prosthetic fabrication more predictable and easier.

COMPONENTS

There are many prosthetic feet, axial rotation devices, knees, and hips available from manufacturers in the United States and other countries. Each component has specific functional features that make it more suitable for particular needs. Some are limited in their use by the level of amputation. The small and very large sizes have a limited availability. The guidelines for component selection are based on the amputee's weight, activity level, and preference after actual testing, the latter possibly being the most important.

The proliferation of prosthetic components has placed a complete description beyond the scope of this chapter; however, some of the more important components will be discussed.

Feet

New developments in prosthetic feet center on the concept of energy storage. Energy storage as described here is the ability of the foot piece to store gravity-generated energy (potential energy) when the amputee shifts the body weight to the foot, thereby deflecting and compressing the internal material; this stored energy is then progressively returned to the amputee by rebound reaction (kinetic energy) as the foot moves through toe-off.[5] The transfer of stored energy into dynamic energy aids in developing a natural walking gait. There are several prosthetic feet designed to store energy (Fig. 24–24).

The important factors that determine which foot is appropriate for the individual amputee include the activity level and lifestyle of the individual, the proper biomechanical alignment of the prosthesis, and the individual's preference after gait trials. It is most beneficial for amputees to test several feet that might meet the demands of their lifestyles. The author has found that the amputee is the best judge of which foot provides a comfortable walk and a suitable gait. The prosthetist assures proper alignment, maximizing the functional output of the component to achieve the most natural gait. It is often necessary to have different foot alignment positions for different activities and not unusual to have one or more interchangeable foot pieces for various activities.[17] At times, additional complete prostheses (one or more) are required, each designed and biomechanically aligned for a specific purpose (see Fig. 24–24).

Axial Torque Absorbers

Axial-torque–absorbing devices are a relatively new development in prosthetic components.[19, 30] They are designed to replace rotation lost as a consequence of amputation, to relieve shear force on the residual limb tissues, and to improve the range of motion during weight bearing.

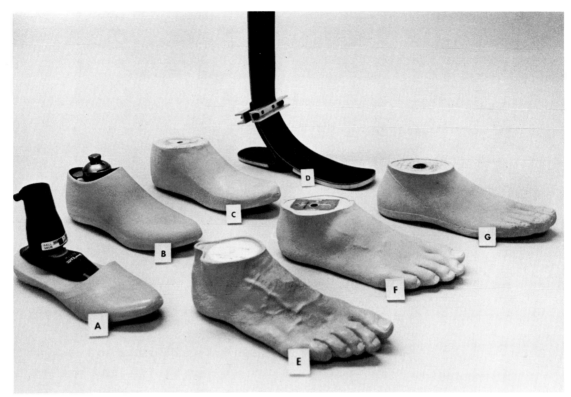

FIGURE 24–24. Designs of interchangeable prosthetic foot pieces: A, Multiflex; B, Multiaxial; C, stationary ankle, flexible endoskeleton (SAFE); D, Flex-foot; E, Seattle foot; F, Carbon Copy II; G, Stored Energy (STEN).

The best mechanical range of motion is provided by a component with 20° of passive axial rotation along a longitudinal axis and with an automatic return capability.[19, 30] One design offers manual adjustment of rotation resistance to accommodate the needs of the individual amputee. In many cases, improved gait symmetry and increased freedom of movement when changing direction of motion are experienced with the use of axial torque absorbers in a prosthetic limb (Fig. 24–25).

Knees

New developments in prosthetic knees focus on achieving (1) greater stability in stance phase, (2) greater variability in controlling the foot and shin during swing phase, (3) greater modularity (ease of exchange to another knee module for gait trials), (4) alignment adjustability, (5) light weight, and (6) a minimal distance above the actual center of rotation (for attaching hardware that accommodates long femoral lengths, including those from knee disarticulations).

Some knees offer stance-phase stability by making it mechanically very difficult, or impossible, for the knee to bend when the amputee has weight on the prosthesis. Other knee units use hydraulic resistance. Improved pneumatic and hydraulic systems achieve smoother swing-phase control during varied walking speeds. Some units incorporate a polycentric design, mimicking anatomical knee action.

There is a tendency toward greater modularity and alignment adjustability along with lighter weight materials in newer knee designs. Such design variability allows the amputee to test different knees and the prosthetist to optimize the biomechanical alignment of each knee to the particular gait of the amputee (Fig. 24–26).

Position Rotators

Position rotators allow active rotation of the prosthesis along the longitudinal axis. This option is chosen primarily by persons with an amputation above the knee so that they can externally or internally rotate the

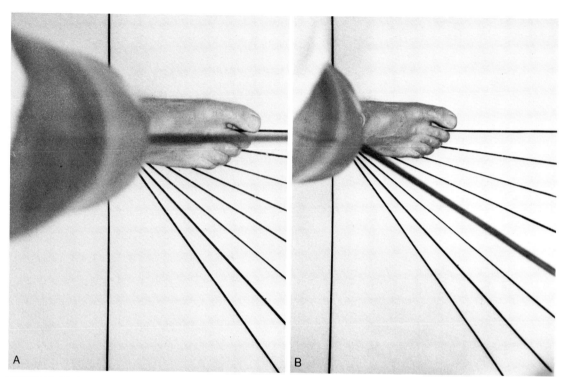

FIGURE 24–25. Action of the axial torque absorber. Amputee standing in prosthesis in neutral position *(A)* and twisting the knee outward *(B)*

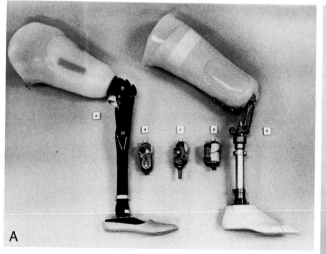
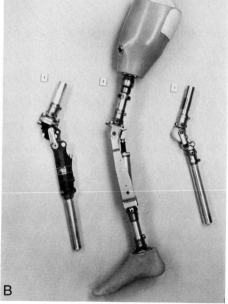

FIGURE 24–26. Modular system for quick and easy exchange of prosthetic leg components.

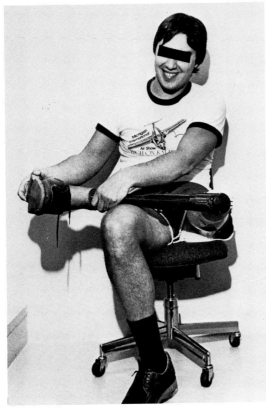

FIGURE 24-27. Action of the position rotator.

prosthesis from the knee down. It is very helpful for sitting cross-legged in a chair or on the floor, for changing shoes, and for getting in and out of a car, a plane, or some other vehicle (Fig. 24-27).

MATERIALS

Materials research in the aerospace, defense, and automotive industries has developed new generations of plastics and exotic metals that benefit the prosthetic field and amputees. Depending on the components used and the size of the residual limb, a below-knee prosthesis will weigh from 1.8 to 4.3 pounds, and an above-knee prosthesis will weigh from 4.5 to 6.5 pounds (for adults).

The prosthetist uses basic criteria, such as the material's weight, flexibility, stability, shrinkage, elasticity, shear strength, tensile strength, and rigidity, to utilize and combine various materials creatively in meeting the specific requirement of the individual amputee. The prosthetist is no longer concerned with blocks of wood, but rather with sheet plastics, resins, foams, silicones, and composite materials. The goal is to design a limb that will not only fit the patient comfortably but also provide stability, flexibility, elasticity, and durability. The first group of new materials includes the sheet plastics that are used in socket formation. Polyethylene, polypropylene, and Surlyn (all thermoplastic polymers) are vacuum-formed over a positive cast to create a socket. The advantage of these thermoplastics over previous designs is the lightweight property they exhibit while still meeting basic design criteria. The weight of conventional prostheses can be double that of those incorporating new materials. Prosthetic limb weight plays an important role in the amputee's energy expenditure. Decreased prosthetic weight allows increased prosthetic function.

Composite materials also mark a major part of the new wave being incorporated into prostheses. Carbon, graphite, and Kevlar, used in the lamination phase of fabrication, aid in providing rigidity for socket design. Kevlar (the lightest of the composites), carbon, graphite, and fiberglass have unique properties that enable them, when used in various combinations, to form sockets highly resistant to fracture.[2]

The field of prosthetic materials will continue to develop rapidly as long as there is an interest in improving the lives of the amputees. Lighter weight supportive designs will require less energy consumption while achieving higher activity levels. Innovation, along with a working knowledge of material properties, will further aid in future developments.

ACKNOWLEDGMENTS

I am indebted to Drs. Moore and Malone for the honor of making a contribution to this much-needed text. I wish to further express my thanks for their unbelievable patience with me in submitting the manuscript.

I extend my sincere gratitude to Craig Starnaman for creating illustrations that give greater meaning to the written word, to Ethel Huntwork and Noreen for typing and editing the manuscript, to Glenn Schober and Dale Conlin for providing the photographs, to Bill Potter for assisting invaluably in processing the film, to Jeff Peterman for photographing and being very patient with all the changes, and to Pam and Kent Turnbow for helping with the components and materials section.

REFERENCES

1. American Academy of Orthopaedic Surgeons: Socket functions and basic classifications. *In* Orthopaedic Appliance Atlas, Vol 2, Artificial Limbs, Prosthetic Devices. Ann Arbor, JW Edwards, 1960, pp 268–312.
2. Berry D: Composite materials for orthotics and prosthetics. Orthot Prosthet 40:38, 1987.
3. Boyd C: Videotape feedback and gait re-education of new unilateral above knee amputees. 5th World Congress of the International Society for Prosthetics and Orthotics, Copenhagen, June 29–July 4, 1986.
4. Burgess EM: Amputations. Surg Clin North Am 63:749, 1983.
5. Burgess EM, Poggi DL, Hittenberger DA, et al: Development and preliminary evaluation of the VA Seattle foot. Rehabil Res Dev 22:75, 1985.
6. Chino N, Pearson JR, Cockrell JL, et al: Negative pressures during swing phase in below-knee prostheses with rubber sleeve suspension. Arch Phys Med Rehabil 56:22, 1975.
7. Deffer PA: More on the Ertl osteoplasty. *In* Committee on Prosthetic-Orthotic Education: Newsletter: Amputee Clinics 2:7, 1970.
8. Deffer PA, Moll JH, LaNoue AM: The Ertl osteoplastic below-knee amputation. Presented to the American College of Orthopaedic Surgeons, Phoenixville, Pennsylvania, 1971.
9. Effeney DJ, Skinner HB, Abrahamson MA, et al: Development, testing, and evaluation of new prosthetic devices. J Rehabil Res Dev Prog Rep. San Francisco, Veterans Administration Medical Center, 1983, pp 4–5.
10. Ertl J: Regeneration: Ihre Anwendung in der Chirurgie. Leipzig, Verlag Johann Ambrosius Barth, 1939.
11. Ertl J: Ertl osteogenic lower limb amputation. The American Academy of Orthotists and Prosthetists Annual Meeting and Scientific Symposium, Las Vegas, January 30, 1986.
12. Ertl W: Ertl amputation technique. Presented to the American Surgery Association, Sarasota, Florida, October 19, 1979.
13. Ferner H, Staubesand J (eds): Sobotta Atlas of Human Anatomy, Vol 2. Baltimore, Urban & Schwarzenberg, 1983, pp 246–251.
14. Grevsten S, Marsh L: Suction-type prosthesis for below-knee amputees, a preliminary report. Artif Limbs 15:78, 1972.
15. Hoaglund FT, Jergesen HE, Wilson L, et al: Evaluation of problems and needs of veteran lower-limb amputees in the San Francisco Bay Area during the period 1977–1980. J Rehabil Res Dev 20:57, 1983.
16. Katz K, Susak Z, Seliktar R, Najenson T: End-bearing characteristics of patellar-tendon–bearing prosthesis— a preliminary report. Bull Prosthet Res 16:55, 1979.
17. Kegel B: Sports for the Leg Amputee. Redmond, Washington, Medic, 1986.
18. Klopsteg PE, Wilson PD: The amputee and the problem. *In* Klopsteg PE, Wilson PD (eds): Human Limbs and Their Substitutes. New York, McGraw-Hill, 1954, p 1.
19. Lamoureux LW, Radcliffe CW: Functional analysis of the UC-BL shank axial rotation device. Prosthet Orthot Int 1:114, 1977.
20. Levy SW: Skin problems of the amputee. St Louis, Warren H Green, 1983, p 48.
21. Lippert FG 3d, Burgess EM, Starr TW: Physiologic suspension factors in below-knee amputees evaluated. J Rehabil Res Dev Prog Rep. Seattle, Veterans Administration Medical Center, 1983, p 5.
22. Long IA: Normal shape-normal alignment (NSNA) above-knee prosthesis. Clin Prosthet Orthot 9:9, 1985.
23. Loon HE: Biological and biomechanical principles in amputation surgery. *In* Prosthetics International: Proceedings of the Second International Prosthetics Course, Committee on Prostheses, Braces, and Technical Aids, International Society for the Welfare of Cripples, Copenhagen, 1960, p 46.
24. Loon HE: Below-knee amputation surgery. Artif Limbs 6:86, 1962.
25. Malone JM, Moore W, Leal JM, Childers SJ: Rehabilitation for lower extremity amputation. Arch Surg 116:93, 1981.
26. Murdoch G: Research and development within surgical amputee management. Acta Orthop Scand 46:531, 1975.
27. Murphy EF: The fitting of below-knee prostheses. *In* Klopsteg PE, Wilson PD (eds): Human Limbs and Their Substitutes. New York, McGraw-Hill, 1954, p 711.
28. Norkin C, Levangie PK: Joint Structure and Function: A Comprehensive Analysis. Philadelphia, FA Davis Co, 1983, p 259.
29. Persson BM, Liedberg E: Measurement of maximal end–weight-bearing in lower limb amputees. Prosthet Orthot Int 6:147, 1982.
30. Racette W, Breakey JW: Clinical experience and functional considerations of axial rotators for the amputee. Orthot Prosthet 31:29, 1977.
31. Radcliffe CW, Foort J: The patellar-tendon–bearing below-knee prosthesis. Biomechanics Laboratory, School of Medicine, University of California, Department of Engineering, Berkeley, 1961.
32. Redhead RG: Total surface bearing self suspending above-knee sockets. Prosthet Orthot Int 3:126, 1979.
33. Rose HG: VA prosthetics . . . views of a medical investigator. DAV Mag 24:8, 1982.
34. Sabolich J: Contoured adducted trocanteric-controlled alignment method (CAT-CAM): Introduction and basic principles. Clin Prosthet Orthot 9:15, 1985.
35. Schwartz SI (ed): Principles of Surgery, 3rd Ed. New York, McGraw-Hill, 1979, p 2023.
36. Staats TB: Advanced prosthetic techniques for below knee amputations. Orthopedics 8:249, 1985.
37. Stokosa JJ: Prosthetics of the whole person. Presented at the Annual Conference of the Michigan Rehabilitation Association, Kalamazoo, Michigan, October 12, 1979.
38. Stokosa JJ: Prosthetics for lower limb amputees. *In* Haimovici H (ed): Vascular Surgery—Principles and Techniques. Norwalk, Connecticut, Appleton-Century-Crofts, 1984, pp 1143–1162.
39. Varnau D, Vinnecour KE, Luth M, et al: The enhancement of prosthetics through xeroradiography. Orthot Prosthet 39:14, 1985.
40. Williams P, Warwick R (eds): Gray's Anatomy, 36th Br Ed. Philadelphia, WB Saunders Co, 1980, pp 378–390.
41. Wilson AB Jr: To fill a void. Newsletter Prosthet Orthot Clin 4:7, 1980.

25

Amputation for Trauma

James M. Malone, M.D.
Kenneth E. McIntyre, Jr., M.D.
Jeffrey R. Rubin, M.D.
Jeffrey Ballard, M.D.

Before the development of modern orthopedic and vascular surgery reconstructive techniques, amputation was the best treatment for severely injured extremities. Limb amputation is perhaps one of the oldest surgical procedures on record, dating back to the Samnite Wars of 300 BC.[30] Many innovations were first described by military surgeons, whose most common battlefield operation was limb amputation. As military weaponry became more sophisticated, the incidence and magnitude of extremity injuries increased, which resulted in a greater number of major limb amputations and higher levels of amputation. Until the twentieth century, most wartime amputations were performed on the battlefield or in military hospitals where surgical conditions were marginal at best. Anesthesia was not routinely used; therefore, operations were performed as quickly as possible, and a premium was placed on short-duration surgery.

In such a surgical setting, exsanguinating hemorrhage and overwhelming sepsis were common surgical complications after amputation. In the fifth century BC, Hippocrates

recommended that amputation be carried out through devitalized tissues in order to reduce postamputation hemorrhage.[30] Cautery, although probably employed much earlier, was formally introduced as an antiputrefactive by Leonides of Alexandria in the first century AD.[30] There were many modifications of Leonides' "red-hot iron" technique, such as cautery with hot coals, hot stones, hot oil preparations, boiling water, and the "red-hot knife techniques" described by Fabrious Hildanus in 1600.[30] Vessel ligation was probably first practiced by Celsus in the first century AD but was not widely accepted until Ambroise Paré (1545), the renowned French army surgeon, reintroduced this practice and developed instruments such as forceps to assist in limb amputation.[30] The use of tourniquets was probably instituted in the sixteenth century by Botallo and was improved in the eighteenth century by Petit (1718).[30] Tourniquets permitted accurate vessel identification and individual vessel ligation as well as the safer performance of above-knee amputation. All of these developments helped to decrease the incidence and extent of hemorrhage as a complication of traumatic lower extremity amputation.

Controversy concerning the proper timing of amputation and primary versus secondary wound closure probably began in the twelfth century and continues to the present day. Jean Faure, a French army surgeon during the Napoleonic wars, noted higher patient survival when amputations were performed between 29 and 52 days after injury rather than immediately.[30] That observation contradicted the writings of Dominique Larrey, Napoleon's chief surgeon, and George Guthrie, an English surgeon, who described a lower incidence of wound infection and hemorrhage and a lower mortality rate when amputation was performed immediately after femur fracture (musketball injuries) and extensive lower extremity injuries.[2, 30] Larrey, Dupuytren, LisFranc, and Liston stressed the importance of allowing amputation wounds to close by secondary intention, which they felt decreased the incidence of wound infection.[30] During that era, sepsis from infected residual limbs that had been closed primarily remained as the greatest cause for amputation morbidity and mortality. A compromise solution to the dilemma was developed at about that time: delayed primary closure. A waiting period was instituted of several hours to days before residual limb closure. That delay allowed bleeding to cease and the wound to be cleaned. Wounds were then closed with either adhesive tapes or suture material.[30]

Mortality rates due to sepsis after traumatic amputation remained extremely high (20 to 30% for leg amputation and 40 to 60% for high thigh amputation) until improvements in prevention of postsurgical sepsis were achieved.[30] In the 1850s, Florence Nightingale began stressing the importance of cleanliness in the field hospitals of the Crimean War.[30] At that time, military hospitals were considered "death houses" because of the excessive postsurgical mortality resulting from surgical and traumatic infection.

Two scientific innovations that served to decrease amputation morbidity and mortality were the development of anesthesia and the evolution and acceptance of Lister's principles of antisepsis. In 1844, Wells used nitrous oxide as an anesthetic agent, and in 1846, Morton used ether for the same purpose.[30] Amputations could now be performed without speed being the primary criterion of

surgical success; therefore, more attention could be paid to the technical details of the surgical procedure. With the implementation of the antiseptic operating room and surgical techniques, postsurgical infection rates decreased, and postsurgical morbidity and mortality due to infection similarly decreased.

Myocutaneous flaps and myoplasty for residual limb coverage were first described by Oribasius (403) and later described and popularized by Yonge (1679) and Verduin (1697).[30] Many surgeons in the 1700s and 1800s recommended high bone division to prevent erosion of the distal bone through the healed residual limb.[30] In addition to improving postsurgical healing, these operative innovations in residual limb closure allowed the easier application of prosthetic devices and facilitated patient rehabilitation. The most recent advances in amputation surgery have involved innovation in surgical techniques to create the "ideal" residual limb and have accompanied the evolution of the field of prosthetics from a cottage industry to an allied health profession.

There are approximately 500 thousand amputees in the United States, and it is estimated that 30 to 50 thousand new lower extremity amputations are performed each year.[13] Over one half of all lower extremity amputations are performed for complications of peripheral vascular disease or diabetes mellitus, and the remaining amputations are performed for tumor, congenital anomalies, or infection.[11–15, 17, 25] Approximately 10 to 20% of these amputations are performed after traumatic injury. Traumatic lower extremity amputation occurs most frequently in healthy young men as a result of industrial or motor vehicle accidents. The psychosocial and economic impact of traumatic amputation is difficult to evaluate and quantitate but must be measured in terms of the functional status of the patient before injury. The primary goal of the amputation surgeon should be to achieve early ambulation and rehabilitation, thus permitting the patient with a traumatic amputation an early return to society, employment, or education and the ability to function independently.[3, 12–15, 24]

The following sections address the preoperative, intraoperative and postoperative assessment and management of patients who are undergoing amputations for traumatic injury. The results of the author's management of traumatic amputations at the University of Arizona and at the Maricopa Medical Center are discussed, with emphasis on those factors that are important in the overall successful rehabilitation of the individual who has sustained a traumatic injury resulting in the loss of a lower limb.

PATIENT MANAGEMENT

Treatment of patients with severe lower extremity trauma begins with a complete evaluation (history, physical examination, and appropriate laboratory and X-ray studies) after resuscitation in the emergency room. Severe extremity trauma is often associated with other life-threatening injuries involving the abdominal cavity, chest, or head. Injury to vital structures or life-threatening injuries require priority in the treatment of the patient with multiple injuries. Once life-threatening injuries have been addressed, attention can be turned to the traumatized extremity. The five components of the extremity—skin, nerves, blood vessels, muscle, and bone—must be evaluated both individually and as a functional unit. Important considerations in the evaluation are the mechanism of injury (avulsion, crushing, or degloving), the interval from injury to treatment, and the status of the wound (clean, contaminated, or filthy). Functional restoration of the limb should be the primary treatment goal. If functional restoration of the lower extremity cannot be achieved because of the irretrievable loss of three or more of the major components of the limb, amputation rather than limb salvage is usually a more appropriate course of action.

Skin

Viable skin is of paramount importance for wound closure in extremity injuries.[10] Frequently, major crushing or degloving injuries create large areas of traumatized skin, thereby producing significant problems in wound closure and coverage of vital structures in the extremity. There is a relative paucity of spare skin in the lower extremities, which makes mobilization of the remaining

healthy skin quite difficult. A problem that frequently develops after wound debridement is that skin closure may only be accomplished with significant tension. The skin closure may then be further stressed by postoperative edema from soft tissue injury or compartment syndromes. The end result may be tissue necrosis, wound dehiscence, and exposure of underlying arterial, venous, nervous, or orthopedic repairs. Obviously, this loss of protective skin coverage compromises vital structures exposed to the environment. Other more chronic problems may include delayed or failed union of fractures or arterial or nerve repair disruption due to chronic infection. If primary wound closure cannot be easily accomplished, free-skin grafting or coverage with a myocutaneous flap may be a reasonable alternative.[10] Another temporary alternative is the use of porcine heterografts for coverage of large defects until more definitive plastic reconstructive procedures can be accomplished. Regardless of the type and mechanism of wound coverage, it is clear that limb salvage depends on protection of vital structures and coverage by either skin or other biological substitutes.

Muscle and Tendon

Muscle and tendon, like the integument, must be inspected for tissue viability and the potential for structural and functional support of the extremity. Ischemic or severely traumatized muscle that is allowed to remain in the wound may undergo necrosis, providing an excellent bacterial culture medium. Also, release of myoglobin from injured muscle may induce acute renal failure. It is therefore important to debride aggressively all injured and nonfunctional muscle and tendon to reduce the chance of subsequent infection or myoglobinuric renal dysfunction.[13] Attempts to close muscle by suture techniques should be avoided, since muscle will not hold sutures and such surgical efforts will actually result in more muscle trauma. Closure of fascial defects is not desirable, since elevated compartment pressures may ensue postoperatively. Tendon repairs must be accomplished meticulously, be kept immobile, and be covered with skin in order to ensure maximal functional recovery.

Bone

The goal of orthopedic trauma treatment should be a functional and essentially pain-free extremity. The ability to restore function effectively after a severely comminuted or displaced fracture depends on many factors; the status of the blood supply to the fracture site, the degree of joint injury, the anticipated amount of limb shortening that will result from repair, and the ability to achieve fixation of the comminuted fracture segments all are equally important factors that influence the final outcome. Because of the prolonged period required to ensure that satisfactory healing has occurred, many salvage failures will not be noticed until months after the injury. The decision to pursue aggressive orthopedic reconstruction assumes that the final functional outcome for the traumatized extremity will be *better* than that with primary amputation.

Nerve

Accurate assessment of neurological injury in the traumatized lower extremity is extremely important for determining the proper management of the patient. Nerve regeneration in the lower extremity is poor in comparison with that in the upper extremity. Therefore, the prognosis for neurological recovery in the injured lower extremity is not good, despite the quality of the operative nerve repair. Performing a sophisticated vascular repair or attempting limb reimplantation without a good prospect for nerve recovery would produce a viable but non-functional limb. Therefore, one must determine whether the nerve has been divided (neurotmesis), whether only axons have been interrupted while the supporting nerve structures have been left intact (axonotmesis), or whether the nerve has been functionally interrupted without loss of axonal integrity (neurapraxia). Neurotmesis is commonly associated with penetrating arterial injuries, whereas axonotmesis is more likely to occur with blunt trauma. Neurapraxia occurs more commonly with stretching injuries such as fractures. The prognosis for recovery depends on the anatomical integrity of the nerve and is best for neurapraxia, average for axonotmesis, and poor for neurotmesis.[26, 32] To achieve the best results, microscopic fascicular nerve repair must be performed without anastomotic tension.[28] Even with the microscopic technique, the long-term results of lower extremity nerve repair have been disappointing in most series.

Vasculature

Evaluation of the arterial system should include an adequate preoperative history in order to exclude prior vascular occlusive disease. The physical examination should assess the color, temperature, sensation, and motor function of the extremity as well as the status of pulses. Intact distal pulses do *not* guarantee the absence of proximal arterial injury. The noninvasive vascular laboratory may also help to diagnose an injury or assess postoperative results. Doppler-derived pressure measurements are easily obtainable and are quite accurate. Finally, if time permits, arteriography is still the definitive test of vascular integrity;[18] however, the surgeon must be aware that a normal arteriogram does not exclude a significant venous injury. Unfortunately, with the exception of arteriovenous fistulas or major venous injuries (i.e., of the iliac or vena cava), preoperative radiographic evaluation for suspected venous injuries is not helpful.[27]

With the current techniques of vascular reconstruction, primary amputation solely due to vascular injury is unusual in the absence of significant surgical delay and prolonged ischemia (more than 6 hours). Amputation is more common when nerve, bone, and soft tissue trauma accompanies the vascular injury (irreparable injury to three or more structures in the limb). The timing of arterial and venous repair with respect to the time elapsed since injury is important in order to avoid delays that might result in irreversible nerve or muscle ischemia. Bone fixation, usually with external fixators, should be completed before vascular repair. Indwelling arterial and venous shunts can be placed in order to restore circulation as soon as possible and allow arterial reperfusion during prolonged orthopedic repair.[8] Venous injuries should be repaired before re-establishing arterial inflow. In general, arterial flow should be re-established (by repair or with shunts) within 6 hours of injury. Longer delays in arterial reperfusion significantly increase the risk of amputation.[16]

External bleeding should be controlled to prevent unnecessary blood loss. This is best accomplished with digital pressure or compression dressings rather than with tourniquets. Prolonged tourniquet time may further embarrass the circulation of the extremity. Blind clamping of vessels or attempts at suture ligation should not be performed in the emergency room. Penetrating foreign bodies, hematomas, and blood clots found in the wound should not be disturbed until the patient is in the controlled environment of the operating room. Once the patient is in the operating room, an operative plan, which is often multidisciplinary, should be instituted in a logical and sequential manner.

Arterial repair may be accomplished by primary arteriorrhaphy, bypass grafting, or arterial ligation.[7, 19-21, 29] Grafting is preferably performed with autogenous tissue, such as saphenous vein, provided it is of adequate caliber, it is not diseased, and the ipsilateral deep venous system is intact.[18] If suitable vein is not available, synthetic material such as polytetrafluoroethylene (PTFE) may be used, but this is less desirable because of the theoretical risk of placing prosthetic material in contaminated wounds.[21] However, Vaughn and associates have reported excellent results using PTFE for vascular reconstruction in contaminated fields.[29] Arterial ligation is rarely required and is acceptable in only very limited circumstances.

The repair of injured lower extremity deep system veins is important in order to decrease the incidence of postphlebitic leg syndrome.[22, 23] Also, a patent deep venous system helps to reduce edema in the traumatized extremity and helps increase tissue perfusion with combined arterial and venous injuries. Venous repair may be accomplished with lateral venography, with interposition saphenous vein grafts or patches, or with ring PTFE.

Summary

The decision to amputate or attempt limb reconstruction is a complex one that will try the judgment of even the most experienced surgical teams. The decision almost always involves input from general and vascular surgeons, orthopedic surgeons, and occasionally hand surgeons or neurosurgeons. The integrity of all five components of the extremity—skin, bone, muscle, nerves, and blood vessels—must be carefully evaluated before a decision can made to reconstruct or amputate. Although some of the decision-making process can take place in the emergency room, most of the evaluation ultimately takes place in the operating room when the injured extremity can be more carefully evaluated. In general, if three or more structures in the lower limb have irreparable damage, amputation is recommended.

Limb reimplantation is not usually attempted for massive traumatic injuries to the lower extremities. This is partly due to the difficulty in achieving a functional and pain-free extremity after lower limb reimplantation. In addition, the state of the art for lower extremity prosthetic rehabilitation is such that amputation with prosthetic fitting may provide superior results to limb replantation in some cases. This approach is in almost direct contrast with that used in upper extremity injuries; however, it must be realized that unlike the case with prosthetic feet, prosthetic hands do not provide an adequate replacement for the human hand.

AMPUTATION AND TIMING OF PROSTHETIC FITTING

The operative management of patients who have experienced traumatic lower extremity amputation or for those who require amputation for irreparably damaged limbs includes debridement, amputation, and either primary or secondary wound closure. Delayed primary wound closure may also be considered in selected cases.

The level of amputation is usually determined by the injury itself, but certain elements must be satisfied to ensure a functional, well-healed residual limb. First, there must be an adequate support for the residual limb; the bony architecture must be able to support ambulation on a prosthesis. For example, even if enough skin and muscle are present to close a below-knee amputation, inadequate tibial length or disruption of the knee joint may preclude satisfactory prosthetic fitting at the below-knee level, thereby necessitating a through-knee or long above-knee amputation. Similarly, amputations of the proximal forefoot (tarsal or calcaneal) may seem more favorable than amputations below the knee, but proximal forefoot amputations pose a challenging problem for prosthetists because of the propensity for forefoot residual limb erosion and the complexity of forefoot prosthetic fabrication. Syme's amputation is an excellent level for very active individuals but, because of the "large" ankles of the prosthesis, is less favorable for persons concerned with cosmetic appearance.

Controversy also exists concerning the closure of these contaminated or potentially contaminated wounds and the timing of prosthetic fitting. Since traumatic limb loss is unquestionably psychologically devastating,[3, 9] the goal of treatment should be rapid successful rehabilitation on a prosthesis.[9, 12–15]

At the University of Arizona Health Science Center and at the Maricopa Medical Center, the authors have used a multidisciplinary approach to the patient with massive lower extremity injury. When appropriate, patients undergo limb salvage and limb-sparing procedures such as those described in preceding sections. For the patient with a nonsalvageable lower extremity injury, the authors prefer to treat the patient with amputation and immediate postoperative prosthetic fitting (IPPF, IPOP, or IPSF).[12–15]

The authors' success rate of IPPF has been excellent for elective amputations in both dysvascular and nonvascular amputees,[3, 13–15] but not all authors have achieved similar results.[6] IPPF techniques have not been widely applied in a trauma setting outside of large centers specializing in amputation surgery. IPPF techniques have not been applied to those patients who should almost always become rehabilitated successfully, young traumatic amputees; this is primarily because it has been assumed that early weight bearing might hinder the healing of the residual limb of a traumatic amputation. In addition, there is valid concern that primary wound closure (with immediate postsurgical prosthetic fitting) might lead to a high incidence of residual limb infection. The latter problem can be for the most part eliminated by using delayed primary or secondary wound closure and early prosthetic fitting when wound healing has occurred. The former problem has not occurred in the authors' series.

Clinical Experience

A review of the traumatic amputations performed at the University of Arizona Health Science Center and at the Maricopa Medical

Center revealed 47 amputations performed in 42 patients between January 1977 and March 1988. The group was composed of 37 males and five females, with a mean age of 30.2 years (a range of 4 to 72 years). There were 18 upper extremity amputations (12 below the elbow, four above the elbow, and two shoulder disarticulations) and 29 lower extremity amputations (one Syme's, 19 below the knee, eight above the knee, and one hip disarticulation). The authors' experience with traumatic upper extremity amputation and prosthetic rehabilitation has been reported elsewhere.[12] The remainder of this chapter deals specifically with lower extremity amputation.

A review of the mechanism of injury in 29 lower extremity amputations in 26 patients reveals the following incidence: eight train accidents involving a pedestrian, six motorcycle accidents, five motor vehicle accidents, three car accidents involving a pedestrian, three work-related accidents, two garden machinery accidents, and two gunshot wounds. There were associated injuries in 10 of 26 patients (38%) and an average of 2.7 associated injuries per patient. Twenty of 27 associated injuries (74%) were orthopedic in nature.

Patient Management

The overall principles of management for traumatic lower extremity amputation included priority concern for life-threatening injuries; preservation of maximal limb length; careful debridement with a Waterpik; primary or delayed primary closure, if possible; immediate or early prosthetic fitting; and early aggressive prosthetic rehabilitation.

When amputation was deemed necessary, an attempt was made to preserve maximal limb length consistent with prosthetic rehabilitation. For partial foot injuries, an attempt was made to salvage either a distal transmetatarsal amputation or a Syme's amputation. The proximal limit for salvage of a below-knee amputation was 5 cm of the tibia inferior to the tibial tubercle after debridement of devitalized tissue; however, in order to perform a below-knee amputation, an adequate length of posterior, medial, or lateral skin was mandatory in order to allow construction of a myocutaneous flap for residual limb closure (although the traditional below-knee amputation for the dysvascular patient involves a posterior myocutaneous flap, in young trauma patients [in whom vascular insufficiency is not usually a problem] a posterior, medial, or lateral flap can be used for residual limb closure). Knee joint salvage was not attempted if an amputation could not be performed at the below-knee level. In such instances, a long above-knee amputation (a modified knee disarticulation) was performed.[13] For a traumatic injury above the knee, an attempt was made to preserve maximal femur length. In one patient, a hip disarticulation was required, and in that case, a posterior myocutaneous flap was constructed with the posterolateral aspect of the thigh.

Wounds were copiously irrigated with a cephalosporin-saline solution (1 g/1000 ml) to remove foreign debris and devitalized tissue. Debridement was aided by Water-pik irrigation and conventional sharp debridement. Vascular structures were carefully suture ligated. Tendons were gently pulled down into the wound, sharply divided, and allowed to retract out of the wound. Major motor and sensory nerves were similarly retracted into the wound, suture ligated, transected distal to the suture, and allowed to retract out of the wound. Wound closure consisted of approximation of the fascia with interrupted absorbable sutures, and the skin was either left open (9 patients) or closed primarily (20 patients), depending on the degree of contamination and the judgment of the surgeon. If skin closure was performed, skin was approximated using either stainless steel staples or 3-0 monofilament interrupted sutures. Because of "wet wounds," 13 amputations (45%) required residual limb drainage with closed suction Silastic drains. Although there was no significant difference between the number of complications in drained and undrained wounds, postoperative edema resolved at a more rapid rate in those limbs that were drained.

Immediate Postoperative Prosthetic Fitting

Standard IPPF techniques were used for all patients.[4, 5, 12–15] The surgical wound was covered with Owen's silk soaked in a 1%

cephapirin sodium (Cefadyl) solution or with Xeroform gauze. The end of the residual limb was then padded with sterile lamb's wool before the application of a sterile Spandex residual limb sock. Bony prominences were padded with felt pressure-relief pads that were glued to the Spandex sock before casting. The cast shell was fashioned with an inner layer of elastic plaster (Orthoflex)* and an outer layer of Scotchcast.† The pylon/foot assembly was secured to the residual limb cast with Scotchcast. A waist suspension belt aided cast suspension in all cases. When drains were used, they were usually brought out laterally through the cast to facilitate easy removal. Drains were removed when drainage subsided, usually 2 to 3 days after surgery.

Normally, the first cast change and wound inspection occurred at 7 to 10 days after surgery; however, if there was concern about a residual limb infection (increased temperature or elevated white blood cell count) or inappropriate pain (increased *not* decreased pain during the first few days after surgery) the cast was removed, and the wound was inspected. If the wound and residual limb were unremarkable, the cast and prosthesis were replaced. If, however, there was concern about residual limb infection or skin healing problems, the limb was wrapped with an Ace bandage, and the wound was carefully evaluated over the ensuing days. If the wound appeared to be healing well at 7 to 10 days, a second cast was applied that remained in place for another 7 to 10 days. After the second cast change (14 to 20 days), patients were fitted with a lightweight removable, temporary or "throwaway" prosthesis. These prostheses were constructed with Scotchcast and a United States Manufacturing Company Aqualite lower extremity kit, using techniques that have been described previously.[13] Because of the expense of a permanent prosthetic device and the 3 to 6 months required to achieve residual limb maturity (even with IPPF), it is impractical to prescribe a permanent prosthesis until approximately 6 months after amputation. The use of temporary, removable ("throwaway") prostheses allows continued rehabilitation

---

*Johnson & Johnson Co., New Brunswick, New Jersey.
†3M, St Paul, Minnesota.

and physical therapy without the expense of multiple permanent artificial legs.

Postoperative rehabilitation began immediately after surgery. On the first day after surgery, patients were taught touchdown weight bearing at bedside. During the first 7 to 10 days, they walked between parallel bars in physical therapy with only partial (10%) weight bearing. During the second 7 to 10 days, patients progressed to 50% weight bearing between parallel bars. At the time of the second cast change (14 to 20 days after surgery), the patients were fitted with a temporary, removable prosthesis, and they were advanced to full weight bearing with careful repeated residual limb inspection. When the patients could ambulate satisfactorily with either partial or full weight bearing between parallel bars, they were taught the use of crutches or a walker and then were rapidly progressed to independent ambulation when they achieved full weight bearing. The postoperative rehabilitation process was carefully followed up by the surgeon, the prosthetist, and the rehabilitation therapist.[12–15]

Those patients who were not treated with immediate postoperative prosthesis because of open surgical wounds (four above-knee and five below-knee amputees) were sent to rehabilitation as rapidly as possible for upper extremity strengthening and passive and active lower extremity range of motion exercises. After either delayed primary closure or secondary wound closure, those nine patients were fitted with an early postsurgical prosthesis (constructed as an IPPF prosthesis) and were advanced through the rehabilitation process as previously described for the IPPF patients.

Results

For the 29 traumatic lower extremity amputations reviewed in the authors' series, 20 (five above-knee, 14-below-knee, and one Syme's amputation) were closed primarily and fitted with immediate postoperative prostheses; and nine (four above-knee and five below-knee amputations) underwent delayed primary closure or secondary closure, and the patients were rehabilitated as soon as their wounds permitted application of prostheses. The interval between injury and operation ranged from half an hour to 17 days (the latter was a patient in whom knee salvage was attempted), with a mean of 42.5 hours. Most patients received definitive treatment less than 2 hours from the time of injury. There were no postoperative deaths. Five of nine (56%) above-knee amputations were closed primarily. There were no infections or residual limb breakdowns in the group with primary wound closure. Three of the remaining four above-knee amputations were closed without complication several days after initial debridement and amputation. Fourteen of 19 (74%) below-knee amputations were closed primarily, and there were no wound complications. Five wounds were left open because of concerns about gross contamination, and all five required formal secondary revision for eventual wound closure, which occurred without complication.

Twenty-six patients with 29 lower extremity amputations were available for long-term follow-up, with a mean of more than 4 years. Three patients were lost to long-term follow-up. Patients were not classified as being fully rehabilitated unless they continued to use their prostheses for most activities of daily living or work.

Three of 26 patients (15%) undergoing traumatic lower extremity amputation required subsequent surgery at times ranging from 2 days to 11 months after amputation. One patient required revision for a neuroma at 11 months, and one patient required wound revision because of necrotic skin edges at 3 weeks; one patient required neuroma excision twice, at 4 months and at 6 months.

Twenty-one of 23 patients (91%) were successfully rehabilitated with a prosthesis: one of one hip disarticulation, five of six (83%) above-knee amputations, 14 of 15 (93%) below-knee amputations, and one of one Syme's amputation. The patients were placed in one of three categories on the basis of their activities before injury: those at work, those in school, and those either retired or unemployed. More than 80% of the patients at work or at school returned to their previous activities.

There were no complications due to the immediate postoperative prosthesis (0/20). The length of hospitalization ranged from 8 to 58 days, with a mean hospital stay of approximately 3 weeks. Most patients left the hospital ambulatory with crutches or a walker, and several patients left after 3 weeks, walking independently.

SUMMARY

A review of the data suggests that

1. Primary closure of *selected* traumatic lower extremity amputation results in a low incidence of infection and a high incidence of primary healing and allows early aggressive rehabilitation.

2. Patients with below-knee amputations appear to have the best chance for full rehabilitation and return to work.

3. A team approach to the treatment of a person with a traumatic amputation has the best chance of achieving overall rapid rehabilitation. If a full rehabilitation team is not available, a team of three (the surgeon, prosthetist, and physical therapist) can be expected to achieve results similar to those of the full team.[13]

Amputation after trauma will have the best results if certain principles are followed. This chapter has outlined these principles and stressed the importance of a team approach. The rehabilitation program's goal is to restore the patient to a state of functional independence as soon as possible. That goal is best achieved by immediate postoperative prosthetic techniques combined with early aggressive wound management to allow prosthetic fitting as soon as possible. It should be emphasized that if there is a long delay between accident and operative intervention or if there is a significant degree of wound contamination (such as from water-related or farm accidents), primary wound closure and IPPF should not be attempted. In these latter cases, delayed primary closure or secondary residual limb closure with early prosthetic fitting should be used.

REFERENCES

1. Berlemont M: Notre expérience de l'appareillage précoce des amputés des membres inférieurs aux établissements helio Marins de Berk. Ann Med Phys 5:4, 1961.
2. Bodemer CW: Baron Dominique Jean Larrey, Napoleon's surgeon. Am Coll Surg Bull July 1982, pp 18–21.
3. Bradway J, Racy J, Malone JM: Psychological adaptation to amputation. Orthot Prosthet 38:45, 1984.
4. Burgess EM, Romano RL: The management of lower extremity amputees using immediate post-surgical prosthesis. Clin Orthop 57:137, 1968.
5. Burgess EM, Tramb JE, Wilson AB Jr: Immediate post-surgical prosthetics in the management of lower extremity amputees. Bulletin TR 10-5. Washington, DC, Veterans Administration, 1967.
6. Cohen SI, Goldman LO, Salzman EW, Glotzer DJ: The deleterious effect of immediate postoperative prosthesis in below-knee amputation for ischemic disease. Surgery 761:992, 1974.
7. DeBakey ME, Simeone FA: Battle injuries of the arteries in WW II. Ann Surg 123:534, 1946.
8. Eger M, Gokman L, Goldstein A, Hirsch M: The use of a temporary shunt in the management of arterial vascular injuries. Surg Gynecol Obstet 132:67, 1971.
9. Engstrand JL: Rehabilitation of the patient with a lower extremity amputation. Nurs Clin North Am 11:659, 1976.
10. Hoopes JE, Jabaley ME: Soft tissue injuries of the extremities. *In* Ballinger WF, Rutherford R, Zuidema G (eds): The Management of Trauma. Philadelphia, WB Saunders Co, 1973, pp 496–524.
11. Huston CC, Bivins BA, Ernst CB, Griffin WO Jr: Morbid implications of above-knee amputations. Report of a series and review of the literature. Arch Surg 115:165, 1980.
12. Malone JM, Fleming LL, Roberson J, et al: Immediate, early and late post-surgical management of upper extremity amputation. J Rehabil Res Dev 21:33, 1984.
13. Malone JM, Goldstone J: Lower extremity amputation. *In* Moore WS (ed): A Comprehensive Review of Vascular Surgery, 2nd Ed. Philadelphia, WB Saunders Co, 1986, pp 1139–1208.
14. Malone JM, Moore WS, Goldstone J, Malone SJ: Therapeutic and economic impact of a modern amputation program. Ann Surg 189:798, 1979.
15. Malone JM, Moore WS, Leal JM, Childers SJ: Rehabilitation for lower extremity amputation. Arch Surg 116:93, 1981.
16. Miller HH, Welch CS: Quantitative studies on the time factor in arterial injuries. Ann Surg 130:428, 1949.
17. Otteman MG, Stahlgren LH: Evaluation of factors which influence mortality and morbidity following major lower extremity amputation for arteriosclerosis. Surg Gynecol Obstet 120:1217, 1965.
18. Perry MO: Management of Acute Vascular Injuries. Baltimore, Williams & Wilkins, 1981, pp 13–42.
19. Rich NM, Baugh JH, Hughes CW: Acute arterial injuries in Vietnam: 1000 cases. J Trauma 10:359, 1970.
20. Rich NM, Hobson RW II, Collins GJ Jr, Anderson CA: The effect of acute popliteal venous interruption. Ann Surg 183:365, 1976.
21. Rich NM, Hughes CW: The fate of prosthetic material used to repair vascular injuries in contaminated wounds. J Trauma 12:459, 1972.
22. Rich NM, Hughes CW, Baugh JH: Management of venous injuries. Ann Surg 171:724, 1970.
23. Rich N, Spencer F: Venous injuries. *In* Rich N, Spencer F (eds): Vascular Trauma. Philadelphia, WB Saunders Co, 1978, pp 55–190.
24. Roon AJ, Moore WS, Goldstone J: Below-knee amputation: A modern approach. Am J Surg 134:153, 1977.
25. Ruby LK: Acute traumatic amputation of an extremity. Orthop Clin North Am 9:679, 1978.

26. Seddon HJ: Three types of nerve injury. Brain 66:238, 1943.

27. Shumaker HB, Wayson EE: Spontaneous cure of aneurysms and arteriovenous fistulas with some notes on intravascular thrombosis. Am J Surg 79:532, 1950.

28. Smith JW: Microsurgery of peripheral nerves. Plast Reconstr Surg 33:317, 1964.

29. Vaughn GD, Mattox KL, Feliciano DV, et al: Surgical experience with expanded polytetrafluoroethylene (PTFE) as a replacement graft for traumatized vessels. J Trauma 19:403, 1979.

30. Wangensteen OH, Wangensteen SD: The Rise of Surgery from Empiric Craft to Scientific Discipline. Minneapolis, University of Minnesota Press, 1978, pp 18–52, 279, 378.

31. Weiss M: The prosthesis on the operating table from a neurophysical point of view. Report of a workshop panel on lower extremity prosthetic fitting. Committee on Prosthetics Research and Development. National Academy of Sciences, February 1966.

32. Young JZ: The functional repair of nervous tissue. Physiol Rev 22:318, 1942.

26

Psychological Aspects of Amputation

John C. Racy, M.D.

Amputation is a triple threat. It involves a loss of function, a loss of sensation, and a loss of body image. The wonder of it is that so many adapt so well, thanks to their resilience and the ingenuity and dedication of those who care for them. In preparing this chapter, use was made of the experience of many people at the University of Arizona College of Medicine and elsewhere.[1, 13] Furthermore, it was possible to arrange a meeting with an amputee self-help group in the Tucson area. Reference will be made to that group, and quotes from its members will be inserted in the text to illustrate points under consideration.

DETERMINANTS OF PSYCHOLOGICAL RESPONSE

The psychological response observed in amputees is determined by many variables. These can be conveniently grouped into psychosocial variables affecting the individual and medical variables reflecting the health and the medical and surgical management of the amputee.

Psychosocial Variables

Age

It can generally be assumed that the degree of psychological difficulty associated with amputation increases with the age of the amputee, all other considerations being equal.[16, 24, 27] Thus, it is noted that children born with a congenitally missing limb adapt adequately as they make use of their remaining faculties. Losses occurring in childhood have the greatest impact on the sense of identity and self-esteem. Young people in general make an excellent adaptation to the loss of function and are able to manipulate the prostheses and other limbs with great agility. Yet, even the most dedicated support of parents, siblings, professionals, and other amputees is not sufficient in the absence of peer acceptance. Lacking the latter, young people, especially preadolescents and adolescents, remain subject to self-consciousness, social withdrawal, and lower self-esteem.[27] Among young adults, the response to the limb loss depends on its causes and the degree of disability and disfigurement resulting from it. Young adults do, however, have the advantages of physical resilience, financial security, and social confidence; hence, they tend to make an excellent adaptation. Among the elderly, ill health, social isolation (especially after the death of a spouse), and financial limitations all conspire to complicate the adjustment to the limb loss. Thus, for the young, the greatest challenges are in terms of identity and social acceptance, whereas for the elderly, the greatest challenges are in terms of livelihood and functional capacity.[16, 23, 27]

Personality Style

The interaction of personality style and limb loss is in some ways predictable and in other ways unexpected. Individuals who are narcissistically invested in their physical appearance and power tend to react negatively to the loss of the limb. They see it as a major assault upon their dignity and self-worth. Conversely, dependent individuals may cherish the sick role and find in it welcome relief from pressure and responsibility. Thus, for them the loss of limb can be approached with considerable equanimity. Not surprisingly, timid and self-conscious individuals are more likely to suffer from limb loss than others who are less concerned about their social standing.[23]

Unexpected reactions may arise from secondary gain. If the individual becomes better off financially or socially as a result of the disability, the adjustment is likely to be made much easier, especially if that gain is not directly challenged. Should the amputation bring about the resolution of a psychological conflict, be it conscious or otherwise, the individual may indeed be happy that it occurred. Individuals possessed of a rigid personality are reported to have a greater incidence of complications such as phantom pain after surgery.[12] Those tending toward a pessimistic or paranoid outlook are likely to find their worst expectations confirmed, and their rehabilitation may be colored by much bitterness and resentment.[23]

Economic and Vocational Variables

It stands to reason that individuals who earn their living from motor skills that are lost with the amputation are especially vulnerable to adverse reactions. Others, who have a wider range of skills or whose main line of work is not particularly dependent on the function of the lost limb, experience less emotional difficulty. The more physical or menial the task, the more likely it is to be affected by limb loss. Conversely, the more intellectual, administrative, or professional the pursuit, the less likely it is to be disturbed by the loss of a limb. Unemployment is associated with a greater degree of psychological distress and is one of the predictors of phantom pain.[20]

Psychosocial Support

All human beings require a support system throughout life in order to maintain emotional health. However, not all are so blessed, and many find themselves transiently or permanently in a state of isolation. Not surprisingly, single and widowed individuals suffer more psychological distress and difficulty in adapting to amputation than do those who are married and have a family. Particularly helpful in the adjustment of the amputee is the presence of a supportive partner who assumes a flexible approach, taking over functions when needed, cutting back when the amputee is able to manage, but at all times maintaining the amputee's self-esteem.[14, 23] Peer acceptance beyond the family is a factor in the successful adaptation of all amputees and is crucial, as mentioned earlier, for older children and adolescents.

Medical Factors

Health

The previous and present health status of the amputee is a major determinant of adjustment. Hence, healthy, young individuals who lose a limb traumatically have many advantages over older, frail individuals.[23] Among the elderly—who, in fact, constitute the vast majority of amputees—the surgery usually comes after a prolonged period of treatment for peripheral vascular disease, often combined with at least two other medical disorders.[27] These disorders are likely to set a limit on functional restoration and the return to an active lifestyle.

Mental health problems can easily enter into the picture through a complicated series of psychosomatic and somatopsychic responses to the loss. In this regard, depression—with its attendant loss of energy, pessimism, and psychomotor retardation—may delay rehabilitation, a delay that in turn exerts a depressing effect on the individual. Anger, sometimes displaced from the surgeon and the amputation team onto the primary care physician or perhaps a member of the family, can lead to maladaptive behavior.[27] Furthermore, anger often underlies the depressive reaction described earlier. In a study of 46 amputees seen in London, Parkes found that "among the 38 amputees who were thought to have some overall limitation of function attributable to psychological origin, factors inculpated, in order of frequency, were depression, timidity, fear of further self-injury, self-consciousness, low intelligence, senility, anger, resentment of the need to rely on others and secondary gain."[23]

Reason for the Amputation

Much of the earlier work on amputation in this century centered on wartime casualties.[5, 12, 24] The current situation is quite different in that the amputation affects a much older age group and follows either trauma or chronic illness, rather than combat. A wartime situation in which the injury to the limb might lead to evacuation from the front, honorable discharge from the service, and rehabilitation to civilian life is not often seen today.[24] Young adults suffering a traumatic or accidental limb loss sustain a major assault on self-esteem. They tend to react with varying forms of denial and bravado.[19, 27] Because of their youth, agility, and determination, they can achieve an excellent adjustment. Young adults who undergo an elective amputation for the cure of a malignancy present a very different picture. In such cases, there is adequate time for exploration of alternatives and for preparation. The reaction is usually one of realistic acceptance and total cooperation with the treatment team.[27] Such individuals seem to make an excellent adjustment, assuming, of course, that the malignancy has been cured.

For the elderly, surgery usually occurs after a long period of suffering resulting from diabetes and peripheral vascular disease. Most elderly patients accept the surgery with much relief, since it often signals the end of suffering and the return to improved functioning. The rest react indifferently or negatively, sometimes viewing the surgery as the ultimate proof of failure.[22, 27] Amputation

necessitated by the negligent behavior of the patient or someone else is likely to produce persistent feelings of resentment and self-doubt.[24] Litigation for compensation can be a complication that has a major impact on the process of rehabilitation and recovery.

Preparation for the Amputation

There is little doubt that those individuals who have had adequate warning and preparation fare better in the postsurgical period, whereas those who do not receive such preparation tend to react negatively or with massive denial. It is less clear whether these differences are evident in ultimate adaptation, which, after all, is governed by many other variables preceding and following the amputation.[3, 6, 11]

Nature and Magnitude of Loss

It can be assumed that the greater the loss, the greater the difficulty in adjustment. Yet, there are those instances of massive psychological reaction to minor loss—for example the loss of a toe or half of a foot—and of minimal reaction to severe loss of several limbs such that a firm rule correlating response with loss cannot be made.[13] Generally, the more of a limb that is lost, the harder it is for the individual to adapt.[1] There is less of a clear indication whether lower limb loss is harder to accept than upper limb loss, as had been suggested.[22, 24] Above-elbow amputation brings with it great anxiety and frustration, and bilateral above-elbow amputation is perhaps the most difficult situation of all. Contrarily, amputation of one leg below the knee allows relatively good adjustment, with restoration of both function and body image.[1]

Surgical Complications

Those individuals who suffer pain, infection, and residual limb revision tend to develop greater degrees of despair and withdrawal than those who do not.[23] This highlights the importance of surgical skill in the performance of the amputation. As the author has written elsewhere, "A poorly performed amputation almost guarantees poor rehabilitation. While a well-performed amputation does not guarantee a successful rehabilitation outcome, it certainly makes successful rehabilitation more possible."[3]

Prosthetic Rehabilitation

The earlier a prosthesis is applied, the less is the psychological distress observed after amputation. Conversely, if the prosthetic application is absent or delayed, greater degrees of anxiety, sadness, and self-consciousness are noted. The crucial elements appear to be the integration of the prosthesis into the body image and the concentration of attention on future function rather than on past loss.[3, 17]

The Team Approach

Because adaptation to amputation is so multifaceted and because it is an evolving process requiring different kinds of attention at each stage, the team approach has emerged as the norm in the care of the amputee.[3, 8, 14, 17, 18, 27] The range of skills and points of view represented in a team increase the probability that all aspects of rehabilitation are addressed and that none are overlooked. The team sometimes includes members of the family and successfully treated amputees. Amputee self-help groups may indeed be regarded as further extensions of this approach.[10, 15] This topic is discussed more completely in Chapter 20.

Vocational Rehabilitation

Although vocational rehabilitation is not strictly a medical approach, restoration of the capability for gainful employment is an integral part of the patient's recovery. In fact, unemployment is predictive of complications such as residual limb and phantom pain.[20] On the basis of extensive experience with amputees, Kohl observed that "men define this loss of income as a denial of their 'right' to participate in the family's decision-making processes." Furthermore, it is her view that "the success of rehabilitation efforts should not only be measured by return to income-producing work, but rather the return to the person of his decision-making abilities to choose the lifestyle that would be most fulfilling to him."[14]

STAGES OF ADAPTATION

It is useful and customary to think of adaptation as occurring in four stages.[3, 4, 7, 9, 14, 24] With the exception of the clear demarcation between preoperative and postoperative stages, most of the adjustment occurs on a gradual and often invisible continuum. A division into four stages, however, allows for the highlighting of issues that arise most critically at each point in time.

Preoperative Stage

For most amputees today, there is ample opportunity for preparation before surgery. Among those so prepared, approximately one third to one half welcome the amputation as a signal that suffering will be relieved and a new phase of adjustment can begin. Along with this acceptance, there may be varying degrees of anxiety and concern. Such concerns fall into two large groups. First, and perhaps for most persons the more important, are such *practical* issues as the loss of function, loss of income, pain, difficulty in adapting to a prosthesis, and cost of ongoing treatment. Second are more *symbolic* concerns, such as changes in appearance, losses in sexual intimacy, perception by others, and disposal of the limb. Most individuals informed of the need for amputation go through the early stages of a grief reaction, which may not be completed until well after their return home. Such a grief response often starts with a "numbing" of feelings and progresses after a few days to profound sadness and "pining" for the part about to be lost, along with varying degrees of anxiety and anger.[21] The manner in which the surgery is presented by the surgeon can have much bearing on the magnitude and kind of affective response. Labeling it as a reconstructive prelude to an improved life is a much different matter from implying that it is a mutilation and a failure. Furthermore, detailed explanation of all aspects of the surgery and the rehabilitative response, maintenance of a hopeful attitude, and answering all questions (especially those that seem trivial) appear to diminish anxiety, anger, and despair.

One member of the self-help group interviewed for this report spoke of her impending amputation as "losing a member of my family." She felt scared "out of my wits" and was repeatedly "horrified." She reported that her surgeon had described her as his "failure" and told her very little about the details of the surgery and the process beyond. Another group member described her reaction as one of ambivalence and oscillation. She switched repeatedly from acknowledging that the amputation was to be expected, and even desirable, to great fear and dread. "Like a ghost in my closet," she said, "I took it out now and then to scare myself with it." A third group member, when informed that she would lose her leg, reacted with the thought, "They might as well take off my head." A 13-year-old reacted to the news that a leg amputation was necessary to cure her osteogenic sarcoma with the statement, "No boy is going to look at me." She wanted her limb to be well cared for because 'it was really a good leg." An older veteran responded with the thought, "I would have to sell pencils for the rest of my life in front of the post office." The last two responses fit in with the general view that for the young, the concern is about body image and peer acceptance, whereas for older individuals, it is about function and livelihood. Those group members who did have the opportunity to receive adequate preparation before the surgery commented on it as having contributed materially to their peace of mind after the event.

Immediate Postoperative Stage

The immediate postoperative stage is the period between the surgery and the start of the rehabilitative process. It may last a matter of hours or days, depending, among other things, on the reason for the amputation, the extent and condition of the residual limb, and the kind of rehabilitation thought to be feasible. Among the psychological reactions noted in this phase are concerns about safety, fear of complications and pain, and, in some instances, loss of alertness and orientation.[14] In general, those who sustain the amputation after a period of preparation react more positively than those who sustain their surgery after trauma or accident. Most individuals are, to a certain degree, "numb," partly as a result of the anesthesia and partly as a way of handling the trauma of loss. For those who have suffered considerable pain before

the surgery, the feeling after amputation may be one of vast relief. This was true for four of the eight members of the self-help group interviewed for this report.

In-Hospital Rehabilitation

In-hospital rehabilitation, in many ways, is the most critical phase, presenting the greatest challenges to the patient, the family, and the amputation team. Among other things, it calls for a flexible approach addressed to the rapidly evolving needs of the individual. Early on, concerns are about safety, pain, and disfigurement. Later on, the emphasis shifts to social reintegration and vocational adjustment.[14, 27] Some individuals in this phase experience and express various kinds of denial shown through bravado and competitiveness. A few resort to humor and minimization. Mild euphoric states may be reflected in increased motor activity, racing through the corridors in wheelchairs, and over-talkativeness. Others make wisecracks, such as, "You see more when you walk slowly."[19] Later, sadness may return or may occur for the first time if there has not been any period of preparation.

Parkes describes the grief response as similar to that seen in widows.[21] He indicates that the process of realization entails four phases: from (1) "numbness," in which outside stimuli are shut out or denied, to (2) "pining" for what is lost, to (3) disorganization, in which all hope of recovering the lost part is given up, and on to (4) reorganization. The degree to which individuals go through these four phases of realization varies from individual to individual, and, indeed, the process often lasts well beyond the period of in-hospital rehabilitation. It is also during this time that individuals experience phantom limb sensations and phantom pain (see the discussion that follows). Factors that are noted to facilitate adjustment and rehabilitation in this phase are early prosthetic fitting, acceptance of the amputation and the prosthesis by family and friends, and introduction of a successfully rehabilitated amputee to the recovering patient.[1, 3, 6, 13, 14, 18, 22, 24, 27]

Almost all the members of the group interviewed for this report agreed that early prosthetic introduction was of the highest importance. For two women who sustained below-knee amputation, awakening to find that they had, indeed, two "legs" in bed was most reassuring and lifted their morale. The 13-year-old delighted in throwing back the bedclothes and flaunting her artificial leg to her adolescent visitors. Those who did not, for one reason or another, obtain a prosthesis, looked forward to it and often fantasized about it. One young man who lost his upper arm as a result of an electrical injury dreamed of becoming a "bionic man."

Sadness, though keenly felt, may also be concealed. A young mother who lost her hand in a paper shredder tried to put on a happy face for her family. "Sometimes," she said, "we have to joke so that people around us can deal with it."

At-Home Rehabilitation

By all accounts, the amputee's return home can be a particularly taxing period because of the loss of the familiar surroundings of the hospital and, more importantly, the attenuation of the ongoing guidance and support provided by the rehabilitation team. Clearly, the attitude of the family becomes a major determinant of the amputee's course beyond this point.[23]

It is during this phase that the full impact of the loss becomes evident. A number of individuals experience a "second realization," with attendant sadness and grief.[22] Varying degrees of regressive behavior may be evident, such as a reluctance to give up the sick role and a tendency to lean on others beyond what is justified by the disability. Some resent any pressure put upon them to resume normal functioning. Others may go to the other extreme and vehemently reject any suggestion that they might be disabled or require help in any way. An excessive show of sympathy generally fosters the notion that one is to be pitied. In this phase, three areas of concern come to the fore: return to gainful employment, social acceptance, and sexual adjustment. Of immense value in all of these matters is the availability of a significant other or family member who can provide support without damaging self-esteem.[14, 23]

The mother of the young man who lost his arm as the result of an electrical injury spoke of the profound change that occurred in his behavior on his return home. He regressed to the point that she felt she "had another baby in the house." The young mother who lost her arm in the paper shredder was con-

cerned that people would look at her as though she were a "freak" but found her anxiety in this regard greatly relieved when both her children and their schoolmates took her amputation in stride and asked matter-of-factly about it. A middle-aged woman who sustained her amputation after a prolonged period of disability resulting from poliomyelitis found herself one day facing a sinkful of dishes and a request from her husband that she wash them. She did wash the dishes, but with tears running down her face and thoughts running through her mind of her husband as cruel and mean. Later she recognized that it was the best thing that he could have done for her and was rather amused to learn that the scenario was contrived by her surgeon and her husband in order to encourage her independence. Equally helpful to her was her children's startled response on learning that their mother was receiving disability benefits. To them, she did not seem to be disabled and therefore did not need benefits. In fact, they were intrigued by her new leg prosthesis and expressed the wish that perhaps they too could don and remove their limbs when they grew up.

The group members were unanimous in rejecting the "handicapped" label, and each thought that his or her affliction was lighter than those of the others. One of them said, "Most well-adjusted people prefer to accept what happened to them" and thus "would not trade with another amputee." All conceded that the adaptation would have been immensely more difficult without the active support of members of their families.

A subtle but often overlooked issue is the ease with which the disability can be concealed. One group member, for example, remarked that one advantage of a leg amputation over an upper limb loss was that it could escape detection in social settings.

Not surprisingly, those amputees able to resume a full and productive life tend to fare best; this is much easier for those with marketable skills who sustain the amputation while still in vigorous health. For elderly amputees who have limited skills, particularly if they have other medical disorders, the probability of full return to an active life is considerably diminished. This can be partially or fully balanced by a more philosophical acceptance of a new, more leisurely way of living and by reduced responsibility and pressure to produce.[14]

SPECIAL AREAS OF CONCERN

Phantom Limb Sensations

The feeling that the amputated limb is present and moving is so common as to be regarded a universal occurrence after surgery.[5, 12, 20] It tends to disappear rapidly, however, so that only a few individuals continue to perceive their limbs as still present and active a year after surgery. Many, however, continue to have *occasional* experiences of itching or locomotion, sometimes after residual limb stimulation. Phantom limb experience has not been noted in those who are born congenitally missing a limb and in those who sustain the limb loss at a very early age.

In general, phantom limb sensations present no particular problem. The members of the self-help group had all experienced them at one time or another. Some of them still do, 10 or 15 years after amputation. For the most part, the phantom limb is experienced in the form of an intermittent itch that, curiously, is relieved by scratching the prosthesis.

Phantom Pain

Pain experienced in the missing limb is a much more serious issue than phantom limb sensations and, fortunately, is much rarer. In the author's experience at the University of Arizona, phantom pain occurs in less than 2% of amputees (also see Chapter 18).

Phantom pain has defied explanation. In all probability, it is an extension or variant of phantom limb sensations, but with added somatic and psychological disturbances. Parkes found that phantom pain could be predicted by certain immediate postoperative phenomena, such as the presence of residual limb pain, prior illness of more than one year, the development of residual limb complications, and, interestingly, other factors not related to surgery (e.g., continued unemployment and a rigid personality).[20] Some amputees experience phantom pain in association with micturition, climatic changes, and emotionally disturbing events.[12] Kolb and Brodie found an association between phantom pain and incomplete mourning for the lost limb.[12] In the series of 2284 amputees studied by Ewalt and colleagues at the end

of World War II, phantom pain was extremely rare and was noted in individuals who also showed psychopathology. The authors wrote that pain "tended to come and to go with psychopathological symptoms, irrespective of what type of external treatment was carried on."[5] Thus, phantom pain, although unusual, can be a serious and disabling condition that is evidently related to the antecedent and concurrent medical states and to environmental and psychological factors.

In the self-help group, only one member described persistent phantom pain accompanied by residual limb pain. This individual had suffered long and complicated procedures after the initial amputation, all designed to relieve his phantom pain. These included nerve stimulation, acupuncture, residual limb revision, and even spinal block. At the time of the interview, his only relief came from the use of oxycodone (Percodan) on a regular basis. So distressed was he by his pain that he had repeatedly entertained the fantasy of taking a gun and shooting his "leg" off in order to rid himself of it. Other members experienced *fleeting* episodes of pain described as an electric shock sensation, or, as one put it, "like putting your finger in a 220 [volt] outlet." A few described cramping sensations and feelings of constriction that diminished over time. Two mentioned aching when the weather changed and rain was approaching. Several members of the group spontaneously volunteered the view that the support of the family members was of great help in reducing phantom pain when it occurred.

Body Image

Amputation, of necessity, requires a revision of body image. This is reflected in dreams and in the Draw-A-Person Test. It has been reported that amputees who adapt well draw a person with a foreshortened limb, or without any limb at all, whereas those who adapt poorly draw the missing limb larger than the opposite limb or with increased markings.[19] Similarly, dreams that incorporate the prosthesis or do not particularly dwell on the missing part are consistent with a more positive adaptation to the amputation rather than a preoccupation with it.[13] It has been suggested that the amputee, in a sense, must contend with three body images: intact, amputated, and with prosthesis. Individuals who are unable to accept their body image either as an amputee or as someone with a prosthesis are likely to reject the use of the prosthesis and to experience difficulty in functional and social adjustment.[13] Related to the issue of revised body image is concern with social appearances and acceptance by others. Even when considerable success is achieved in functional restoration, there often remains some shyness about revealing the amputated body to others.

The members of the group confirmed these observations and saw a connection between accepting one's new bodily configuration and accepting a prosthesis. One viewed her body more positively after amputation because her prosthetic leg worked better than the leg that she had lost. Most had come to regard their prosthesis as part of themselves, as was occasionally revealed in dreams. Nonetheless, despite their successful adaptation and acceptance of the new body image, all of them continue to experience self-consciousness in social situations. For example, they tend to walk more clumsily when they feel observed by other people in public. The group members described a recent pool party to which they had invited their friends and relatives. Significantly, the only people at the party who actually did go into the pool were the nonamputees.

Sexuality

This is an area of some anxiety for most amputees, especially those who are young and in the prime of life.[13, 14, 25] Concern arises from the following sources:

1. A distorted body image and the fear that the body would not be accepted by the partner
2. The loss of a functioning body part, such as the hand
3. The loss of an area of sensation

Whereas a prosthesis can provide functional restoration and some return to normal appearance in most situations, it is absolutely of no use in the sexual area. A comparison with the sexual experience of paraplegics is instructive. Those who suffer paralysis still enjoy sensation from the affected part and continue to see their body as intact. They may also entertain hope of a return of func-

tion in the affected part. The amputee enjoys none of these advantages.[13]

Among the members of the group, sexuality was an important issue that had to be faced by each of them. Most reported success in facing it. Such success was mainly attributed to the supportive response of the partner. Yet despite the verbal and behavioral reassurance of the partner, several individuals spoke of lingering difficulty in seeing themselves as adequate sexual partners rather than as repulsive sexual "freaks." As one group member put it, "There is still a small part that doesn't accept." It would appear that the passage of time aids in this adjustment; one group member stated that 15 years after the event, her missing limb was "a nonissue" in the sexual sense. This was not the case for the 13-year-old, who had expressed the concern that no boy would ever look at her. She lived for 2 years after her surgery but did not have occasion to go out on a date. She did maintain the hope that one day she would do so and was greatly comforted by her brother-in-law, who told her that her amputation would "weed out the creeps."

MANAGEMENT

The principles of successful psychological management of the amputee are implied in the foregoing discussion. Although the involvement of a psychiatrist or psychologist can greatly enrich the therapeutic team and provide guidance and support for those individuals who are intimately involved in the day-to-day care of the amputee, rarely is a psychiatric consultation required.[1, 3, 13, 14] Six principles of management emerge from the foregoing discussion.

Preparation

Although it is hard to prove statistically that preparation has a bearing on ultimate outcome,[3, 6] common sense, clinical observation, and the reports of amputees all suggest that proper preparation is highly desirable.[11, 13, 14, 18] Such preparation must include a clear explanation of the reasons for the amputation; the viable alternatives, if any; the exact surgical procedure; and the rehabilitative process following it. To the extent that it is possible to do so, anticipating and dealing with the various issues that patients will face, even if these are not raised by the patients themselves, is of great help. Such issues include disposal of the limb, the anticipated relationship with friends and family, degree of functional loss and return, work capability, costs of surgery and of rehabilitation, sexual adjustment, and social impact.

It is important to present the amputation as a desirable life-saving or life-improving option rather than as a last resort or an indication of failure. There is indeed some evidence in the literature that the quality of life can sometimes be improved by an amputation as compared with limb-sparing treatments.[26] In connection with this, it has been suggested that the term "reconstructive surgery" is preferable to "amputation" and can certainly be used along with it.[2] It should go without saying that much of the preparation should be conducted by the operating surgeon; although the information is widely available and may be imparted by any member of the team, no other person can communicate the same degree of authority and confidence that patients need as they contemplate the imminent loss.

Surgical Technique

It should be obvious to the readers of this book that good technique is of the essence. What perhaps is not so obvious is the need for the senior surgeon to perform the surgery or to be involved intimately in its performance. It is an error to relegate this procedure to inexperienced hands. As Bradway and associates wrote, "In our program, the senior surgical attending is directly involved in the performance of all amputations and supervises the entire process of amputation rehabilitation."[3]

Early Prosthetic Fitting and Mobilization

There is little doubt that the earlier the prosthesis is applied, the better are the results in terms of functional capacity and psychological adaptation.[6, 17] As Bradway and associates wrote, "Early prosthetic fitting and re-

habilitation enable the patient to incorporate all of his physical and emotional efforts into recovery from the earliest possible moment, rather than allowing the patient to focus only on disabilities and pain."[3] Introducing the patient to a successfully rehabilitated amputee may be of great assistance in this effort.[18]

The Team Approach

A team approach is optimal in amputee rehabilitation and should include the surgeon, surgical nurses, prosthetist, physical therapist, occupational therapist, social worker, vocational counselor, and, if indicated, a psychiatrist or psychologist.[1, 3, 8, 13, 14, 22, 24, 27] With this variety, each member of the team is in a position to address one aspect or another of the patient's needs. Even more importantly, as these needs evolve, flexibility and adaptation to new realities are required not only of amputees but also of those who help them. To the extent that it is possible to do so, the involvement of members of the family at all of these stages can be of tremendous help to the amputees and to those who are caring for them (also see Chapter 20).

Vocational Rehabilitation

No approach to amputation can be considered successful without some resolution of the issue presented by loss of skill, job, and livelihood. Even in the absence of pressing financial need, the loss of earning capacity may entail a profound loss of self-esteem, which brings with it a variety of adverse psychological phenomena. It is not essential that the person resume work, but it is essential that the person accept whatever new role and capacity that can now be enjoyed.[14] This is an issue to be approached with an open mind. Some, for example, prefer to return to employment, with all the security, stimulation, and structure that it presents. Others may find that, thanks to personal wealth or to disability and retirement benefits, they are in a position to stay away from work. As Kohl wrote, "It is important that there not be a judgmental response from the staff toward those patients who do not seek paid employment."[14]

Special Approaches

Increasingly, group support is part of the help being provided to amputees.[10, 15, 27] One such modality is Schwartz's Situation-Transition (ST) group, which is different from other self-help groups for alcoholics, smokers, and overeaters in that "members are *not* required to espouse a particular moral or behavioral value system."[27] Whether a trained person leads the group or it is conducted entirely by its own members, the group experience is likely to be of great value to both the participants and their families. It has been noted that amputee self-help groups shy away from self-pity or self-designation in terms of disability, and emphasize strength and participation in a full and healthy life.[27]

Psychotherapy may be indicated for individuals who suffer difficulty in any of the stages previously described and who are unable to resume a normal existence that otherwise should be possible for them. It is important to recall in this connection that the various stages of grief described by Parkes and others may not be accomplished in the predictable sequence or within the expected time. There are those individuals who may continue to mourn the loss of their limbs for a long time or who, having shelved the issue, return to it at a much later date (delayed grief reaction). In aiding this process, the opportunity to ventilate feelings is a crucial phase that should not be aborted. Feelings of sorrow, anger, and anxiety must be expressed before further therapeutic work can be accomplished. Occasionally, family therapy may be indicated to assist in reaching the proper balance between the legitimate support amputees need and the independence that they must regain. It is, of course, perfectly possible for psychological problems that have been avoided or disregarded in the past to surface after surgery and, indeed, to be blamed on it. This might be the case, for example, in long-standing marital discord, chronic depression, anxiety disorder, drug dependence, alcohol abuse, and antisocial behavior.

These psychiatric challenges can be addressed therapeutically on their own merit, without the necessity of determining the degree to which they are related to the amputation. If and when such a determination becomes desirable, such as in complicated legal situations, the individual's previous history and former level of adjustment can be of great value in clarifying the issue. For most individuals, however, psychiatric consultation and therapy are not indicated. Psychological sophistication and sensitivity on the part of members of the team, however, are indispensable.

In the self-help group that was interviewed for this report, there was unanimous agreement with these principles of management. Furthermore, most individuals noted an improvement in the quality of their lives after surgery. As one member put it, "You become a more compassionate and less critical person towards others." Another, who had suffered greatly both before and after his amputation, said, "When you become an amputee, you become a better person, because you have to work for everything."

ACKNOWLEDGMENTS

Many individuals have assisted materially in all aspects of preparing this report. I wish in particular to acknowledge my debt of gratitude to John Bradway, M.D., who, as a third-year clinical clerk in psychiatry, piqued my interest in this area by preparing a paper on psychological adaptation to amputation, which in turn formed the basis of a report written by him, myself, and a number of others;[3] to James Malone, M.D., for sharing his extensive knowledge and experience; to Joseph Leal, C.P., who put me in touch with the amputee self-help group in Tucson; to Sharon Stites, leader and organizer of the self-help group; to Diane Atkins, occupational therapist and coordinator for the University of Colorado Center for Amputee Services, who shared a wealth of experience with hundreds of amputees at that center; to Sybil Kohl, social worker at the Houston Center for Amputee Services, for her profound observations and reflections on the lives of amputees; to Jan Pankey and Sandy Levitt, third-year clinical clerks, who assisted me greatly in my meeting with the self-help group in Tucson; and to the eight members of the group who, though unnamed, were and are the source of information, guidance, and inspiration to all who study amputation and those who must adapt to it.

REFERENCES

1. Atkins D: Personal communication, 1984.
2. Bowker JH: Amputation rehabilitation: Critical factors in outcome. J Arkansas Med Soc 78:181, 1981.
3. Bradway JK, Malone JM, Racy J, et al: Psychological

adaption to amputation: An overview. Orthot Prosthet 38:46, 1984.
4. Caine D: Psychological considerations affecting rehabilitation after amputation. Med J Aust 2:818, 1973.
5. Ewalt JR, Randall GC, Morris H: The phantom limb. Psychosom Med 9:118, 1947.
6. Friedmann LW: The Psychological Rehabilitation of the Amputee. Springfield, Illinois, Charles C Thomas, 1978, pp 17–67.
7. Gingras G, Mongeau M, Susset V, et al: Psychosocial and rehabilitative aspects of upper extremity amputees. Can Med Assoc J 75:819, 1956.
8. Hamilton A: Rehabilitation of the leg amputee in the community. Practitioner 225:1487, 1981.
9. Hughes J, White WL: Emotional reactions and adjustments of amputees to their injury. US Naval Med Bull (Suppl) March:157, 1946.
10. Kerstein MD: Group rehabilitation for the vascular disease amputee. J Am Geriatr Soc 28:40, 1980.
11. Kessler HH: Psychological preparation of the amputee. Ind Med Surg 20:107, 1951.
12. Kolb L, Brodie K: Modern Clinical Psychiatry, 10th Ed. Philadelphia, WB Saunders Co, 1984, pp 574–576.
13. Kohl S: Personal communication, 1984.
14. Kohl S: The process of psychological adaptation to traumatic limb loss. In Krueger DW (ed): Emotional Rehabilitation of Physical Trauma and Disability. New York, SP Medical and Scientific Books, 1984, pp 113–148.
15. Lipp M, Malone SJ: Group rehabilitation of vascular surgery patients. Arch Phys Med Rehabil 57:180, 1976.
16. MacBride A, Rogers J, Whylie B, Greeman SJJ: Psychosocial factors in the rehabilitation of elderly amputees. Psychosomatics 12:258, 1980.
17. Malone JM, Moore WS, Goldstone J, et al: Thera-peutic and economic impact of a modern amputation program. Ann Surg 189:798, 1979.
18. May CH, McPhee MC, Pritchard DJ: An amputee visitor program as an adjunct to rehabilitation of the lower limb amputee. Mayo Clin Proc 54:774, 1979.
19. Noble D, Price D, Gilder R, Jr: Psychiatric disturbances following amputation. Am J Psychiatry 110:609, 1954.
20. Parkes CM: Factors determining the persistence of phantom pain in the amputee. J Psychosom Res 17:97, 1973.
21. Parkes CM: Psychosocial transitions: Comparison between reactions to loss of a limb and loss of a spouse. Br J Psychiatry 127:204, 1975.
22. Parkes CM: The psychological reactions to loss of a limb: The first year after amputation. In Howells JG (ed): Modern Perspectives in the Psychiatric Aspects of Surgery. New York, Brunner-Mazel, 1976, pp 515–532.
23. Parkes CM: Determinants of disablement after loss of a limb. In Krueger DW (ed): Emotional Rehabilitation of Physical Trauma and Disability. New York, SP Medical and Scientific Books, 1984, pp 105–111.
24. Randall GC, Ewalt JR, Blair H: Psychiatric reaction to amputation. JAMA 128:645, 1945.
25. Reinstein L, Ashley J, Miller KH: Sexual adjustment after lower extremity amputation. Arch Phys Med Rehabil 59:504, 1978.
26. Sugarbaker PH, Barofsky I, Rosenberg SA, Gianola FJ: Quality of life assessment of patients in extremity sarcoma clinical trials. Surgery 91:17, 1982.
27. Whylie B: Social and psychological problems of the adult amputee. In Kostuik JP (ed): Amputation Surgery and Rehabilitation: The Toronto Experience. New York, Churchill Livingstone, 1981, pp 387–393.

Index

Note: Page numbers in *italics* refer to illustrations;
page numbers followed by the letter *t* refer to tables.

341

American Society of Anesthesiologists, patient
classification of, 82–84, 83*t*
Amputation. See also *Lower extremity amputation.*
  above-knee. See *Above-knee amputation.*
  anesthesia considerations in, 74–91
    atherosclerotic disease and, 79–90
    decompensated diabetic and, 76–77
    insulin-dependent diabetic and, 74–75
    intraoperative glucose and, 77–78
    preoperative assessment and, 75–76
    preoperative glucose and, 77–78
  anesthetic technique in, selection of, 78–79
  below-ankle, Doppler-derived pressures
    and, 34
  below-elbow, prosthetic fitting for, 195–197
  below-knee. See *Below-knee amputation.*
  diabetes and, 19
    anesthetic technique for, 78–79
    ankle block in, 78
    general anesthesia in, 78–79
    mortality rate in, 19–20
    peridural block in, 78
    sciatic-femoral nerve block in, 78
    spinal block in, 78
    subarachnoid block in, 78
  guillotine, for foot infection, 26
  healing of, fluorescein and, 53
    skin temperature measurement and, 71*t*
    transcutaneous oxygen pressure and, 72*t*
  immediate postsurgical prosthetic fitting and
    above-knee, 186–192, *187, 188, 189,
      190, 191, 192,* 235–237, *238, 239, 240*
    below-knee, 183–186, *184, 185, 186,
      187,* 239–240, *240, 241*
  of ankle, 93–116
  of foot, 93–116
    causes of, 96
    healing of, 35*t*
    major reasons for, 93
    partial, modern socket design theory and,
      305, *305*
    prosthetic fitting and, 182–183
  of forefoot, Doppler-derived pressures and,
    34–35
    healing of, 35*t*
  of forequarter, prosthetic fitting for,
    197–198
  of toe, Doppler-derived pressures and, 35
    healing of, 36*t*
    techniques for, 96–99
  postoperative weight bearing and, 198, *199*
  preparation for, psychological response and,
    332
  primary, gangrene and, 7
    in limb-threatening arterial insufficiency, 7
  psychological aspects of, 330–339
    adaptive stages and, 333–335
      at-home adaptive rehabilitation and,
        335–336
      in-hospital rehabilitation and, 334–335
      postoperative, 334
      preoperative, 333–334
    age and, 330–331
    body image and, 336–337
    determinants of, 330–333
    limb loss and, magnitude of, 332
      nature of, 332
    management of, 337–339

Amputation *(Continued)*
    psychological aspects of, medical factors in,
      331–333
    mobilization and, 338
    personality and, 331
    phantom limb pain and, 336
    prosthetic fitting and early, 338
    prosthetic rehabilitation and, 333
    psychosocial support and, 331
    sexuality and, 337
    special approaches and, 338
    surgical complications and, 332–333
    surgical technique and, 338
    team approach and, 333, 338
    variables in, 330–331
      economic, 331
      vocational, 331
    vocational rehabilitation and, 333, 338
  reasons for, psychological response and, 332
  translumbar, 168–176. See also *Translum-
    bar amputation.*
  transmetatarsal, 99–101
    Chopart's disarticulation and, 101, *102,
      103, 103,* 104
    completed, *101*
    following bypass graft, *101*
    Lisfranc's disarticulation and, 101, *102,
      103, 103,* 104
  traumatic, 320–328
    above-knee, 140–141
    amputation level and, 324–325
    anesthesia considerations in, 90–91
    axonotmesis and, 323
    bones and, 323
    foot and, 96
    history of, 320–321
    immediate postsurgical prosthetic fitting
      and, 325, 326–327
    muscle viability and, 322
    nerve assessment and, 323
    neurapraxia and, 323
    neurotmesis and, 323
    patient management in, 322–324,
      325–326
    prosthetic fitting for, clinical experience
      with, 325
      timing of, 324–328
    results of, 327–328
    skin in, 322
    tendon viability and, 322
    tourniquet use in, 324
    vasculature and, 323–324
Amputation level, functional loss and,
    271–272
  partial foot, 291–293, *291*
  prosthetic fitting and, procedures for,
    180–198
  socket shape and, 314
  uncommon, 291–293
Amputation level selection, arteriography and,
    30
  by Doppler assessment, 32–37
  by isotope clearance techniques, 38–42
  by laser Doppler flowmetry, 64–68
    calibration of, 66
    experience with, 66–68
    instrumentation for, 65, *65*
    theoretical principles of, 64–65
  by skin fluorescence, 50–61